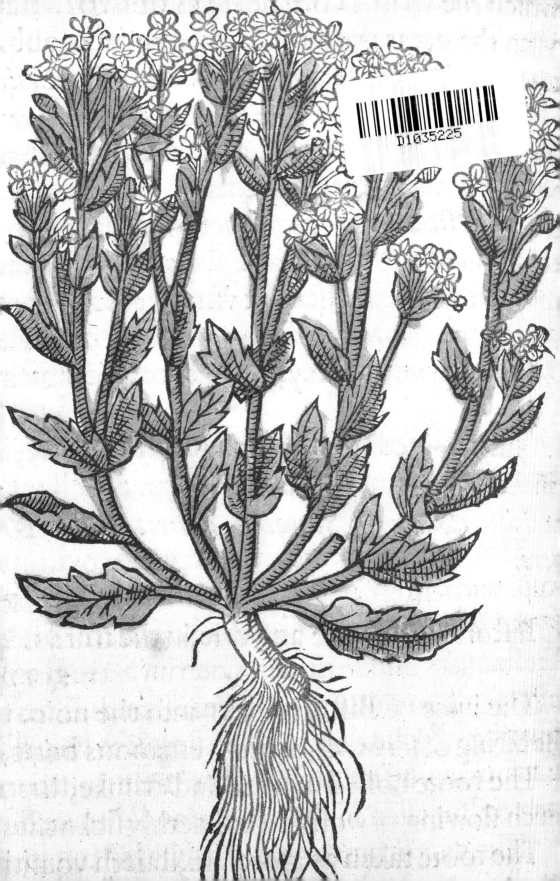

John Hall, Master of Physicke

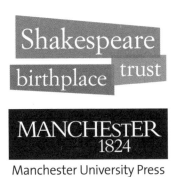

Manchester University Press

John Hall, Master of Physicke

A casebook from Shakespeare's Stratford

Greg Wells

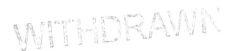

Manchester University Press

Published by Manchester University Press
in association with the Shakespeare Birthplace Trust
Altrincham Street, Manchester M1 7JA
www.manchesteruniversitypress.co.uk

Shakespeare Birthplace Trust
Registered Charity Number 209302
Every purchase supports the vital care and conservation of the Shakespeare Houses and Collections
www.shakespeare.org.uk

British Library Cataloguing-in-Publication Data
A catalogue record for this book is available from the British Library

ISBN 978 1 5261 3453 0 hardback

First published 2020

Typeset by Servis Filmsetting Limited, Stockport, Cheshire
Printed in Great Britain by Bell and Bain Ltd, Glasgow

For Mary Wells

Contents

Figures

Figures

Plates

Plates

7 *Sena orientalis*, senna of the east. From John Gerard, *The Herball or Generall Historie of Plantes* (1597), p. 1114. Reproduced by permission of the Shakespeare Birthplace Trust. SBT OS 97.7.

8 *Borago hortensis*, garden borage. From John Gerard, *The Herball or Generall Historie of Plantes* (1597), p. 653. Reproduced by permission of the Shakespeare Birthplace Trust. SBT OS 97.7.

9 *Burglossa vulgaris*, common bugloss. From John Gerard, *The Herball or Generall Historie of Plantes* (1597), p. 655. Reproduced by permission of the Shakespeare Birthplace Trust. SBT OS 97.7.

10 *Capparis folio acuto*, sharp-leaved capers. From John Gerard, *The Herball or Generall Historie of Plantes* (1597), p. 748. Reproduced by permission of the Shakespeare Birthplace Trust. SBT OS 97.7.

11 *Cochlearia Britannica*, common English scurvy-grass. From John Gerard, *The Herball or Generall Historie of Plantes* (1597), p. 324. Reproduced by permission of the Shakespeare Birthplace Trust. SBT OS 97.7.

12 *Rha capitatum l'obelii*, Turkey rhubarb. From John Gerard, *The Herball or Generall Historie of Plantes* (1597), p. 316. Reproduced by permission of the Shakespeare Birthplace Trust. SBT OS 97.7.

13 *Absinthium iatifolium suie ponticum*, broad-leaved wormwood. From John Gerard, *The Herball or Generall Historie of Plantes* (1597), p. 937. Reproduced by permission of the Shakespeare Birthplace Trust. SBT OS 97.7.

14 *Malus granata siue punica*, pomegranate tree. From John Gerard, *The Herball or Generall Historie of Plantes* (1597), p. 1262. Reproduced by permission of the Shakespeare Birthplace Trust. SBT OS 97.7.

15 *Canelle folium e bacillus*, cinnamon leaf and bark. From John Gerard, *The Herball or Generall Historie of Plantes* (1597), p. 1348. Reproduced by permission of the Shakespeare Birthplace Trust. SBT OS 97.7.

Plates

16 *Helenium*, elecampane. From John Gerard, *The Herball or Generall Historie of Plantes* (1597), p. 649. Reproduced by permission of the Shakespeare Birthplace Trust. SBT OS 97.7.

17 *Althaea ibiscus*, marsh mallow. From John Gerard, *The Herball or Generall Historie of Plantes* (1597), p. 787. Reproduced by permission of the Shakespeare Birthplace Trust. SBT OS 97.7.

18 *Capillus veneris verus*, true maidenhair. From John Gerard, *The Herball or Generall Historie of Plantes* (1597), p. 982. Reproduced by permission of the Shakespeare Birthplace Trust. SBT OS 97.7.

19 *Crocus florens*, saffron flower. From John Gerard, *The Herball or Generall Historie of Plantes* (1597), p. 123. Reproduced by permission of the Shakespeare Birthplace Trust. SBT OS 97.7.

20 *Bellis hortensis multiplex flore albo*, double white daisy. From John Gerard, *The Herball or Generall Historie of Plantes* (1597), p. 510. Reproduced by permission of the Shakespeare Birthplace Trust. SBT OS 97.7.

21 Seventeenth-century majolica drug jar from Venice. Reproduced by permission of the Shakespeare Birthplace Trust. SBT 1993-31-46.

22 Mid-seventeenth-century ceramic drug jar from Delft. Reproduced by permission of the Shakespeare Birthplace Trust. SBT 1993-31-57.

23 Sixteenth-century ceramic drug jar from Tuscany. Reproduced by permission of the Shakespeare Birthplace Trust. SBT 1993-31-68.

24 Late sixteenth-century majolica wet-drug jar. Reproduced by permission of the Shakespeare Birthplace Trust. SBT 1993-31-301.

25 Osias Dyck, *A Doctor Casting the Water* (*c.* 1660s). Oil on panel. 34.3 × 30.5 inches. Reproduced by permission of the Shakespeare Birthplace Trust. SBT 1994-17.

Tables

Foreword

This richly illustrated volume offers the first ever complete translation into English of a Latin medical notebook by Shakespeare's
son-in-law, John Hall (1575–1635). Published incompletely in 1657,
Hall's notebook affords an extraordinary keyhole view of life in
Stratford-upon-Avon in the seventeenth century. It was mainly
written between 1634 and 1635, but includes documentation relating to much earlier cases, the earliest being Case 69 (Mrs Boughton
whom Hall treated for swallowing difficulties in 1611). Hall's Latin
manuscript is now preserved in the British Library.

Hall followed in his father's footsteps by training as a doctor, and
graduated from Queens' College, Cambridge in 1593/4, taking his
MA in 1597. He was living and working in Stratford-upon-Avon
as a physician by June 1607, when he married Shakespeare's elder
daughter, Susanna. With their only child, Elizabeth, born nine
months later, they were resident in Old Town by 1613 in, we
believe, the timber-framed house now known as Hall's Croft.

Hall's links with his famous father-in-law were close. They
travelled to London together in 1614, and Hall probably treated
Shakespeare two years later, during his final illness. Shakespeare
named him (along with Susanna) as joint residuary legatee and
executor of his will, for which Hall was granted probate in London
on 22 June 1616. Susanna Hall inherited the bulk of her father's
estate, including the grand house, New Place.

Preface

It has been my pleasure as well as my loving duty to work on this book, which brings to a wider audience the groundbreaking doctoral thesis of my dear, late friend, Dr Greg Wells (1947–2017). For as long as Greg had made Stratford-upon-Avon his home (since 1985), he was devoted to Hall's Croft, and to learning about the medical practice of John Hall. Like Hall himself, Greg dedicated his life to the improvement and progress of his fellow humans.

Greg transcribed the whole of Hall's Latin manuscript (some 191 pages), and then translated it into English. His bilingual thesis can be consulted at the University of Warwick. In identifying Hall's Latin borrowings from the medical textbooks of his contemporaries, Greg's original work makes a substantial contribution to our knowledge of early-modern libraries, and establishes the first of its kind in Stratford-upon-Avon.

This first complete translation of Hall's *Little Book of Cures* reinstates material omitted by earlier editions. There is, for example, the Bishop of Worcester, whom Hall treated for 'scorbutic arthritis' (Case 164) – but also for extreme melancholy (earlier editions omit the reason for this: the bishop's son had committed murder). For the first time, it is now possible to read about Hall's conversations with his patients, his prayers for their recovery, and his thanksgivings for their cures. Of Richard Wilmore of Norton Curlieu, Budbrooke (whom Hall had treated for 'astonishing worms' when

Preface

Wilmore was 14 years old), Hall writes: 'I saw him in passing two years later and asked whether he ever felt any corrosion of the stomach or passed worms. He replied that he had been free of all pain and torment since that time. Praise God' (Case 77).

Although he relied on the recipes and remedies of others, Hall occasionally made his own potions. To Mrs Richardson (suffering from uterine wind, Case 122), he administered, among other things, 'snail water (my own compound)', and records, 'she recovered her lost strength wonderfully, and said this divine water far surpassed potable gold, and she wished never to be without it because, she said, it was the equal of anything. She was thus completely cured, and after the death of her husband remarried and bore an heir six years later.'

This volume is published in association with the Shakespeare Birthplace Trust whose charitable objectives include conserving and presenting the family homes of William Shakespeare, including those sites most associated with John Hall: Hall's Croft and New Place. We are delighted and proud to be presenting a book which brings to life the work, intellect, faith and social interactions of Shakespeare's son-in-law.

Revd Dr Paul Edmondson
Head of Research, the Shakespeare Birthplace Trust

Acknowledgements

In preparing this book I am particularly grateful to Greg Wells's dear friend, John Heavens, for his work in helping to separate the Latin and English texts; to my colleague and photographer Andrew Thomas for his work in supplying all of the images from the collections of the Shakespeare Birthplace Trust; to Oscar Lake, Greg's grandson, for his work on the list of images, and for his having identified the herbs and plants that Hall most frequently used; to Robert Bearman for reading and commenting on the introductory chapters; to Nicholas Molyneux for information about Westwood Park, Huddington Court and Warwick Priory; to Nick de Somogyi for the tripartite index; and especially to Mary Wells, Greg's widow, for all of her help in preparing the notes on Hall's patients, and for her assistance and encouragement.

Note on the text

Chapter 1, 'Introducing John Hall, Master of Physicke', draws on material from Greg's own essay, 'His son-in-law John Hall', in *The Shakespeare Circle: An Alternative Biography*, edited by Paul Edmondson and Stanley Wells (Cambridge: Cambridge University Press, 2015), material which is reproduced here with the special permission of the publisher.

Arabic numerals printed in bold in square brackets mark the page numbers of Hall's Latin manuscript. So, for example, '**[p. 3]** I prescribed antiscorbutic beer of this sort' indicates that Hall started that prescription on page three of his manuscript.

Hall's many borrowings from his sources are easily identifiable in this edition. They are set in italics and their source is identified at the foot of the page. Unless otherwise stated, all translations are Greg's own.

A full list of the sources Hall regularly used (his personal, working library) immediately follows the text of the casebook. Mary Wells, Greg's widow, has provided the thumbnail sketches of Hall's patients for each of the cases. This information is indebted to Joan Lane's *John Hall and His Patients: The Medical Practice of Shakespeare's Son-in-Law* (1996), where more detailed, contextual information about Hall's patients can be found. Lane, however, was not without her occasional errors in some of her identifications, partly because she was following James Cooke's influential but long out-of-date abridged and partial version of Hall's *Little Book of Cures* (from 1679). Greg's corrections of Cooke's and Lane's misidentifications of patients are included in the footnotes. The index aims to open up Greg's work as much as possible and is in three parts: 'Names and works', 'Places' and 'Ailments and treatments.'

I

Introducing John Hall, Master of Physicke

The earliest reference to John Hall is his admission to Queens' College, Cambridge, aged 14, in 1589. The last is his will dated 25 November 1635. His *Little Book of Cures, Described in Case Histories and Empirically Proven, Tried and Tested in Certain Places and on Noted People* forms the most substantial account of his life and work among his patients in the locale made famous by Hall's father-in-law, William Shakespeare. Most of the records relating to Hall concern his life in Stratford-upon-Avon, starting with his marriage to Susanna, the Shakespeares' eldest child, in June 1607.

Hall was born in Carlton, Bedfordshire, the son of William Hall. John Taplin has written importantly and extensively on Hall's family background in *Shakespeare's Country Families* (Taplin 2018: 85–112). Taplin's book is not widely known but is available for consultation in the Shakespeare Centre Library. Hall received his BA in 1593/4 and his MA in 1597. A doctorate in medicine was required for licensing by the College of Physicians of London or to teach at a university, but not otherwise. An academic doctorate was no more necessary as a medical qualification then than it is now. Although Hall never obtained, or claimed to have, the degree of Doctor of Medicine, his MA made him better qualified than most physicians in England at this time. Hall never used the title of Dr, nor was he addressed so by his contemporaries, though he has frequently and confusingly been granted it *post mortem*.

1 The signature of John Hall, churchwarden, Holy Trinity Church, Stratford-upon-Avon, 20 April 1621. Hall's is the third signature down, just below Thomas Wilson (the vicar). Seventh down is July Shaw (who lived next door but one to New Place and who was one of the witnesses of Shakespeare's will), and ninth down is Bartholomew Hathaway (Anne Shakespeare's brother).

Of the 814 physicians practising outside London between 1603 and 1643, only 78 per cent had formally matriculated at a university (Raach 1962: 250). Of that 78 per cent, 40 per cent held BAs, 34 per cent MAs and 30 per cent were Doctors of Medicine. Hall may, like many English students, have travelled around the Continent and studied for a few weeks or months at one or more universities. If so, the purpose was to gain wider experience rather than a further degree. But short-term, unregistered students who paid their bills, and stayed out of trouble, commonly left no records behind them.

Outside London, physicians were supposed to be licensed by the local bishop but this was not, in practice, essential, and the records are patchy. A physician often applied for a licence only when a dispute arose with a patient or colleague, for the extra status it gave. There are no records of licences in the Worcester diocese before 1661, so either they have been lost, or none were granted. John was recognised as 'professor of medicine' (that is, practising medicine as a profession) by Stratford's Church Court in 1622 (Brinkworth 1972: 148). This was a 'Peculiar' Court, sharing some responsibilities with the bishop but independent of him in two years out of three, so the recognition is equivalent to an episcopal licence.

Hall would have studied medical textbooks as part of his MA, but in addition 'often a young physician would acquire practical bedside knowledge by working with an established physician' (Wear 2000: 122). We know that Hall had access to medical books. As executor of his father's will he received 'all my books of physic' (Marcham 1931: 25). This may indicate that Hall's father was also a physician, but medical books were commonly owned by householders. In fact it tended to be their wives who provided the first line of medical care for the family and servants. Hall's father, William, bequeathed books of astronomy, astrology and alchemy to his servant Matthew Morrys, but only on condition that Matthew should instruct John in these arts, if he wished to learn them. These kinds of books were far less common in a standard household library, and might be indicative of William Hall's main interests. At some point, Morrys, too, moved to Stratford-upon-Avon and seems to have maintained friendly contact with the Halls; he named two of his children Susanna and John, after them. Two years after Shakespeare's death, in 1618, John made Morrys a trustee, along with John Greene, of the gatehouse in Blackfriars that Susanna had inherited from her father (Schoenbaum 1987: 275).

3

2 On 14 May 1622, John Hall was recorded as a 'professor of medicine' (i.e. a practitioner of medicine) in the records of the Stratford-upon-Avon Ecclesiastical Court (also known as the Bawdy Court). This is evidence of Hall being licensed in medicine by a court which had authority to license him when the bishop was not present. The record includes 'He did not appear. Pardoned.' Immediately below Hall's name are three 'professors of surgery': Isaac Hitchcox, John Nason (similarly 'pardoned') and Edward Wilkes ('Let him be cited for the next court.'). They would all have had to present their licences before the ecclesiastical authorities in order to continue their practice.

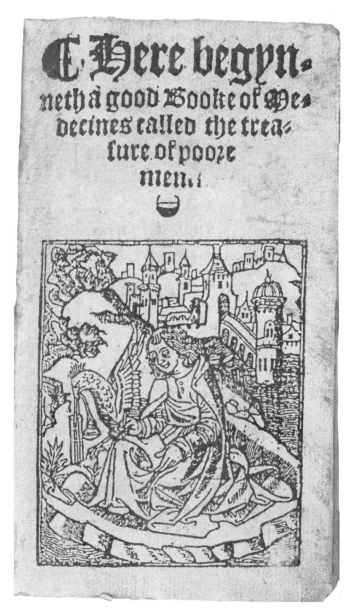

3 Title-page of *The Treasurie of Poor Men* (1560), a popular medical book of the day, written in English, and which emphasises by contrast Hall's own motivation for writing. His text was in Latin and drew freely on other Latin medical texts. Hall wanted to demonstrate that he was a learned physician who was conversant with the best minds of his time.

John Hall, Master of Physicke

It is likely that Hall also learned about medicine from his brother-in-law, William Sheppard, who had gained his MA at King's College, Cambridge in 1590, and his doctorate in medicine in 1597. After marrying John's sister, Sara, Sheppard moved to Leicester in 1599. It is likely that Sara had met William in Cambridge through her brother (since no other connection between the families is known), and that Sheppard invited John to accompany him to Leicester as his medical assistant. If so, then Hall would have had time for four or five years of supervised practice, and a visit to the Continent, before setting up on his own.

Settling in Stratford-upon-Avon

The reasons behind Hall's move to Stratford-upon-Avon are unknown. Stratford was prosperous and had no resident physician, but the same applied to other small towns. The only identified link is through Abraham Sturley, estate agent to the Lucy family at nearby Hampton Lucy. The Lucys had estates near Carlton, so there might have been contact between Sturley and the Hall family there (Mitchell 1947: 10). There is no way of knowing whether John had met the Shakespeare family before his move.

John and Susanna Shakespeare married in Holy Trinity Church on 5 June 1607. Elizabeth, who was to be their only child, was christened on 21 February the following year. It is not known for certain where they lived before Susanna inherited New Place on the death of her father. Hall's Croft was alluded to by the renowned Stratford-upon-Avon antiquarian Robert Bell Wheler in 1814. He says that he has seen 'in some old paper relating the town, that Dr Hall resided in that part of Old Town which is in the parish of Old Stratford' (Halliwell-Phillipps 1886: 321).

Dendrochronological evidence, commissioned by the Shakespeare Birthplace Trust, shows that the oldest part of Hall's Croft, facing on to the road, was built from trees felled in the

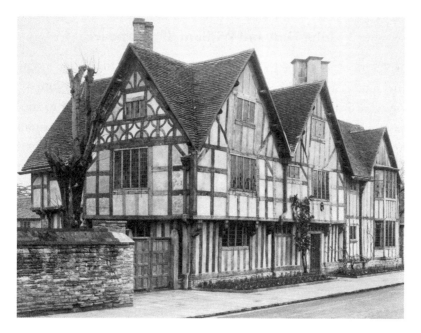

4 The house known as Hall's Croft, the only surviving dwelling of the right period in Old Town that could have belonged to John Hall. The front of the building can be dated to around 1613. It is possible that the present house replaced an earlier dwelling on the same site, which might also have been the home of the Halls from the time of their marriage in 1607. This photo was taken in 1951 when the Shakespeare Birthplace Trust bought the house in order to preserve it for the nation.

summer of 1613 (Anon. 1990). If they did live there for a while, it is likely that they rented it rather than owned it, since there is no record of sale, and the house is not mentioned in Hall's will with his other two properties (a house in London and a house in Acton, Middlesex). Hall did own a 'close on Evesham Way', for which he paid a charge to the Stratford Corporation from 1612 to 1616 (Stratford-upon-Avon Corporation Chamberlain's Accounts 1585–1619: 228, 245, 263, 276). It is likely that Hall used the close as a meadow for the horse he needed in order to visit his patients.

John Hall and William Shakespeare

References to contacts between John Hall and his father-in-law are sparse. In 1611 their names appeared (with sixty-nine others) on what is thought to be a subscription list raising money to support a bill in Parliament for repairs to the highways (Bearman 1994: 44). The Halls would eventually inherit the 107 acres of land purchased by Shakespeare in 1602, land which would have been affected by the proposed enclosure at Welcombe in 1614. The clerk of the Stratford Corporation, Thomas Greene (a distant kinsman of Shakespeare), records a meeting in London on 17 November 1614, commonly assumed to have been with both Shakespeare and Hall, though Greene did not unequivocally state this. Greene visited 'my cousin Shakespeare', 'to see him how he did'. In the conversation that followed, 'He [Shakespeare] told me that they assured him they meant to enclose no further than to Gospel Bush

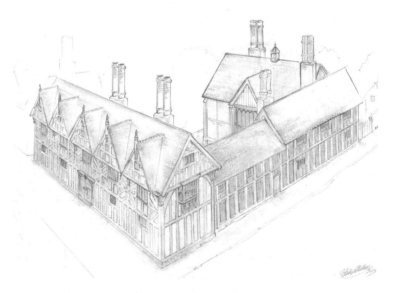

5 An artist's reconstruction of New Place. Hall and his family moved in from 1616 on his wife having inherited on the death of her father, William Shakespeare.

[...] and he and Mr Hall say they think there will be nothing done at all' (Ingleby 1885: iii). Shakespeare was probably reporting Hall's views based on prior discussions in Stratford, to emphasise their agreement on the issue.

In his will of 1616, Shakespeare made Hall joint residuary legatee and executor, along with Susanna (the main executor). Hall proved Shakespeare's will on 22 June 1616 and seems to have discharged his duties satisfactorily (Schoenbaum 1987: 306).

Physicians in Shakespeare's plays

The relationship between Hall and Shakespeare becomes important when considering whether Hall influenced Shakespeare's portrayal of physicians in his plays, a debate that started in 1860 and has continued ever since (Bucknill 1860: 36). The occasionally disputed consensus is, first, that medical matters occur more frequently and are dealt with more seriously in the later plays, and, secondly, that Hall's influence explains this. Two considerations rarely mentioned in this respect are that Shakespeare's subjects and style changed over time, and that his characters are on stage for dramatic purposes, wider issues (such as the accuracy of medical references) being subordinated to the immediate pressures of plot and situation.

One does not need to invoke Hall's influence to see that a physician like Dr Caius (*The Merry Wives of Windsor*, 1597–98) would be inappropriate in the later tragedies. Dr Pinch (*The Comedy of Errors*, 1594) is a schoolmaster, therefore a cleric not a physician. The scenes with a doctor in *The Two Noble Kinsmen* (1613–14) are by John Fletcher, not Shakespeare. Helen's circumstances in *All's Well That Ends Well* (1604–05) were uncommon but not unknown. Wives or daughters did sometimes inherit a practice and, with conditions, continue to practise physic (Pelling and Webster 1979: 183). In the medical marketplace of London or Norwich, about a quarter of unlicensed practitioners (excluding nurses and midwives), or one-eighth of all, were women. The dialogue between the Doctor and Cordelia in *King Lear* (1605–06) serves to slow down the action and build up tension before Lear's wakening. The advice given to Cordelia as her father regains consciousness is general enough to be given by a Doctor in the 1608 quarto, but by a Gentleman in the First Folio. The Scottish Doctor in *Macbeth* (1606) has been criticised for political and medical fearfulness and for avoiding any positive medical action in the sleepwalking scene. That, however, is not his dramatic function. He provides half a dialogue without which the sleepwalking scene would be a dumb show. A brisk statement that he would be back in the morning with a purge, a cupping glass and a remedy for melancholy might sound better professionally, but hardly fits the plot.

Pericles has attracted most attention, having been written around the time of John and Susanna's wedding. In a play in which the astonishing and the everyday are juxtaposed, Cerimon the physician is remarkably down to earth. He enters with the most practical medical exchanges that Shakespeare wrote. He says to a servant, 'Your master will be dead ere you return./ There's nothing can be ministered to nature/ That can recover him'; and to a poor man, 'Give this to th' pothecary/ And tell me how it works' (*Pericles* scene 12.7–10). Cerimon here performs the two key functions of a physician: to pronounce a prognosis, and if possible, prescribe treatment.

Cerimon's speech about his practice has been read as a description of an ideal physician, and perhaps as praise of Shakespeare's new son-in-law:

> I ever
> Have studied physic, through which secret art,
> By turning o'er authorities, I have,
> Together with my practice, made familiar
> To me and to my aid the blest infusions
> That dwells in vegetives, in metals, stones; (*Pericles* scene 12.28–33)

The 'secret art' should not be heard too literally. Supposedly secret remedies are a commonplace in the medical literature of the time. Hall quoted the *Thresor des remedes secrets pour les maladies des femmes* in his *Little Book* (Liébault 1585). The reference to metals and stones has been taken as indicating the influence of the highly influential early-modern Swiss physician, Paracelsus (the inference being that Shakespeare would have known more about medical treatments through his son-in-law), but the parallel with Friar Laurence in *Romeo and Juliet* (1594–95), 'O mickle is the powerful grace that lies / In plants, herbs, stones, and their true qualities' (*Romeo and Juliet* 2.2.15–16), shows that Shakespeare's use of this kind of language cannot be attributed to his relationship with Hall.

Whereas it might be pleasant to think of the depiction of Cerimon as Shakespeare's wedding tribute to Hall, Cerimon's referring to 'authorities' and 'practice' may be more significant. He claims to have both a traditional book-based university education, and practical proof from his own experience that his treatments work. Hall based the title of his manuscript, *A Little Book of Cures, Described in Case Histories and Empirically Proven, Tried and Tested in Specified Places and on Identified People*, on that of his favourite author, Martin Ruland the Elder (1569–1611). The pairing of 'practice' with 'authorities' was still relatively new and Ruland felt the need to explain it: 'I call those cures empiric, not because they are based on experience only as the empiric sect declares, but those which combine simultaneously rational teaching with practice, and are managed by method' (Ruland 1628: Sig.a3v). This is the most likely, perhaps only, point at which we see can Hall's influence on Shakespeare's writing.

John Hall in Stratford-upon-Avon's civic and religious life

Between 1616 and his death, Hall is mentioned in various records relating to civic life. He was elected to the Corporation in 1617 and 1623, but was excused from taking up the position on both occasions. In 1625 he sold most of his share of the tithes to the Corporation (Eccles 1963: 105). The following year he was fined £10 for not having turned up to Charles I's coronation (which gentlemen in ownership of lands valued above £40 were required to do, in order to be created knights – one of the new king's ways of raising extra money). In 1628 he was elected churchwarden, and in 1629 presented a new pulpit to the church (Lane 1996: xxv); the pulpit was eventually replaced. In the same year, trouble over his brother Dive's will meant that Hall agreed that he had given up executorship of their father's will because it would be 'a hindrance … in his practice being a physician' (Eccles 1963: 112).

Hall is usually described as a Puritan, a contested word that meant something very different in the early seventeenth century to the circumstances of the post-war Commonwealth period. Hall would more likely have described himself as one of the 'Godly', an evangelical strand of the Church of England tending to Calvinism, emphasising preaching of the word, and consciously aiming to improve society as well as personal morality. Detractors used 'Puritan' to label behaviour that they saw as hypocritical, self-serving and prurient prying into other people's affairs (Marshall 2012: 146). Alternatively, 'Puritanism did not involve particular, exclusive positions, but rather the holding of conventional Protestant positions in an especially zealous and committed form' (Hughes 1994: 62). Hall was certainly committed to the Episcopal Church of England, and showed no sympathy for Presbyterianism or non-conformism. If Susanna's absence from Easter Communion in 1606 was due to Puritan rather than Catholic leanings, she may have been the more radical of the two (Greer 2007: 239).

From around 1625 onwards, Hall was increasingly caught in a conflict between the Corporation and the vicar of Holy Trinity (Hughes 1994: 69–74). If his behaviour was difficult, even intemperate, he was not alone. He and other leading citizens faced a set of insoluble problems within a confusion of overlapping

responsibilities and jurisdictions. The Corporation was responsible for the vicar's and schoolmaster's salaries, but the Lord
of the Manor held the presentation to the living. The Puritan-
dominated Corporation took advantage of confusion over the
Lordship in 1619 to appoint a new, learned vicar. Opponents of
Thomas Wilson's appointment (including John Lane, who had
accused Susanna of adultery in 1613) disrupted his installation by
rioting around and in Holy Trinity, and publishing libels which
led to a Star Chamber suit.

At first the Corporation supported the vicar, increasing his
stipend from £20 to £60 (a very considerable sum) in recognition
of his preaching. They supported each other against the Bishop
of Worcester's complaint that Wilson was taking more powers
to the Church Court than he should. Relationships must have
started to sour before 1629, when Wilson's stipend was cut and
another preacher appointed following a dispute about the profits
of the churchyard. Hall sided with Wilson, claiming that his sale of
the tithes in 1625 had been intended to enhance the stipends of
the vicar and schoolmaster. He finally agreed to election on to
the Corporation in July 1632, but in October 1633 was displaced
for breach of orders and non-attendance. The same year he was
briefly and irregularly reappointed churchwarden, and was associated with Wilson's Chancery suit against the Corporation for restoration of his stipend. Hall's relationships with the Corporation
soured to the point that in 1634 the members met to discuss and
deny Hall's charge that they were 'foresworn villains' (Hughes
1994: 68).

The animosities spilled over into an unseemly personal row
about the allocation of pews in Holy Trinity, which had to be
resolved by Bishop Thornborough of Worcester. Wilson had
granted Hall and his family a pew which it was claimed had always
been used by the burgesses' wives. Hall had the advantage of
having successfully treated Thornborough in February 1633. The
bishop supported Hall's case, writing the letter to 'Mr John Hall

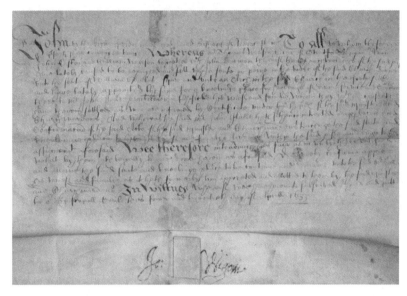

6 The Bishop of Worcester's grant to John Hall for a family pew, February 1633, in which he is very clear about referring to Hall by his profession: 'that Mr. Thomas Willson, Vicar of Stratford-upon-Avon together with John Easton, William Willson, and John Burman the three Churchwardens of the Parish Church of Stratford-upon-Avon had lately caused to be repaired and set up a seat or pew in the Body of the said Church, adjoining to the seat of William Combe, Esquire and to an arch on the North side of the Church and had lately appointed the same for a kneeling place for hearing Divine Service and Sermons to Mr. John Hall, practitioner of Physik, his wife and family whom they without consent have settled. It was thereby witnessed that the Bishop of Worcester confirmed to John Hall and Susanna, his wife the said seat.'

practitioner of physic' – not a licence, but clear episcopal recognition of his status (Thornborough 1635).

This growing antagonism may be behind the odd timing of Hall's agreement to join the Corporation in 1632, when relationships were already soured. It might have suited the vicar to have an ally there, while at the same time the burgesses could feel that Hall had at last recognised their importance. If this was an attempt to manage the problem, it failed, as did all other attempts. The bitter quarrel continued until Wilson's death in 1638. The underlying causes may have been tensions within Puritanism itself, and a growing gap between clerical and lay understandings of their roles (Hughes 1994: 71). Stratford was not unique in experiencing such tensions, and the change of Church policies under Charles I and Archbishop Laud may have created other hidden tensions (Marshall 2012: 149). Whatever the reason, when Hall was forced to make a choice he was more committed to his Church than to his civic responsibilities.

John Hall's medicines

Hall's references to physiology and pathology follow the traditional Galenic and Hippocratic model of four humours – blood, phlegm, yellow bile and black bile – which had to be balanced individually for good health. Imbalances might be due to incorrect diet, improper digestion, or blockage of excretion via the digestive system, urine, menstruation or through the skin. Corrupted humours were thought to accumulate beneath the skin until they broke out, as in smallpox or measles.

Hall's therapies, though, were taken from both Galenic and chemical texts. In the terms of his period, he was neither a Galeno-Hippocratic dogmatist nor a Paracelsian, but a Chymiatrist, drawing on both (Moran 2005: 82). Galenic and chemical remedies were both derived from minerals as well as animals and vegetables, but more important than the ingredients was the method of preparation. The chemical system favoured distillation to produce essences from raw materials, while traditional methods relied more on extraction with water or oil (Moran 2005: 12).

Hall was neither greatly advanced nor conservative in his practice. He saw himself as a specialist in scurvy, more knowledgeable about diagnosis than his colleagues. He bled fewer of his patients than most of his textbooks recommended, but purged almost everyone who was not elderly, pregnant or a child, before starting specific treatments. He relied on uroscopy (visual examination of the urine) a great deal, though this was already becoming old-fashioned. He went on buying new medical books all his life.

Physicians were trained in the use of simples prepared from a single ingredient, as well as compounds containing perhaps dozens of simples. Hall used traditional European simples and newer ones from the Americas and Far East such as guaiacum and sarsaparilla. The *Pharmacopoeia Londinensis* in 1618 listed 680 simples, 47 of which are metals. About 80 per cent of Hall's compound remedies are listed in the *Pharmacopoeia*. He also used several chemical pharmacopoeias, such as *Basilica chymica* (Croll 1609).

It is obvious from reading Hall's *Little Book of Cures* that he kept a certain amount of essential herbs in stock for, as it were, immediate use. If he went out to see a patient in the neighbourhood, he used a standardised treatment very often on the first day: a purgative, to clear the humours, for which he must have had the most relevant herbs and ingredients close to hand in order to refill his travelling bag as required. These included mainly senna and rhubarb. Hall would not have mixed these himself, but instead would have sought the services of a local apothecary. His family would have grown some herbs, and collected some for use, but a herb garden would have been mainly for their own domestic use and pleasure. The local apothecaries would have been responsible for buying ingredients and having them sent up from London. The records show that some things were not always instantly available, which meant that an alternative was used instead. Hall would not have undertaken any kind of surgery on a patient; there were surgeons in the locale.

It is worth considering his wife Susanna's role in Hall's medical practice. It was automatically the job of the wife of the head of the household to provide first-aid care for her family, servants and anybody else who became became part of the household. It is reasonable to imagine a division of labour. Hall would have had his professional medicines, Susanna her own preparation of

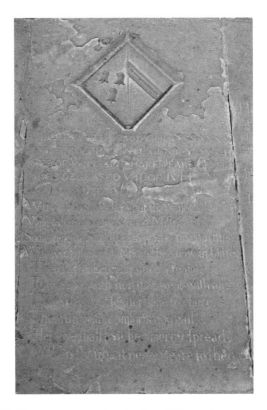

7 Susanna Hall's gravestone and epitaph, which reads:

> Witty above her sex, but that's not all,
> Wise to salvation was good Mistress Hall,
> Something of Shakespeare was in that, but this
> Wholly of him with whom she's now in bliss.
> Then, passenger, ha'st ne'er a tear,
> To weep with her that wept with all?
> That wept, yet set herself to cheer
> Them up with comforts cordial.
> Her love shall live, her mercy spread,
> When thou ha'st ne'er a tear to shed.

Cordials of the kind for which she is remembered were used during recovery, the third phase of treatment (after purgation and treatment for the specific illness). They strengthened the patient's heart, and would probably have been delivered from London in the form of crushed powder (and bought by Hall from a local apothecary).

herbs and distillations which she would use initially to look after the household. This suggestion is emphatically borne out by the inscription on her gravestone. It seems pretty clear that she cared for a community, and 'with comforts cordial'; in other words she had a good reputation for knowing how to use certain kinds of medicines and administering these to the townspeople. Part of her profile in the town was probably that of the well-to-do wife of a physician, with something of an elevated wise woman about her. People would have known that they could consult her and ask for her help and advice: the famous local poet's daughter, and the physician's wife. No doubt this kind of consultancy continued after Hall's death (she outlived him by fourteen years).

Opening up John Hall's *Little Book of Cures*

Hall would be a significant figure in the history of medicine even without the Shakespeare connection, for physicians' records from the early seventeenth century are rare. Hall's *Little Book of Cures* is in many respects unique, being a detailed record of the practice of a provincial physician, associated with neither the Court nor the London College. He composed it in Latin, mostly between 1634 and his death in 1635. Hall's choice of Latin is curious. If he planned to publish the book, it suggests a desire to emulate Continental writers rather than add to the, by then, growing number of English-language medical texts.

The small notebook, now in the British Library, contains 178 case reports of varying length, dated between 1611 and 1635, in roughly chronological order. Hall must have gone through his original notes, looking for and copying out cases of interest. Most were cases with successful outcomes, as was customary in the current medical literature, but he included some which puzzled him, including unexpected deaths. James Cooke, a Warwick surgeon, obtained the manuscript from Susanna in 1642, translated it and eventually published it in 1657, and a second edition followed (Hall

1679). Cooke was a surgeon with the Parliamentary forces based in Warwick during the Civil War, and already the author of a text-book on military surgery: *Mellificium chirurgiae, or the Marrow of Many Good Authors, wherein is briefly and faithfully handled the Art of Chirurgery* (1648). Cooke was eager to play down Hall's indebtedness to tradition and to emphasise his originality, so he left out material that contradicted this view, including several of Hall's references to his sources. Cooke's second edition has been reproduced twice in facsimile (Joseph 1964; Lane 1996). Joan Lane's commentary is particularly useful for her detailed social studies of Hall's patients. These editions have made Hall's notes relatively accessible, and useful to historians of medicine (Beier 1987; Nagy 1988; Wear 2000). The vividness of his clinical descriptions has also made him a popular source for medical writers with an interest in history (Moschowitz 1918; Betts and Betts 1998; Pearce 2006; Fernandez-Florez 2010).

Hall's *Little Book of Cures* refers to several of Shakespeare's family members and friends. Within the family Hall treated himself, his wife Susanna and daughter Elizabeth, Elizabeth's mother-in-law Mary Nash, and George Quiney, Judith Shakespeare's brother-in-law. He also treated Richard Tyler, Thomas Russell's daughter and son-in-law, Francis Collins's daughter Alice and Thomas Greene's daughter Anne, several members of the Rainsford family at Clifford Chambers, their friend the poet Michael Drayton, and William Combe's mother-in-law, wife and daughter. It is likely that he also treated his father-in-law, but the clinical details did not strike him as worth recording.

Hall's cases in the *Little Book of Cures* are mostly drawn from the middling well-to-do tradesmen and more educated citizens of Stratford (teachers, clergy and lawyers), and the gentry (including some Roman Catholics) in the surrounding countryside. Among the nobility, he treated the families of the Earls of Northampton and Shrewsbury, and of Lord Saye and Sele near Banbury. Naming important patients was commonplace in medical literature at the time, a way of providing evidence for a physician's success. Payment is only rarely mentioned. The Countess of Shrewsbury gave him 'great thanks, with a large payment' for successfully treating her son, and Lady Puckering's companion, Mrs Iremonger, rewarded him 'so that I might help others' (Hall 1635: 54, 91; see pp. 131 and 171). He also treated Mr Nash's serving maid and a poor man named Hudson, along with many others who cannot be identified. We should not assume that the patients he recorded are typical of his practice as a whole.

Hall composed his manuscript in an unusual way, perhaps because his Latin was limited outside of professional study. Over a third of his text is made up of phrases, sentences or whole paragraphs borrowed from his medical textbooks and rearranged to suit the circumstances of his own patients. Throughout the English translation, these borrowings are printed in italics and their sources referenced at the foot of the page. He used this method to describe patients, illnesses and outcomes, as well as for details of remedies. Usually he gave no reference, and it is only the existence of searchable online databases that has enabled his sources to be identified. The cases of his daughter and wife are good examples of his methods of composition and practice.

Elizabeth suffered from *tortura oris* (spasm of one side of the mouth) in January 1624. Hall gives a reference for the signs, then started her treatment with a purge and an ointment (Valesco 1560: 88–90; Platter 1602: 387). Elizabeth recovered after further purging, anointing and treatment for absence of menstruation. The condition recurred in April, and Hall referred to chapters on the disease and its treatment in several texts (Houllier 1611: 96–99; Platter 1602: 375; Rondelet 1574: 101v–102v; Amatus Lusitanus 1556: 394–396). Treatment continued with ointments and purgatives and was eventually successful. Cooke's bald translation that 'she eat [*sic*] nutmegs often' has been taken as Elizabeth's personal quirk, but he omitted Hall's statement that this was 'as Platter strongly recommends', as well as all the other references (Hall

1679: 33; Hall 1635: 36; see p. 113). The case report concludes 'all her symptoms diminished, and daily over a few days she reached complete health, freed from death and deadly illness' (Ruland 1628: 217; Hall 1635: 37; see p. 119).

Hall treated his wife, Susanna, for scurvy, a disease for which he regarded himself as a specialist. He relied mainly on two standard textbooks: Eugalenus's *De scorbuto morbo liber* (1604) and Sennert's *De scorbuto tractatus* (1624). Scurvy was at that time thought to be a severe disease of the spleen due to excess of black bile (melancholy). It had been described in travellers' accounts and medical texts from the early sixteenth century onwards, and treatment with antiscorbutic herbs such as scurvy-grass, watercress and brooklime was standard by the 1590s. There was nothing particularly advanced in Hall's treatments, though Cooke made much of them. Rather, Hall prided himself on his ability to diagnose a notoriously tricky disease that often mimicked other conditions. In his report on Bishop Thornborough's scorbutic arthritis he borrowed a sentence from Eugalenus: 'The false appearance of the arthritis deceived and made sport of his physicians' – even though Hall regarded them as 'experienced and learned in traditional medicine' (Eugalenus 1604: 97; Hall 1635: 161; see p. 252).

Susanna suffered from 'lower backache, convulsions, diseased gums, foul-smelling breath, wind, melancholy, heartburn, spontaneous tiredness, difficulty in breathing, fear of choking, tightness and torment of the abdomen', all of which together pointed to scurvy (Hall 1635: 115; see p. 198). Hall applied plasters and liniments to her abdomen and lower back, and prescribed an antiscorbutic electuary (Sennert 1624: 674). The cure was completed with steeled wine (wine boiled with steel filings) mixed with a large number of antiscorbutic herbs, the recipe of a leading French chemical physician (Du Chesne 1607: 74).

A few independent witnesses indicate how Hall was regarded by his patients. Lady Tyrrell wrote an undated letter to her friend Lady Temple sympathising with her husband's mischance, and

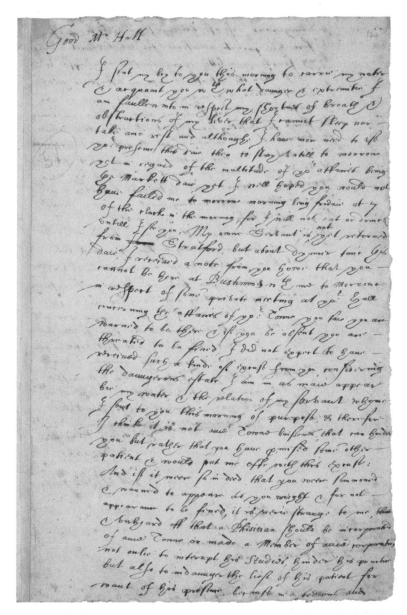

8 and 9 A letter of complaint from Sidrick Davenport to John Hall remonstrating with him for sending an excuse for not coming to see him on the morrow. He says that he is dangerously ill (though he was apparently well enough to write a 616-word letter). A full transcript can be found on pp. 24–25.

& dangerous diseaſe his preſſure is to be preferred
before his private occaſions, for what cannot a daie
bring foorth & a little error cauſely a relapſe w'ch
is worſe then the diseaſe, I know my diseaſe is gilous
& proc̃aſtination is dangerous, I haue relied on you
& truſt you will not faile me now, I know you cannot
be fined for viſiting me patiently, Neither the Towne
ſo barren of able men nor the Magiſtrates ſo
indiſcreet to lay this burthen vppon you wheſe p̃titio̅
is to be moſt abroad & cannot be effected by an
apprentice as theirs was, & for you to be teyed to y'e
Towne buſineſſe whoſe calling is out of Towne it might
ſeeme a great folly in you & more malliciouſ then to
inquire. Therefore I councell you as a friend never be
bounde; as long as you may be free, you shall but
derogat from y' ſelfe, Haue a great deale of troubles
vppon you diſtract you from y'e Studio w'ch deſtroyes
the wholſe imployment of any Man, had he a 100
yeares to liue longer. Therefore I pray you all
excuſes ſet a part that you wille here to morrow
morning by 7 of y'e clock for I will faſt tile you come
and I know you cannot inc̃urr any danger hauing
ſo lawfull a calling. Thus with my beſt wiſſes &
hartie loue remembred to y'r ſelfe & y'e reſt of my
good freinds to Eyper I commit you to Gods helie
protection & euer remaine.

                  Yo'r truely loving frend
                  & Seruant

           Sid. Dauenport.

My brother Colmores Phiſick is ended
& all is taken he starteth at home
purpoſly to speak with you tomorrow
morning for further directions. /

Buſhwood. thurſdaie 8° July 1632

praising his intention to consult Hall: 'I know by experience that he is most excellent'; Sidrick Davenport, however, wrote to Hall on 5 July 1632 complaining of his tardiness, and requesting an urgent visit: 'it is very strange to me, and unheard off that a physician should be incorporated of any Town or made a member of any corporation, not only to interrupt his studies but also endanger the life of his patient for want of his presence' (Joseph 1964: xi, 27–28). Patients sometimes refused to follow Hall's advice, and several in particular refused to be bled.

A full transcription of Davenport's letter reads as follows:

Good Mr Hall I sne my boy to you this morning to carrie my water & acquaint you with what daunger & extremitie I am faullen into in respect of my shortness of breath & obstructions of my liver, that I cannot sleep nor take anie rest, and although I have more need of yr presence this diae than to stay untill to morrow yet in regard of the multitude of yr affairs being ye Markett daie yet I well hoped you would not have failed me to morrow morning being fridaie at 7 of the clock in the morning, for I will not eat and drink until I see you, My owne Servante is not yet returned from Stratford, but about dynner time this daie I received a note from you howe that you cannot be here at Bushwood with me to morrow in respect of some private meeting at yr hall concerning the affairs of yr Towne you saie you are warned to be there & if you be absent you are threatened to be fined, I did not expect to receive such a kinde of excuse from you, considering the daungerous estate I am in, as maie appear bie my water, & the relation of my servant whome I sent to you this morning of purpose, & therefore I think it is not anie Town business, that can hinder you but rather that you have promised some other patient & would put me off with this excuse: And if it were so indeed that you are summoned & warned to appear as wright & for not appearance to be fined, it is verie strange to me. & unheard off that a Phisitian should be incorporated of anie Towne or made a Member of anie corporation, not onlie to interrupt his Studies, hinder his practice but also to indaunger the liefe of his patient for want of his presence, because in a tedious & dangerous disease his presence is to be preffered before his private occasions, for what cannot a daie bring fourth & a little error causeth a relapse wch is worse than the disease, I know my disease is p[ar]lous & procrastination is daungerous. I have relied on you I trust you will not faile me now, I know you cannot be fined for visiting yr patients. Neither the Towne so barren of able men, nor the Magistrates so indiscreet to lay this burthen uppon you whose profession is to be most abroad & cannot be effected by an apprentice as theirs maie, & for you to be vexed with Towne buissenes whose calling is out of Towne it would seem a great folly in you & more malice in them to require. Therefore I councell you as a friend never be bounde as long as you may be free you shall but derogate from yr selfe, heap a great deale of troubles upon you distract you from yr Studie wch deserveth the whole employment of anie Man, had he a 100 yeres to lyve longer: Therefore I pray you all excuses set apart that you wilbe here to morrow morning by 7 of ye clock for I will fast until ye come, and I know you cannot incur anie daunger having so lawfull a calling. Thus with my best wishes & hartie love remembered to yr self & ye rest of my good friends with you I commit you to God holie protection & ever remain

Yor trewly loving friend and Servant
Sid Davenport

My Brother Colemores Phisick is ended & all is taken he staieth at home purposely to speak with you tomorrow morning for futher directions.
Bushwood. thursdaie 5 July 1632 (Lane 1996: xxvi–xxvii)

The end of Hall's life

John Hall's ledger-stone in Holy Trinity Church, Stratford-upon-Avon, records that he died on 25 November 1635, aged 60. Hall's death was presumably unexpected, as he made a nuncupative will (orally in front of witnesses) the same day. His wife and daughter inherited everything except his 'study of books' which went to his son-in-law, Thomas Nash, 'to dispose of them as you see good' (Marcham 1931: 25). His manuscripts would have gone to one Mr Boles 'if he had been here', but as he was not 'you may son Nash burn them or do with them what you please'.

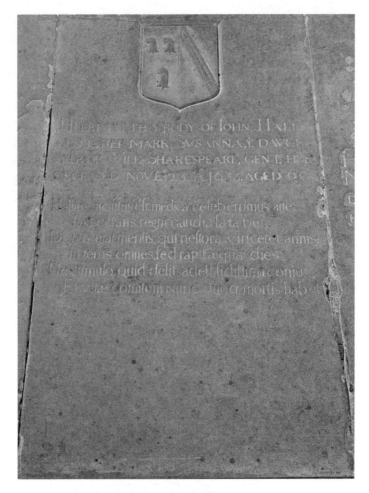

10 John Hall's gravestone and Latin epitaph, which can be translated as:

> Here is sited Hall, most renowned in the medical art,
> Awaiting the happy joys of the Kingdom of God.
> Such were his merits that he deserved to outlive Nestor in years,
> But indiscriminate time snatches away everyone on Earth.
> So that nothing may be lacking in his tomb,
> His most faithful wife is here,
> And he has her, his companion in life, now also in death.

Hall's epitaph reads almost like a tribute from Stratford-upon-Avon's citizens. The last three lines anticipate Susanna's being buried alongside him, and suggest that a place for her was already reserved.

Hall's will was dictated too hastily for the usual preamble expressing his faith, but the introduction to his own illness in the *Little Book of Cures* used texts from the Vulgate Old Testament and the physicians Valleriola and Ruland to the same purpose (Hall 1635: 150; see p. 239):

> Thou Lord, *hast power of life and death; thou leadest to the gates of hell, and bringest up again* [1 Samuel 2:6]. I confess *neither by human work, nor help from the art, nor advice, but only by your goodness and mercy you made me whole, and recovered me beyond all hope and expectation from the most severe and deadliest signs of a lethal fever, as if rescued from the jaws of hell and restored to perfect health* [Valleriola 1573: 1]. For this *I give thanks to you, most merciful God and Father of our Lord Jesus Christ, who through your fatherly mercy has made me whole. Give me grace, that I may recognise and remember your blessings with a grateful mind* [Ruland 1628: 231].

The combination of texts stressing divine rather than human works, and the thanks for God's mercy, reflect the evangelical element in Hall's beliefs. In other cases too, he frequently attributed cures to divine grace, even when treating his Catholic patients.

This edition marks the first time that a full translation of Hall's *Little Book of Cures* has been made available. It is here that we come closest to Hall's medical and intellectual outlook, and his pastoral care, including prayers for his patients' recovery, and thanksgivings when they were cured.

2

John Hall's working library

Hall's library was a dynamic creation. Its changing character over time reflects changes in his interests at different stages of his life. This edition makes it possible for the first time to identify the books Hall was using, the extent of his borrowings from them, and to understand how they contributed to his medical knowledge and practice. Knowing about Hall's books encourages questions about how he might have acquired them, and about the significance that his own working library has when considered in the context of his time. Hall used his books to identify therapies for his patients and to help him turn his initial notes into a draft for his own Latin case-book. There is no reason to believe that the books Hall used were the only ones he possessed. What can be put together is a partial list of the books Hall chose to use. His working library reflects two aspects of his working life: the sources of the remedies he used in treating his patients, and his wider sense of medical literature that helped him to compose his *Little Book of Cures*. It is only possible to reconstruct Hall's library through the close study of his Latin manuscript because of the extent to which he borrowed from Latin textbooks.

This borrowing has been hitherto unrecognised because of our reliance on James Cooke's partial English translation, *Select Observations of English Bodies*. Hall's borrowings make up between 30 and 40 per cent of the whole of his manuscript, a remarkable proportion. Although so significant a use of sources has not been described in any other casebook from Hall's period, Hall's borrowing from other texts was not unique. It should not be surprising that learned physicians, educated through the use of Latin textbooks, should use them in their daily practice. For historians of early modern English medicine, Hall's casebook is a reminder that appropriate attention should be given to the influence of these Latin texts. In fact, any use of Latin in a medical casebook should be considered as possibly deriving from a published Latin source, even if there is no explicit reference to it.

A greater understanding of medical libraries is one of the tools with which to study the development of early seventeenth-century medical practice.

Early modern medical libraries

The two major sources for understanding English libraries, *Books in Cambridge Inventories* and the *Private Libraries of Renaissance England* series (PLRE), are considerably more sparse for the early seventeenth century than they are for the sixteenth. Cambridge inventories with medical content jump from Thomas Lorkin (Professor of Physic at Cambridge, 1564–90) to John Nidd (*c.* 1620/30–1659). Nidd was not medically qualified but bequeathed over a hundred medical texts. The PLRE volumes (up to volume 8 at the time of writing) contain no medical collections of relevance for the last decade of the sixteenth century or later. Identifying a library such as John Hall's – even a partial one – for the years 1600 to 1650 contributes important new information.

It is a commonplace in the history of early modern medicine that Latin was the language in which learned, university-educated physicians received their education. The texts required in medical curricula were in Latin, though English ones might have had a supporting role (Siraisi 1990: 50; Jones 2000: 117). Yet much of the secondary literature on libraries implicitly or explicitly excludes

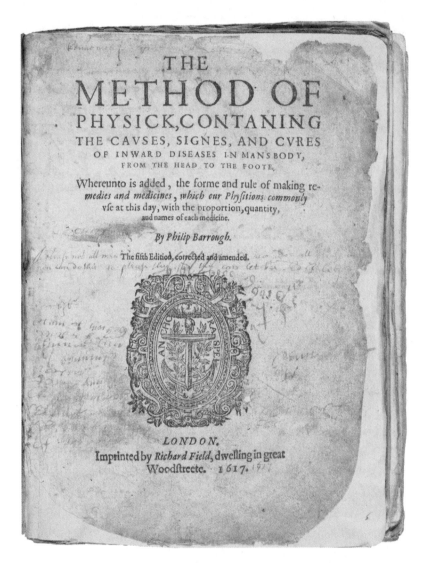

11 Title-page of Philip Barrough's *The Method of Physick* (1617). Philip Barrough was active from around 1590. This book was widely used, and published by Richard Field (the printer of Shakespeare's narrative poems), who was born in Stratford-upon-Avon. Barrough's reference work has helped to inform the glossary on pp. 288–297.

Latin texts in favour of the vernacular (Slack 1979: 238). Even when the importance of Latin for medical education is recognised, the subsequent use of it in medical practice is underplayed by comparison with vernacular texts. Hall relied almost entirely on Latin texts in his practice and in writing his manuscript. This is not to say that he did not own or read English medical texts, but for professional purposes the Latin texts were the important ones.

John Hall's library

What might we surmise about Hall's books? We know that he inherited his father's medical books on his death in 1607. John Hall was a medical student at Cambridge from 1589 to 1597. An anonymous Cambridge bookseller's probate inventory of 1588/89 gives an idea of the kind of books which appealed to the medical readers at the time. It contains works by Hippocrates and Galen, epitomes and commentaries on them and books in both Latin and English by sixteenth-century authors. Such books might be shared and borrowed by students as well as bought, but all these and others were available to the student with deep pockets, generous parents, or helpful tutors (Jones 2000: 467).

So far this could apply as a generality to any student of the period, but in Hall's case we can turn for a more personal view to *Select Observations*. James Cooke, translator and editor of *Select Observations*, visited Susanna Hall specifically to see her late husband's books in 1642, suggesting a collection worth viewing. He referred to Hall's interest in scurvy and claimed that he was ahead of his time in its treatment. The literature on scurvy was extensive by Hall's time, so he would have had a wide range of texts to choose from. Cooke added that Hall had travelled abroad and knew some French, so might have owned one or more books in that language (Hall 1657: sig. A3r–A4v).

Twenty authors and twenty-two books are named in Hall's manuscript and in Cooke's *Select Observations* (see Table 1). One

Table 1   Sources named in *Select Observations* and Hall's manuscript. The
dates following the publication details give the range of publication dates
of editions to which Hall might have had access. If no date range is given,
there is evidence that Hall used the specific edition listed.

Author	Title
Amatus Lusitanus	*Curationum medicinalium centuriae quatuor, quarum duae priores ab auctore sunt recognite, duae posteriores nunc primum edite* (Basel: Froben, 1556). 1556–57.
College of Physicians of London	*Pharmacopoeia Londinensis*, 2nd edn (London: John Marriot, 1618).
Johannes Crato	*Consiliorum et epistolarum medicinalium*, 6 vols (Frankfurt: Wechel, Marnius et Aubrius, 1591–1611).
Oswald Croll	*Basilica chymica* (Frankfurt: Marnius et heredes Aubrii, 1609). 1600–34.
Tobias Dornkrell	*Dispensatorium novum continens descriptiones et usum praecipuorum medicamentum* (Ultzen: Cröner, 1600). 1600–23.
Joseph Du Chesne	*Diaeteticon polyhistoricon* (Frankfurt: Schönwetter, 1607).
Severinus Eugalenus	*De scorbuto morbo liber* (Leipzig: Michael Rantzenberger, 1604). 1588–1624.
Gregor Horst	*Observationum medicinalium singularium libri quatuor* (Ulm: Saurius, 1625).
Jacques Houllier	*De morbis internis libri II* (Frankfurt: Wechel, 1589). 1570–1623.
John of Gaddesden	*Praxis medica, rosa anglica dicta* (Augsburg: Michael Manger, 1595).
Jean Liébault	*Thresor des remedes secrets pour les maladies des femmes* (Paris: Jacques du Puys, 1585).
Giovanni Battista da Monte	*Consultationum medicinalium centuria prima* (Venice: Valgrisius, 1556). 1554–69.
Bernard Penot	*De denario medico, quo decem medicaminibus, omnibus morbis internis medendi via docetur* (Berne: Ioannis le Preux, 1608). 1608–18.
Felix Platter	*Praxeos: Tractatus de functionem laesionibus* (Basel: Conrad Waldkirch, 1602). 1602–25. *Praxeos: tractatus secundus de doloribus* (Basel: Conrad Waldkirch, 1603). 1603–25. *Praxeos: tractatus tertius et ultimus de vitiis* (Basel: Conrad Waldkirch, 1608). 1608–25.

Table 1   *continued*

Author	Title
Rodrigo de Fonseca	*Consultationes medicae singularibus remediis refertae* (Venice: Ioannis Guerilius, 1620). 161–25.
Guillaume Rondelet	*Methodus curandorum omnium morborum corporis humani in tres libros distincta* (Paris: Carolus Macaeus, 1574). 1553–67.
Martin Ruland the Elder	*Balnearium restauratum, in quo curantur morbi tam externi quam interni* (Basel: 1579). 1556–1613. *Curationum empyricarum et historicarum, in certis locis et notis personis optime expertarum, et rite probatarum, centuriae decem* (Lyons: Pierre Ravaud, 1628). 1577–1628.
Daniel Sennert	*De scorbuto tractatus* (Wittenberg: Zacharia Shürer, 1624).
Valesco de Taranta	*Epitome operis perquam utilis morbis curandi* (Lyons: Ioan. Tornaesius: Gulielmus Gazeius, 1560).
François Valleriola	*Observationum medicinalium libri sex* (Lyons: Gryphius, 1573).

unusual book is *Thresor de remedes secrets pour les maladies des femmes* by Jean Liébault (*c.* 1535–96). This is in French, which must have been Hall's choice as it was also available in Latin. This is the only evidence to support Cooke's claim that Hall 'had been a traveller, acquainted with the French tongue' (Hall 1657: sig. A4r). Judging from Hall's manuscript, his acquaintance with French was slight: he added a translation in a mixture of English and Latin between the lines of the French text he borrowed. Perhaps he bought a copy of Liébaut's book as much to practise his French while travelling as for its medical content.

The differences between the list of authors identified in *Select Observations* and the full list of authors discernible through Hall's *Little Book of Cures* throw some light on Cooke's activities as an editor and his deliberate creation of Hall as a physician driven by empirical observation. Likewise, John Bird's foreword to *Select Observations*, 'To the Judicious Reader', underplays the importance of books in Hall's practice. Prescriptions from learned sources fell 'short in performing the cures they promise' and were not as trustworthy as first-hand experience (Hall 1657: sig. A6r–A6v). Cooke's and Bird's words should not be taken as entirely disinterested. They were in effect writing advertising copy for Cooke's own edition, rather than neutral appraisals.

Cooke removed all references to texts except those by Du Chesne, Sennert and Eugalenus (and in fact removed most references to the latter two). The excisions were not random. Most were from sixteenth-century sources, while those retained were from seventeenth-century books. There are exceptions in both directions. For example, John of Gaddesden remained in *Select Observations* despite his *Praxis medica rosa anglica* dating from the fourteenth century. Several references to the *Pharmacopoeia Londinensis* (published 1618) were removed. Their presence would have undercut Cooke's claim that Hall was not interested in authorities.

There is written evidence in Hall's manuscript for all the titles listed above. To these books must be added the final set of sources, the anonymous borrowings identified by online searches (see Table 2). This brings the complete list of Hall's working library to forty-three authors and sixty titles, at a conservative count.

Identifying John Hall's borrowings from other books

The process of identifying the borrowings grew from some chance findings, and was a lengthy and complicated task. It started simply enough, with a few online searches to check the spellings of technical words, but then became a process of checking Hall's manuscript from beginning to end. The most accessible if not the most reliable database for doing this was books.google.co.uk. Other significant supplementary sources were the digital collection of the Bayerische Staatsbibliothek (digitale-sammlung.de) and of the Bibliothèque nationale de France (bnf.fr). The Early European Books database (eeb.chadwyck.co.uk) was (at the time of writing) too recent a development to have been much help, but must be an important resource in the future.

The first few searches on single words showed by chance that they were frequently embedded in longer passages. Trial and error showed that searching for two- or three-word strings produced the most matches, though it was not adequate as a strategy on its own. In some cases Hall had changed the word order of his source, and these passages could only be identified by searching on groups of separate words. Growing familiarity with Hall's own Latin helped to identify certain phrases or expressions as probable borrowings (gerunds and gerundives are uncommon in his own words, but quite frequent in borrowings for example).

Spelling variations and the limitations of Google's Optical Character Recognition (OCR) software also created problems. Hall sometimes abbreviated words in a different way from his source, or expanded words which had been abbreviated and vice versa. Abbreviations were not standardised and varied between authors and editions. Sometimes the sexes and ages of patients in Hall's source differed from his own patient, so that the Latin grammatical endings changed. In addition, Google OCR struggled to cope with the poor quality of print in many of the sources, and with early modern printing conventions. Long esses are usually rendered as f, and ligatures are often unrecognised; 'v' and 'u' had their early modern values. The essential questions were, first, how might the original text have been spelled compared to Hall's, and then, how might that text appear when digitised? Sometimes several trials of different combinations of spellings, abbreviations and possible OCR readings were needed to produce a result.

Unfortunately, one important section of text was almost entirely unsearchable: the recipes. These are almost always abbreviated in the originals, but in no standard way even within a single book. They also contain non-standard characters such as pharmaceutical and quantity symbols which the OCR did not recognise.

The recipes I have identified were usually found by searching on adjacent plain text such as preparation instructions.

A few borrowings were identified directly from the sources. Hall had a tendency to borrow several texts from pages in close proximity, so that a search forward and back from an identified text did sometimes reveal others.

For my standard searches I set year limits of 1550 to 1635. The choice of 1550 was a pragmatic one based on experience, and 1635 was the year of Hall's death. In no case did test searches prior to 1550 find a text which could not be identified after that, and it seemed unlikely though not impossible that Hall's library would have gone that far back. This timescale also had the benefit of covering the probable lifespan of John's father William, and therefore including books he might have acquired and passed on to his son. The end point was useful as a standard cut-off, but was not definitive. Several texts were identified by searching later periods, on texts with better-quality printing, and then working backwards to an edition in Hall's lifetime. The borrowing from Thomas Adams in the epigraph, for example, was initially found in a nineteenth-century volume of collected sermons.

I have not included as borrowings any identical texts from two or more sources. This is a conservative approach, as Hall might well have owned one or more of them, but in the absence of a firm identification they have all been excluded. Fortunately different editions often had slight differences of words which allowed one or other to be identified as Hall's. My approach throughout has been conservative, and it is very likely that there are other unidentified borrowings still to be found. A method of searching for recipes which is not overly time-consuming would certainly reveal more. On the other hand, I am confident that I have not to any serious extent misidentified any borrowings or their sources.

Table 2   Authors and texts identified from anonymous borrowings in Hall's manuscript

Author	Title
Thomas Adams	*Mystical Bedlam*
Amatus Lusitanus	*Curationum centuriae quinta et sexta*
Jean Béguin	*Tyrocinium chymicum*
Bernard de Gordon	*Lilium medicinae*
Gualtherus Bruele	*Praxis medicinae*
Robert Burton	*Anatomy of Melancholy*
Rodrigo de Castro	*De universa mulierum medicina*
Girolamo Cardano	*Ars curandi parva*
Johannes Crato	*Consiliorum … liber secundus*
	Consiliorum … liber quartus
	Consiliorum … liber quintus
	Consiliorum … liber sextus
da Monte	*Consultationes medicae*
John Donne	*Devotions upon Emergent Occasions*
Joseph Du Chesne	*De priscorum philosophicorum materia*
	Pharmacopoea dogmaticorum
Thaddaeus Dunus	*De curandi … per venae sectionem*
Pieter van Foreest	*Observationum … de febribus ephemeris et continuis libri duo*
Jean Feyens	*De flatibus*
Jean Fernel	*Consiliorum liber*
	Therapeutices universalis
Johann Hartmann	*Praxis chymiatrica*
Luigi Luisini	*De morbo Gallico omnia*
Albert Occo	*Pharmacopoeia Augustana*
Pierre Potier	*Insignium curationum*
	Pharmacopoea spagirica
Felix Platter	*Praxeos … de vitiis*
	Observationum … libri tres
Henrik Ranzau	*De conservanda valetudine*
Jacob Rueff	*De conceptu*
Martin Ruland the Younger	*De morbo Ungarico*
Daniel Sennert	*De febribus libri*
	Medicina practica
Reiner Solenander	*Consiliorum medicinalium … Solenandri*
Benedetto Vettori	*Exhortatio ad medicum recte sancteque medicari cupientem*
Leonello Vittori	*De aegritudinibus infantium*
Jodocus Willich	*Urinarum probationes*

The number of texts could have been made much higher by counting each separate century of Ruland the Elder's *Curationes* as a separate publication, the format in which they were published in the 1580s and 1590s. As they were also published in a single volume in 1577 I have counted them as a single book. Similarly, Sennert's *De scorbuto morbo tractatus* contains, as well as his own work, reprints of texts on scurvy by Baudouin Ronsse, Johann Echt, Johannes Wier, Johann Lange, Salomon Alberti and Matthaeus Martini. There is no evidence that Hall used any of these independently of Sennert's volume, so only the latter is included in the library. A different problem is encountered with the borrowings from Crato. As well as appearing in books under his name, several but not all of the borrowings from Crato appear in the massive compendia by Johannes Schenk von Grafenberg (1530–98). These do not provide any additional borrowings not found elsewhere. Relying on Crato's volumes alone gives the lowest number of books needed to cover all Hall's identified borrowings from this author.

The three books with English titles are worth noting. They were all written predominantly in English, but in each case Hall made use only of Latin borrowings. Two of them are religious works by Thomas Adams (1583–1652) and John Donne (1572–1631). Their paths may have crossed around 1621 when Adams was a preacher at St Gregory by St Paul's and Donne was Dean of St Paul's Cathedral. Adams was a Puritan vicar and preacher whose sermon *Mystical Bedlam* used madness as an allegory of different ways of falling away from godliness. Hall used as one of his epigraphs a sentence from 'The Impatient' who, 'when the ties of softer afflictions will not hold him, he must be manacled with the chaines of judgements' (Adams 1615: 68).

John Donne's *Devotions upon Emergent Occasions and Several Steps in my Sickness* describes his physical and spiritual course through a severe illness. Hall used a line from the *Devotions* to describe a treatment he received during his own illness, the application of a live pigeon to his feet to draw down the humours (Donne 1624: 284).

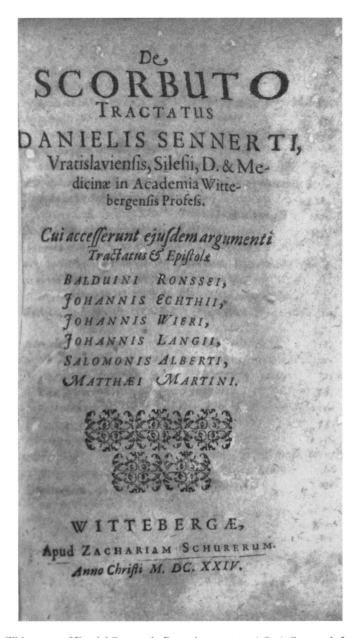

12 Title-page of Daniel Sennert's *De scorbuto tractatus* (1624). Sennert's Latin textbook, to which Hall often referred, includes reprints of texts on scurvy by Baudouin Ronsse, Johann Echt, Johannes Wier, Johann Lange, Salomon Alberti and Matthaeus Martini.

Descriptions of this therapy were available in standard medical texts, but Donne's more religious expression of what it was to be seriously ill must have spoken directly to Hall's own circumstances and religious beliefs.

The third English book which Hall used was that monumental work, *The Anatomy of Melancholy* by Robert Burton (1577–1640). In the Second Partition, Section 1, Member 4, subsection II, Burton considered the need for patients to be 'conformable, and content to be ruled' by their physician. Among the authorities he quoted are da Monte, giving an English translation in the main text and Latin paraphrases in two footnotes. Hall used Burton's footnotes rather than da Monte's original text (Burton 2001: 302). The context was a conversation with a patient, in which Hall asked for and received assurances of the patient's cooperation during a long and difficult treatment. It demonstrates the way Hall used concepts from his sources in his discussions with patients, though it does not prove that the words in his text were precisely those he used in conversation.

The extent of Hall's borrowings seems to have been unique, but there is evidence that other physicians did the same but to a lesser degree. Hall himself provides evidence of this. Mrs Delabere (Case 111) went to Bath and was prescribed a sweating decoction to use after bathing. Her remedy was based on a mixture of two recipes taken from Du Chesne's *Pharmacopoea dogmaticorum* (Du Chesne 1607: 53). Hall did not state who prescribed this, but it was clearly not him. From another source, John Symcotts started his 'Observations 1636' with sentences in Latin, the first taken from Sennert's *Opera omnia*: 'Si multi pravi succi in corpore abundant purgationes periculosiores sunt' (If many corrupt humours abound in the body, purgations are more dangerous) (Sennert 1631: 690; Poynter and Bishop 1951: 51). This is followed by a longer extract also from Sennert, expanding on the same subject (Poynter and Bishop 1951: 51). Symcotts went on to describe cases from his own experience exemplifying this problem.

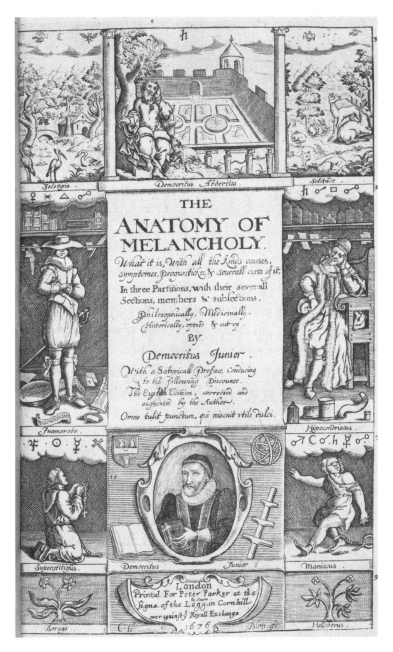

13 Title-page of Robert Burton's *The Anatomy of Melancholy* (1676). One of the most influential books of the age, and an important source that shows how Hall in part understood the emotions and feelings of his patients.

Hall was used as an unattributed source himself by James Cooke in *Mellificium chirurgiae*. Cooke follows the custom of the time by listing in his preface several authorities from whom he took remedies. Among those he mentioned in his address 'to the young Chyrurgeon' and which were also used by Hall are Sennert, Béguin, Potier, Foreest, Houllier, Ruland, Platter and Du Chesne (Cooke 1648: sig. A7r). Cooke continues: 'besides thou hast the secrets of practitioners, whose names are worthy to be mentioned, and should if it were not for fear of offending them, they came unexpectedly into my hands, and are as freely set out for thy benefit' (Cooke 1648: sig. A7r).

One recipe that Cooke very probably borrowed from Hall is his treatment of Mrs Wincoll (Case 10) for a prolapsed anus. Hall took this from Penot's *De denario medico* (Penot 1608: 64). Cooke was writing a textbook, not a series of case reports, so his grammar differs from Hall's manuscript and from *Select Observations*. His remedy (in Latin) is nonetheless almost identical to that of Hall, Penot and his own translation in the first edition of *Select Observations* (Cooke 1648: 308; Hall 1657: 16). The English directions for treatment which follow are clearly from the same source. Further evidence of Cooke's use of Hall is his comment before giving the recipe: 'externally use this fomentation, with which two was cured'. Hall added at the end of his report on Mrs Wincoll that he had successfully treated Mr Broad's tutor in the same way.

When did John Hall acquire his books?

Hall's involvement with physic, from his matriculation at Cambridge in 1589 to his death in 1635, spanned forty-six years. This was a period of change in styles of medical writing and long enough for Hall's own interests to change and develop. Did he replace old practices with new, add new modes of thinking to his repertoire, or rely on tried and tested remedies throughout his career?

Hall's working library at the time he was writing contained books written over eight decades, from 1550 into the 1630s. Such lengthy spans were not unusual. What Hall's library shows is that such older books were not simply sitting on shelves waiting to be inventoried, but were regularly used even in the later years of his practice.

Many books had lengthy publishing histories so that dating an acquisition is not easy. Hall might have acquired a book any time after it was published and before his first dated use of it. The dates of acquiring mid-sixteenth-century books are most difficult to pin down. They might have been purchases from his university years, gifts from his father at that time or inherited from him in 1607. With regard to books published later, particularly those published after 1607, Hall seems to have been using them (and therefore owning them) fairly soon after their publication. An exception to this is Eugalenus's *De scorbuto morbo*, published in 1604 but not mentioned by Hall before a report in 1629. The books in Hall's library first published between 1550 and 1569 are predominantly Galenic and Hippocratic in outlook. Hall's more theoretical texts (by Fernel and Cardano – neither extensively used) come from this period. Da Monte and Rondelet represent important strands in academic teaching, from Padua and Montpellier respectively. Both are authors who would have appealed to medical students as well as practitioners. Several books from this period deal with single topics, including conception, medicinal baths, venesection, the French disease and illnesses in children. They seem to be over-specialised for a student, but perhaps some of them were among the texts Hall inherited from his father. None of them made a major contribution to his borrowings.

Books published between 1570 and 1589 are more of a mix-ture. Houllier represents another important academic strand, this time from Paris, to supplement da Monte and Rondelet. Both Ruland the Elder and Valleriola were important sources for Hall throughout his career, so were perhaps authors whose writings he came to know well while at university. Considering his enormous output and Hall's evident attraction to series of publications (for example, those by Ruland the Elder, Crato and Platter), it seems somewhat strange that Foreest is represented by only a single volume. Hall did use some of Foreest's remedies for scurvy but these were reprinted in other texts Hall owned, such as Sennert's *De scorbuto tractatus*. There is no evidence that Foreest was an original source for Hall's knowledge of scurvy. Ruland the Elder's *Curationum ... centuriae* was first published as a single volume in 1577. The latter would have been cheaper and useful to a student, while the former, if Hall owned it, might have come from his father. Single topic books are again present, dealing with uroscopy, regimens of health and women's illnesses. There is some change in the type of books, but also, more importantly, in their use. Both Ruland the Elder and Valleriola's texts were books Hall knew well and relied on as standards throughout his working years.

The 1590s were the main period of Hall's medical education, followed by a time probably gaining practical experience, before he moved to Stratford-upon-Avon around 1607. An important medical publishing event of this time must have been the series of Crato's *Consiliorum*. Crato and Ruland the Elder were the sources of recipes in Hall's earliest dated case, in 1611. Two authors from this period were used frequently by Hall, Bruele and Crato. Others were used more sparingly.

The final phase of Hall's book-buying comes with his life in Stratford-upon-Avon after 1607. The pattern is quite different from what went before. Almost every medical book he acquired in this period is chymiatric to some degree. Some of Hall's new books were very definitely so: Penot's *De denario medico* is more alchemical than medical, while works by Béguin, Potier and Johann Hartmann (1568–1631) take a strong, more chemically based approach to the body.

Hall was also buying books by authors already on his shelves, including new works by Du Chesne and Platter (both important sources, particularly Platter's *Observationum*). Sennert became important to Hall from the mid-1620s onwards. He was published from early in the seventeenth century, but all of Hall's borrowings come from later books.

Pharmacopoeias make up a good proportion of acquisitions. Hall might have acquired Du Chesne's *Pharmacopoea dogmaticorum* early (it was published in 1607) and there is evidence from remedies used that he owned the 1613 edition of the *Pharmacopoea Augustana*. At some point he updated this with the *Pharmacopoeia Londinensis* (1618). His continuing interest in chemically based approaches is shown by the use of Potier's *Pharmacopoea spagirica* (1622), even though the *Pharmacopoeia Londinensis* was supposed to have become the exclusive standard for England at that time.

Five other books require a mention, two in particular because Hall used them intensively. Ruland the Younger's *De morbo Ungarico* was published in 1610. Hall used it in only five of his cases, but relied on it almost entirely in each of them. It was his standard work on malignant fevers, to the exclusion of other texts. Gregor Horst's *Observationum* was published in 1625, but despite its late date Hall used it often, particularly as a source for treatments of scurvy. The other three are Hall's English books, the aforementioned volumes of devotions by Donne and Adams, and Burton's *Anatomy of Melancholy*. They are a reminder that Hall was much involved in the religious and social life of Stratford-upon-Avon. As a committed Puritan member of the Church of England he almost certainly had an extensive library of religious texts as well as medical ones.

In sum, Hall's working library was not static but grew over decades, reflecting the different stages of his working life. He started with books useful to a student and later in life developed new interests in chymical practice and scurvy. Among the books inherited from his father may have been a small number of theoretical texts and some unusual single-topic texts, perhaps reflecting his father's tastes rather than his own. Once settled in Stratford-upon-Avon he bought new books regularly, mainly ones that combined a practical slant with a chemical interest. In most of his practice he continued to rely on books he had known since his early education.

How did John Hall acquire his books?

This question is most relevant to Hall's time in Stratford, as the earlier periods are relatively straightforward. There were book-shops in Cambridge where he was a student and books could be borrowed from colleges or staff. His father might have provided him with the beginnings of a library before or during his studies, which would explain the presence of several books from around 1550 to 1575.

Once Hall had settled in Stratford-upon-Avon he no longer had a bookseller immediately on hand, but still bought at least twenty books between 1607 and 1635. In some cases there is evidence for him using new books soon after their publication, so he must have been able to choose, purchase, read and apply them quite rapidly. He used the *Consultationes* of Rodrigo de Fonseca (1550–1622) in the year it was published (1619) and Horst's *Observationum* the year after its publication in 1625.

London was the centre of the English book trade and the essential link in the importation of books from Europe – the 'Latin trade'. From 1616 to 1627 this was supposedly a monopoly of the Stationers Guild in London. Most of the imported books came to London from one of the trade fairs in Germany, of which Frankfurt was the most important in Hall's time. Book fair catalogues were published twice yearly and circulated widely. If Hall had access to these he might have been able to make specific requests based on them. Obtaining a specific book could be a complicated and frustrating process for a country gentle-man, whether on personal visits to London or through a trusted intermediary. Pedlars and chapmen formed an extended network for booksellers to distribute their wares outside of London. They might have carried catalogues to tempt wealthier buyers as well as more popular literature. Stratford-upon-Avon had a regular carrier service to and from London from Elizabethan times. It carried letters as well as other goods and might have carried books or catalogues.

There was another, shorter link to booksellers, perhaps more useful for a working physician (though there is no more supporting evidence for it than for a direct connection to London). This would have been through booksellers in Oxford. They had a market among both university staff and students and with the growing Bodleian Library, founded in 1602. In 1615 the Bodleian curators commissioned two London booksellers to visit every Frankfurt fair and also other important outlets on the Continent. The Bodleian committee met soon after the arrival of each fair's catalogue to decide on purchases. It would have been easier and more informative for Hall to visit Oxford twice a year to inspect new purchases at the Bodleian and peruse the catalogues, than to travel to London. He could then have used the same trade links as the Bodleian to order and receive any books he wanted. There is a closer match between the authors in Hall's library and the Bodleian than with any of the other booklists.

Did John Hall's use of books change over time?

Did new books replace old, or did old favourites retain their places throughout Hall's career? Not all of the dating evidence can be used to answer this. A minority of Hall's consultations are datable and not all of Hall's borrowings can be taken as contemporaneous with the original consultation. He might have used borrowings for descriptions of patients or their illnesses without having owned the source at the time of the consultation. The best dating evidence is that of the remedies, which must have been available at the time the patient consulted Hall.

Table 3   Most frequently used texts, with number of consultations they appear in, and dates of earliest and latest known use

Author, title	Number of consultations	Earliest dated consultation	Latest dated consultation
Ruland, *Curationum*	11	1611	1633
Platter, *Observationum*	9	1619	1634
Horst, *Observationum*	8	1626	1633
Sennert, *De scorbuto*	8	1629	1634
Platter, *Praxeos*	5	1617	1634
Valleriola, *Observationum*	5	1619	1633
Crato, *Consiliorum*	4	1613	1626
Eugalenus, *De scorbuto morbo*	4	1629	1633
Du Chesne, *Pharmacopoea dogmaticorum*	3	1611	1630

Table 3 shows how different books or series of books were used in datable consultations and the periods of time over which they were used. Nine books are mentioned three times or more, Ruland the Elder's *Curationum* and Platter's *Observationum* occurring most frequently (eleven and nine times respectively). They are followed by Horst's *Observationum* and Sennert's *De scorbuto* with eight appearances each. Most of the books in this list were first published in the 1590s or later. There are relatively fewer from earlier in the sixteenth century. Ruland the Elder and Valleriola are exceptions, both having been published before 1590. Hall used them consistently from before 1620 into the 1630s. Ruland the Elder and Du Chesne both appeared in Hall's earliest dated consultation in 1611 and remained in use by him for around twenty years. At the other extreme Horst, Sennert and Eugalenus, Hall's main texts on scurvy, only came into use in the late 1620s, though quite intensively from then on.

Hall relied mainly on old favourites, using recently acquired works only occasionally. There is one possible suggestion of a fundamental change. Hall used Crato from 1613 until 1626, which was also the first year in which he used a remedy from Horst. Since he used Horst several times thereafter but not Crato, this may be evidence of Hall abandoning an older text in favour of something newer.

3

John Hall's manuscript of
A Little Book of Cures

John Hall's Latin manuscript is the one record we have of his authentic voice, even if expressed at times in the words of others. It is contained in a small notebook, measuring approximately 18 by 10 centimetres. It is now in a leather binding marked 'British Museum' (from around 1868, before its transfer to the British Library) with a title, 'Case Book of Dr John Hall', on its spine.

The manuscript is complete, with no missing pages. The paper has faded to a light brown with only a few stains and blemishes. The top, bottom and sides of each page have faint ruled margins, and the text, written in ink now faded to a dark brown, mostly stays within them. There are few corrections and no deleted text apart from occasionally corrected words. Hall consistently recorded dates in the new style, with the year starting on 1 January. He wrote in an italic hand, used many abbreviations and made errors in grammar. Hall's writing is on the whole tidy and formal with well-spaced lines. The manuscript is sometimes more crowded and uneven, before Hall returns to his initial tidiness. The writing is consistent throughout with no evidence of deterioration from beginning to end.

The numbering of the manuscript's pages is complex. At the front there are five unnumbered pages, three blank followed by one stamped 'E.G.2065 (Farnb.)' and written below, 'purchased by Mr Paterson 10 Oct. 1868'. There follows another blank page

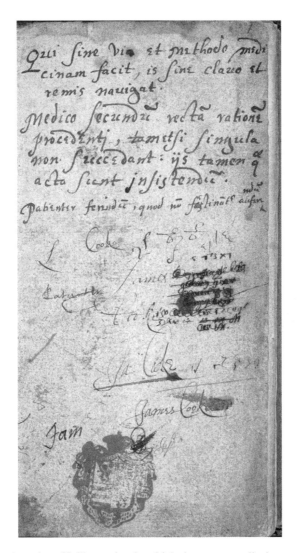

14 The epigraph to Hall's casebook, which draws on medical texts of his
time as well as Hippocrates (and alludes to Marcus Aurelius). Translated
it reads: 'Whoever practises medicine without direction and method,
sails without rudder or oars. When a physician proceeds according to
correct reasoning, even though he does not succeed every time, he should
nevertheless persist in his course of action. One must bear patiently
what one cannot immediately lay aside.' James Cooke, who owned the
manuscript, has signed his name (in whole or in part) on this first page four
times.

15 The first page of Hall's manuscript: *Curationum historicarum et empiricarum, in certis locis et notis personis expertarum et probatarum, Libellus.* Hall's Latin title alludes to the title of a book by his Swiss peer, Martin Ruland the Elder: *Curationum empyricarum et historicarum, in certis locis et notis personis optime expertarum, et rite probatarum, centuriae decem* (1628). Note Hall's legible handwriting with many abbreviations, his original page numbering (1) and that added later (2). The first case report has no separate heading and starts with the patient's identity.

16 Page 35 of Hall's manuscript, showing his correction of 'morbilli' to 'variola'.

before Hall's text starts with an unnumbered page of epigraphs and a further blank page. At the end of the manuscript there are five unnumbered pages, the first bearing a pencilled note, '131 folios HK November 1869'. The remaining four are blank.

The pages of Hall's text in the centre of the manuscript are numbered in two systems. One, in pencil, and in a similar hand to the note dated November 1869, runs from folio 1r (Hall's epi-graph page) to folio 131v. This is presumably an editorial addition from the time of its ownership by the British Museum. Hall's own numbers start with 1 on his title page (f.2r) and run to the end of his text, a total of 191 pages. His numbering went awry towards the end, the last five pages running 187, 187 (duplicated), 188, 199 and 200. Hall did not number his page of epigraphs nor the page after them (ff.1r–1v) preceding his main text. He started an index but left it unfinished, on folios 123r to 129r. I have not included this in the critical edition as it is adds little information.

Several of the other pages of writing can be firmly associated with James Cooke. He wrote his name four times, in whole or part, on the epigraph page. The next page contains two short recipes and a note 'Mr John Sherley Golden Pelican in Little Britain' in a different hand. John Sherley was the publisher of the first edition of Cooke's abridged translation. Between the end of Hall's text and his index are a mixture of consultation and other medical notes in English and Latin. Three reports (folios 105v–106v) are dated 7, 23 and 24 January 1656, when the book was in Cooke's possession. All the patients lived in or near Warwick, where Cooke practised. Further medical notes in Cooke's hand and two pages on the Hebrew alphabet and grammar occupy a few pages after the index and before the final blank pages.

The dates of composition of the manuscript can be quite tightly limited. The consultation with Anne Smith (Case 3) has been dated by Joan Lane to 1634, meaning that the bulk, and probably the whole, of the manuscript was written during 1634 and 1635 (Lane 1996: 9).

17 Page 67 of Hall's manuscript. Note the less tidy handwriting than on page 1, and a separate heading referring to the illness at the start of Case 141.

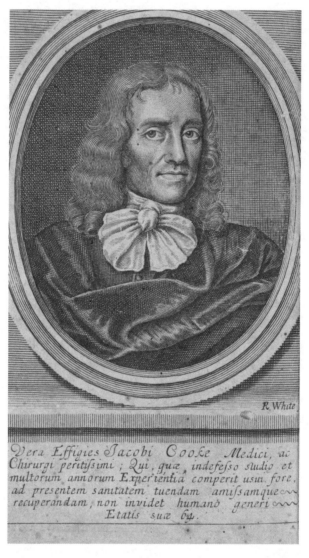

Vera Effigies Jacobi Cooke Medici, ac
Chirurgi peritissimi ; Qui, quæ, indefesso studio et
multorum annorum Experientia comperit usu fore,
ad presentem sanitatem tuendam amissamque
recuperandam, non invidet humano generi
Etatis suæ 64.

18 Portrait of James Cooke, who visited Susanna Hall to procure her
late husband's medical papers, and first published selections from Hall's
casebook in 1657. This portrait is reproduced from the 1683 edition. The
Latin inscription can be rendered: 'A true likeness of James Cooke, doctor
and most skilled surgeon, who does not grudge humanity, who discovers,
by tireless zeal and by experience of many years [things] that are of use
to preserving present health and regaining lost health. The age of 64.'
Translation by Amy Hurst.

The history of Hall's manuscript

John Hall's nuncupative will of 25 November 1635 contains the earliest mention of his books and papers:

> concerning my study of books I leave them (sayd he) to yow my sonn Nash [Hall's son-in-law Thomas Nash] to dispose of them as yow see good. As for my manuscripts I would have given them to Mr Boles [unidentified] if hee had been here but forasmuch as he is not heere present, yow may son Nash burne them or doe with them what yow please. (Prerogative Court of Canterbury, 115 Pile: Marcham 1931: 25)

No probate inventory survives to provide details. The next reference to the manuscript is found in James Cooke's preface to the first edition of *Select Observations*. Some of the books and manuscripts must have remained with Hall's widow Susanna, rather than with Hall's son-in-law, according to James Cooke's description of how he acquired them:

> Being in my art an attendent to parts of some regiments to keep the pass at the bridge of Stratford upon Avon [around 1642], there being with me a mate allyed to the gentleman that writ the following observations in Latin, he invited me to the house of Mrs Hall wife to the deceased, to see the books left by Mr Hall. After a view of them, she told me she had some books left, by one that professed physick, with her husband, for some money. I told her, if I liked them, I would give her the money again; she brought them forth, amongst which there was this with another of the authors, both intended for the presses. I being acquainted with Mr Hall's hand, told her that one or two of them were her husbands, and shewed them her. She denied, I affirmed, till I perceived she began to be offended. At last I returned her the money. (Hall 1657: sig. A3r–A4r).

This passage has caused much debate among Shakespearean scholars: how could Susanna Hall not have known her own husband's writing? And what speculations might we make from that about her literacy? Lachlan Mackinnon argues convincingly that she was literate and simply 'couldn't be bothered with someone fossicking after her husband's papers' (Mackinnon 2015: 81). My own interpretation is that Mrs Hall thought Cooke was only interested in buying printed books and tried to pass her husband's manuscripts off as such. Once it became clear that Cooke was interested mainly in the manuscripts, the misunderstanding was cleared up. He purchased them and perhaps other books as well. Cooke was a surgeon with ambitions to be a physician (he was licensed in 1661), so perhaps he saw translating and publishing a medical text as a step towards this. At any rate he:

> resolved to put it to suffer according to perceived intentions, to which end I sent it to London which after viewed by an able doctor, he returned answer, that it might be usefull, but the Latin was so abbreviated or false that it would require the like pains as to write a new one. (Hall 1657: sig.A3v–B1r)

Fortunately, Cooke 'put it into this garb, being somewhat acquainted with the author's conciseness, especially in the receipts, having had some intimacy with his apothecary' (Hall 1657: sig. B1r).

The next reference to the manuscript is in Edmond Malone's edition of Shakespeare's plays:

> The private note-book of [...] Dr Hall, containing a short state of the cases of his patients, was a few years ago put into my hands by my friend, the late Dr Wright; and as Dr Hall [...] undoubtedly attended Shakspeare in his last illness, being then forty years old, I had hopes this book might have enabled me to gratify the publick curiosity on this subject. (Malone 1821: II, 505–506)

Malone's hopes were dashed: there is no mention of the playwright in the manuscript, an omission that has engendered pages of speculation ever since. According to Joan Lane, the manuscript had been owned by the actor David Garrick prior to Malone (Lane 1996: xxx–xxxi).

John Hall's attitude to his patients

Certain themes in Hall's writing run across more than one case report and it is these more than the details of individual patients which provide an insight into his thinking and attitudes. Many, such as Hall's conversations with patients, his relationships with other practitioners and his uses of theory, were removed by Cooke from *Select Observations*. They are only to be seen by going back to his original text.

A number of Hall's patients were treated by someone else before turning to him. The other practitioners included an empiric (Lady Smith, Case 118), surgeons (William Clavell, Case 76, and Mr Barnes, Case 81) and a midwife (Mrs Fiennes, Case 167). Hall recorded the prior treatment and his own successful therapy for each patient, but made no explicit criticism of the other practitioners involved, nor of their fitness to practise. Nor did he offer overt criticism of patients for consulting them. This contrasts strongly with the views of his Northampton colleague, John Cotta, who strongly disapproved of medical treatment being offered by anyone but a physician. In contrast to his dispassionate view of other practitioners, Hall regularly emphasised his successes where other experienced physicians had failed. Mr Harvey (Case 139) 'received differing opinions from many physicians'. Mrs Woodward (Case 150) was treated by a physician, but 'fell from the continual burning fever into a dangerous bastard tertian'. Mr Kimberley (Case 169) 'took much from physicians, to no avail'. In each case Hall treated the patient successfully. The emphasis on the experience of other physicians is particularly noticeable in relation to the diagnosis of scurvy. Mrs Swift (Case 166) and Mrs Stoughton (Case 175) had both been 'purged by an experienced physician' before Hall made the correct diagnosis. One of his strongest statements relates to Dr Thornborough, Bishop of Worcester (Case 164): 'The deceptive appearance of the arthritis misled and toyed with his physicians, who were experienced and learned in traditional medicine.'

Hall's uneasy relationship with other physicians also comes through in the treatment of his own illness (Case 155) when his wife called in two other physicians. Though he referred to them as friends and took the remedies they prescribed, his summary of their efforts was less than gracious:

> Before the physicians attended me, I took 10oz of blood from the hepatic vein, and the third day after that, leeches were applied to the haemorrhoidal veins [...] but I give thanks first to God, then to the hartshorn decoction, and finally to the venesection.

Hall offered no thanks to the physicians and does not mention their treatments among those he evidently regarded as successful. He comes across as the archetypal practitioner who is a difficult patient when ill himself.

Hall also accepted patients' self-treatment as a normal part of practice. As Elaine Leong and Sara Pennell put it, 'the decision to call on the services of a physician ... or other forms of paid medical practice, usually followed the failure of domestic treatment' (Leong and Pennell 2007: 134). This is evident in Hall's reports on Mrs Kempson (Case 78), Squire Rainsford (Case 80), Mrs Randolph (Case 99) and the schoolmaster John Trapp (Case 177). Patients also sometimes queried or changed Hall's prescriptions, with purgation or bleeding a particular issue. Mr Broad (Case 100) refused venesection and so 'fell into a continual burning fever as I foretold'. On Hall's next visit he was 'in danger of death, unable to say anything. Immediately I cut a vein and bled to 10oz', which worked well enough for Mr Broad to say that he was greatly relieved. The second Countess of Northampton (Case 144) 'does not want to be purged, nor do I wish it'. She also disliked the barberry conserve which Hall prescribed and instead 'took jelly of hartshorn shavings with marigold and crocus flowers'.

As this shows, treatments were sometimes changed from those prescribed. Hall prescribed a mixture with oil of water-lilies for Grace Court (Case 143), 'but since this oil was not to hand' she used a mixture of oils of scorpions and almonds. For Mr Barnes's toothache, 'since I had no remedy to hand, I prescribed cold water held in the mouth and often spat out', which worked well. The Revd Holyoak's son was prescribed a pomegranate syrup described as particularly suitable for measles, but 'this was not to hand' so a different one was used 'with happy effect'.

Recipes were circulated and exchanged among lay people and from physicians to lay people. Hall refers to this explicitly in four reports. Two of them add an extra link to the chain, in that the transmitted recipe came originally from one of Hall's printed sources. Squire Pakington (Case 71) asked for something to restore his appetite and Hall prescribed *pulvis senae Montagnanae* (Montagnana's senna powder), using the recipe given in the 1613 edition of the *Pharmacopoeia Augustana*. Mrs Murden (Case 107) complained of giddiness and headache and was prescribed a laxative remedy taken from the first book of Crato's *Consiliorum et epistolarum*.

Hall recorded several consultations with children. His treatments for either fits or worms are good illustrations of what Hannah Newton calls 'children's physic' in the seventeenth century (Newton 2014: 2–3). They also demonstrate his use of Latin texts to find therapies specifically intended for this age group. The Revd Walker's six-month-old son (Case 35) and two-year-old Lydia Trapp (Case 114) both suffered from fits. They received similar treatments, with sliced peony roots hung round their necks, peony powder sprinkled in their hair and an ointment of Venice treacle and peony root applied over the heart. The source of the latter two treatments was Felix Platter's *Observationum*. The case that these were borrowed from is headed *Epilepsia in infante*, and for both his patients Hall used the exact ingredients and quantities specified by Platter.

Several of Hall's child patients suffered from worm infestations. Newton states that purgatives were generally not used in children, but Hall used them to expel the worms, favouring much milder ones than he used in adults (Newton 2014: 76). Four-year-old Winter (Case 40) and three-year-old Dixwell Brent (Case 94) both had a honey suppository based on a recipe in Platter's *De vitiis*. The one-year-old George Talbot (Case 56) and Mr Bishop's six-year-old son (Case 59) both received a milk and sugar enema. Mr Bishop's son also had a linctus for his chest which contained two mild purgatives, manna and cassia. This recipe was taken, exactly as printed, from Vittori's *De aegritudinibus infantium*.

Hall did not give children modified versions of the much stronger purgatives he used to treat worms in adults. Mrs Bovey (Case 161) and Edith Stoughton (Case 170) received the identical treatment from Amatus Lusitanus, containing wormseed (a vermicide) and strong purgatives. Hester Sylvester (Case 125) was treated with a different recipe from the same source. Mary Heath (Case 17) was treated with wax infused into a cooked apple, a remedy from Valleriola which Hall commended.

Hall occasionally recorded detailed conversations with his patients. The longest record relates to Dr Thornborough (Case 164). This covered the reasons for Hall's diagnosis of scorbutic arthritis (missed by other physicians), some background theory on scurvy which evidently interested the bishop, and the tragic story of his son's suicide. In the consultation with Mrs Mary Talbot (Case 103), Hall's diagnosis of long-standing scurvy led the patient to explain that she had indeed been treated for scurvy previously and 'had been cured in the Archduke's palace in the Low Countries two years previously'. Hall also noted the patient's pride at carrying out his instructions to take exercise. He saw her at a relative's house and 'she thanked me greatly, and said she had walked three miles'. Hall also showed pleasure in treatments which both cured a patient and resulted in a successful outcome to pregnancy. He referred to a 'beautiful baby' twice, in the reports on Mrs Combe (Case 130) and again on the Countess of Northampton (Case 144):

> She bore a beautiful daughter afterwards, and meeting in passing, I
> saw her carrying her beautiful daughter in her arms. She declared
> that she gave thanks to God and to me for her, because she had not
> thought that she could survive.

Here and in similar reports Hall showed a personal and sympathetic interest in his patients' histories and outcomes. This is
also evident in his comments on Lady Browne's condition (Case
106), which 'arose from the death of her beloved, beautiful and
devout daughter, whose life (a year previously) changed to death
in childbirth, and she sleeps peacefully with the Lord'.

A rather different theme in Hall's manuscript is his application
of theory to his diagnoses and treatment. I use theory here in a
fairly wide and general sense, to refer to any writing or theory
on the causes of disease or differential diagnosis, as opposed to
therapy of a specific illness. Readers of *Select Observations* may
be forgiven for thinking that Hall had little interest in this, an
impression which is largely an artefact of Cooke's editing. By my
count the manuscript contains twenty references to medical theory
across fifteen case reports (Cases 4, 16, 106, 112, 113, 121, 133, 150,
154, 162, 164, 165, 167, 174 and 175). Of these, Cooke omitted all
but three (Cases 4, 112 and 175) from *Select Observations* and in only
one (Case 112) translated the passage completely.

Hall made the greatest number of references to theory in
relation to the diagnosis of scurvy, mainly using Sennert and
Eugalenus as his sources. These references are placed in the text
at points where Hall is discussing his diagnosis and before pro-
ceeding to treatment. In two reports Hall gave references to the
causes of scurvy (Cases 154 and 165). In another three he referred
to differential diagnoses, distinguishing between scorbutic symptoms and conditions mimicking them (Cases 106, 150 and 167). A
sixth explains an unusual event, the occurrence of epilepsy during
recovery from scurvy. The final two cases contain borrowings
which describe the pathogenesis of scurvy caused by blockage
of the meseraic veins and how melancholy vapours produced

around the spleen spread the disease to all parts of the body (Cases 150 and 162).

In a different way, Hall appended borrowings relating to theory at the end of three reports. Mr Dyson (Case 16) suffered from abdominal pain relieved by eating, rather than brought on by it. Hall borrowed two paragraphs from a lengthy review of this unusual presentation from da Monte's *Consultationum*. James Ballard's treatment for bloody flux (Case 112) finishes with a borrowing from Croll's *Basilica chymica* listing the differences between dysentery, lyentery and diarrhoea. The report on Katherine Sturley (Case 133), who complained of blood in the urine without pain, concludes with a list of Hippocratic aphorisms commenting on this presentation. Hall's source for these was Willich's *Urinarum probationes*.

What these examples show is that Hall did not draw on more theoretically orientated authors even when including theory in his reports. He took theory from the same practical texts that he used for his therapies. He gave no explanation as to why he wanted to include theory in some reports, so the following suggestions are speculative. In relation to scurvy, Hall's references to Sennert and Eugalenus may have been intended (if his book had been published during his lifetime, as seems to have been his intention) to bolster his standing as a specialist in scurvy compared to other physicians. His borrowings and references emphasise his ownership and use of the best available texts on the subject. However important empirical observation might be, it had to be applied in the context of up-to-date book-learning in the traditional style if it was to play a part in establishing his credibility.

The reports in which Hall appended a text on theory at the end are different in content and style. I suggest that in these Hall is addressing himself in the first place, ensuring that he has not missed any important element in the causation and therefore correct treatment of the patients. This harks back to his epigraph based on one of Hippocrates' aphorisms: 'When a physician proceeds according to correct reasoning, even though he does not succeed every time, he should nevertheless persist in his course of action.' These may be reflective conclusions to reassure himself that in the context of unusual illnesses he has truly proceeded according to correct reason. If these suggestions are correct, Hall used theoretical borrowings and references for two different reasons: to justify his claim to special knowledge of scurvy and to reassure himself (and his putative readers) that he had reasoned correctly.

What these extracts have in common is that they were all either removed entirely or drastically reduced by Cooke in *Select Observations*. Cooke's Hall is impersonal, detached and clinical, while also more empirical and less dependent on texts. In fact, as an understanding and careful reading of Hall's complete manuscript shows, Hall was actually documenting his ability to make correct diagnoses in the correct way. He was recording his emotions and feelings, was concerned for his standing among his fellow physicians, and was sympathetic to his patients in their sorrow and joy.

4

Textual introduction

The need for a new edition

James Cooke's translation in the second edition of *Select Observations* has been the standard version of Hall's manuscript since 1679. Historians have too easily taken it for granted that the translation was both accurate and complete, without comparing it with the original Latin. Joan Lane made more effort than most to compare *Select Observations* with Hall's manuscript, but her main interest was in the identity of his patients. Her comments show that she tended to look only at the opening and closing paragraphs of each report in the Latin which carried most of the information about Hall's patients. Cooke's translation contains both errors and omissions. One error is Cooke's attribution of the cure of the Earl of Northampton (Case 137) to the Oxford physician Dr Clayton rather than to Hall himself. Hall wished to start with immediate venesection, but the Earl refused. Instead Hall applied a plaster, but after a troubled night the Earl requested advice from Dr Clayton of Oxford and 'sent for him at precipitate speed'. Hall then prescribed an unusual plaster, requiring two entire swallows' nests 'including straw, dirt and swallows' droppings', along with other ingredients. This was successful: 'the Earl was satisfied with these prescriptions alone, before the Doctor arrived [...] he breathed and swallowed easily'. Hall's relief at treating the Earl successfully before the arrival of a colleague (or rival) is apparent in the text.

This is not evident in *Select Observations* because Cooke's incorrect translation attributed the recipe and its success to Dr Clayton.

Equally significant are omissions by Cooke that affect the balance of the text. Hall recorded several conversations with patients, either at the time of consultation or at follow up. Cooke radically abridged these, turning consultations into brisk medical summaries, but in the process losing much of Hall's personal views on his relationships with patients. These deletions may be explicable as removing matter of little interest to a late seventeenth-century medical readership, for whom the identities of patients would not have been relevant as evidence of successful therapies.

Two other categories of omission, of references to named authors or books and of theoretical texts, are more likely to be Cooke's editorial policy. The inclusion of these would have weakened Cooke's deliberate presentation of Hall as a physician dependent almost entirely on empirical practice and observation. This is expressed in the words of Cooke's colleague John Bird of Cambridge, in a foreword to the first edition:

> For this book, I have this to say, that as Practice is the last and chiefest part of Physik, so is Observation the surest, and most demonstrating, part of Practice. Hence it cometh to pass through defect of Observations, that so many Prescriptions we meet with in the works of the most learned Practitioners, fall often short in performing the cures they promise, and we took them up for; so often delivering us as their own what they took from other men upon Trust. ('To the Judicious Reader', in Hall 1657: sig. A6r)

Hall's practice was undoubtedly based on 'the works of the most learned practitioners'.

Casebooks are becoming more closely studied and compared, but this will only pay dividends if the texts used are accurate and complete and their mode of composition taken into account. Doreen Nagy used Hall's treatment of acute urinary retention (John Smith, Case 66), with diuretic herbs and local heat applied to the perineum via a hot fried onion as an illustration of cures

Select *Observations*
ON
ENGLISH
BODIES:
OR,
Cures both Empericall and
Hiſtoricall, performed up-
on very eminent Per-
ſons in deſperate
Diſeaſes.

Firſt, written in *Latine*
by Mr. *John Hall* Phyſician,
living at *Stratford* upon *Avon*
in *Warwick-ſhire*, where he
was very famous, as alſo in
the Co nties adjacent, as appeares by theſe Obſervations
drawn out of ſeverall hun-
dreds of his, as choyſeſt.

Now put into Engliſh for com-
mon benefit by *James Cooke*
Practitioner in *Phyſick* and
Chirurgery.

London, Printed for *John Sherley*, at the
Golden Pelican, in *Little-Britain*. 1657.

19 James Cooke records John Hall's fame on the title-page of his first
version of Hall's medical notebook in 1657.

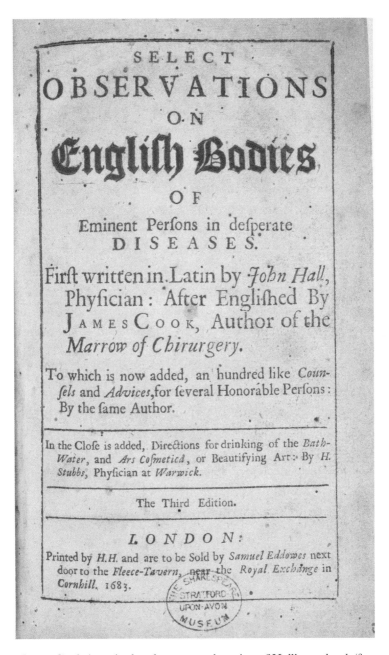

SELECT
OBSERVATIONS
ON
𝕰𝖓𝖌𝖑𝖎𝖘𝖍 𝕭𝖔𝖉𝖎𝖊𝖘,
OF
Eminent Perſons in deſperate
DISEASES.

Firſt written in Latin by *John Hall*,
Phyſician: After Engliſhed By
JAMES COOK, Author of the
Marrow of Chirurgery.

To which is now added, an hundred like *Coun-
ſels* and *Advices,* for ſeveral Honorable Perſons:
By the ſame Author.

In the Cloſe is added, Directions for drinking of the *Bath-
Water,* and *Ars Coſmetica,* or Beautifying Art: By *H.
Stubbs,* Phyſician at *Warwick.*

The Third Edition.

LONDON:
Printed by *H.H.* and are to be Sold by *Samuel Eddowes* next
door to the *Fleece-Tavern,* near the *Royal Exchange* in
Cornhill, 1683.

20 James Cooke's revised and augmented version of Hall's casebook (from
1679 and subsequently, for example in this third edition of 1683) omits
reference to Hall's fame, but draws attention to Cooke's own augmentation.

available to both learned and other practitioners. Nagy wrote of this that 'Doctors' records ... illustrate the striking similarity between their treatments and those used by lay practitioners', but gave no evidence for this treatment being used by anyone other than Hall (Nagy 1988: 43). She seems to have taken it as self-evident that a therapy based on fried onions must be rooted in popular tradition. Hall in fact took this remedy almost verbatim from Ruland the Elder's *Curationum* (1628), so despite appearances it is part of the learned, Latin medical techniques.

Wendy Churchill supports her argument that melancholy and the mother coexisted with a quotation from *Select Observations* (Mrs Peers, Case 123; Churchill 2012: 189). Cooke's words are that 'from her Melancholy she fell into the Mother' ('the mother' means illness caused by supposed movement of the womb from its normal place within the abdomen), but Hall's Latin reads 'ob maerorem in suffocationem matricis incidebat' (on account of grief she fell into a suffocation of the mother). In two other reports Hall used 'maeror' for the emotion of a parent at the loss of a child. Lady Browne's scurvy (Case 162) was brought on by grief at the death of her daughter. Similarly Bishop Thornborough's grief over his son's suicide caused first severe melancholy and then scurvy (Case 164). However, melancholy and grief are not synonymous. The report on Lady Browne's illness describes melancholy in a way which brings out its physicality:

> The source of scurvy in the spleen produces a flatulent melancholy, since the regions of the hypochondria encircle the spleen. The melancholy bubbles up in the meseraic veins around the pancreas and putrefies as if it were fermenting.

In these illnesses, as with Mrs Peers's, the relationship is between a strong emotion (grief) and physical illness (melancholy and/or scurvy). This is not, however, to deny Churchill's argument for a relationship between melancholy and the mother. Another report in Hall's manuscript is much more supportive of this. He made the relationship between the mother and melancholy explicit in the case of Mrs Baker (Case 127), which is headed 'cure of a fit of the mother, that is, melancholy'. Cooke's translation loses this close link ('troubled with the Mother, Melancholy'). The issue is a complex one involving powerful emotions interacting with illnesses which had both physical and psychological components.

Editorial procedures

In order to produce a full, English translation of Hall's manuscript, a careful transcription of the Latin had to be produced first. Punctuation is editorial, though I have tried to be sensitive to Hall's usage. My major change relates to paragraphs. Hall tended to write his text almost continuously throughout a case, except that in about 90 per cent of occurrences the 'recipe' symbol (℞) stands at the start of a line, before a list of ingredients. I have placed all instances of ℞ at the start of a line, otherwise the text is divided into paragraphs following the sense. The ℞ (for 'recipe') is the only pharmaceutical symbol retained, as a marker for remedies in the text, an aspect of the manuscript that was clearly important to Hall.

Hall was not consistent in his methods of indicating pharmaceutical quantities. I have standardised them all as abbreviations.

The styles of writing in Hall's manuscript vary considerably, partly a reflection of the mixture of his own notes with borrowings from texts. Some details, for instance references to the quality of urine and the number and quality of faeces, are given as short phrases rather than complete sentences. The borrowings on the other hand are often lengthy and prolix. I have reflected both these styles in my translation.

Hall's manuscript also varies, sometimes within a single paragraph, in the use of the present or past tense. This may reflect carelessness on Hall's part or alternatively may be the result of combining text from his original patient notes (in the present) with his retrospective rewriting, or of using borrowings which themselves used different tenses. I have mostly put texts into the past, except where the case for the use of the present has felt particularly strong.

Hall's borrowings from Latin texts are shown in italics and their source identified at the foot of the appropriate page, but without indicating Hall's omissions.

Some features of the translation need some explanation. Two relate to his patients' socio-economic status. An unusual feature of Hall's manuscript is his use of 'virgo' or 'virgo intacta' in relation to four female patients, not a usage I have come across in any other casebook. He recorded ages for three of them, all between 20 and 28 years. I have interpreted his phrase as a social reference to unmarried women of marriageable age rather than as a clinical and anatomical finding and have therefore translated it as spinster.

Hall was precise in his use of personal titles and for the most part a precise equivalent is available. A problem arises with the words *Generosus/-a* and *Magister/-ra*. Cooke translated both as Mr and Mrs, but that is to blur a distinction that was still important at Hall's time. I translate them both as Mr or Mrs, but for patients titled *Generosus/-a* , with the addition of 'gentleman' or 'gentlewoman' after the name, to emphasise the social distinction. Hall gave male patients with knighthoods the title 'Eques', which I have translated as 'Squire'.

Two other points are pharmaceutical. The pharmacopoeias of Hall's time made a distinction between powders and species. The former refers to any ingredient which has been dried and powdered. The latter means a mixture of powders ready prepared to be made up into a remedy such as an electuary (a medicine mixed with honey or other sweetener). I have signalled the difference by translating species as 'powder for' rather than just powder. Hall used an antimony cup on occasion to provoke vomiting in his patients. I have translated this as his 'chymical cup' rather than chemical, to make clear that he was not operating within the chemistry systems of later centuries. I have used 'chymical' elsewhere in the same way.

Footnotes have been used to identify the sources of Hall's (here translated) borrowings from Latin medical books and other sources, as well as to provide thumbnail sketches of all of his patients. These are indebted to Joan Lane's work, and some include corrections of her errors.

John Hall's
A Little Book of Cures

[Epigraphs]

Whoever practises medicine without direction and method, *sails without rudder or oars.*[1]

When a physician proceeds according to correct reasoning, even though he does not succeed every time, he should nevertheless persist in his course of action.[2]

One must bear patiently what one cannot immediately lay aside.[3]

[p. 1]

Health is from the Lord.

A Little Book of Cures, Described in Case Histories and Empirically Proven, Tried and Tested in Specified Places and on Identified People[4]

[Case 1]

The [1st] Countess of Northampton:[5] about 44 years old. 6 March 1622. She is pious, good-looking, modest, well endowed and of excellent character though not very talented. While walking in her chamber she fainted suddenly, and lay without any movement or sense for almost half an hour. She bruised and cut her face on the rush flooring, then developed an inflammation leading to a copious and troublesome flow of rheum from the eyes, which rendered her whole face torn and ulcerated, and

---

1 Fernel, *Therapeutices universalis*, p. 38.

2 A reworking of Hippocrates, aphorism 52, book II: the wording differs from all the standard versions, and may be Hall's own. There is an echo of Marcus Aurelius, *De vita sua*, lib. XII.

3 Adams, *Mystical Bedlam: or, the World of Mad-Men*, p. 68.

4 Based on the titles of Ruland the Elder's series of texts: *Curationum empyricarum et historicarum, in certis locis et notis personis optime expertarum, et rite probatarum, centuriae decem.*

5 Elizabeth, Countess of Northampton (1578–1632). Elizabeth Spencer was 21 when she married William Compton, twice her age. She was an heiress, 'pious, beautiful', not very intelligent. She had three children and a large household, and sometimes entertained royalty. Her husband became the 1st Earl of Northampton in 1618. She died in 1632 aged 54.

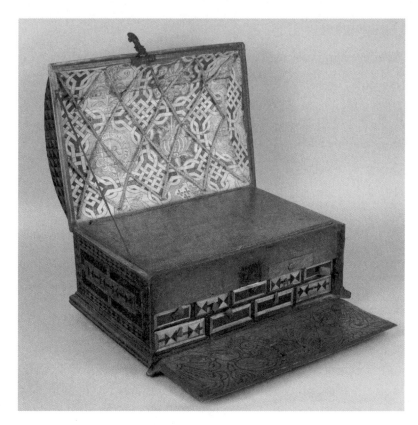

21 A mid-sixteenth to early seventeenth-century medical chest, made by a German immigrant craftsman in Southwark, London. It is probably of a better quality than a provincial physician such as Hall would have used, but he would have needed a chest very like this when travelling to visit his patients. It is 395mm wide, 200mm high and 260mm deep (15.5 × 7.8 × 10.2 in.), so he or a servant could have either carried it on their backs, or in a horse-pack. Its fifteen small drawers would be ample for the pills and medication he would have needed. Hall would have travelled with a few of his medical textbooks as well to help him with diagnoses and cures.

disfigured her. She has suffered from wasting and scurvy for a long time. She was then living at the Welsh Castle in Ludlow. I was summoned to her and freed her entirely, by God's will and the following remedies:

℞: *senna leaves 1oz, agaric 3dr, rhubarb 2dr, cinnamon 1½oz. Infuse according to practice in 3 pints white wine for twelve hours. Then strain six or seven times through a woollen bag and sweeten with ½lb* **[p. 2]** *of good sugar in the form of nectar.*[1] Dose: 5oz twice a day, on an empty stomach in the morning and about four o'clock in the afternoon.[2]

She was purged five or six times, very well and without colic, and continued the course for the next four days. To control the flow of rheum, I instructed her to rub camphorated white ointment on her face. It healed within four days. As her body was not yet adequately purged, she was very well purged again with the following pills:

℞: pills – Ruffus's, Crato's amber, in equal amounts. Make 7 pills from 1dr.

I prescribed 3 to be taken at bedtime (but this was strange, she chewed them. She said she never could swallow a pill, even a small one) and she took them very well in this way. On the following day: six or seven stools, and continue twice a week. On quiet days she used Crato's steeled electuary[3] with salts of scurvy-grass, wormwood and coral. Every third night she chewed the above pills without disgust or nausea. These antiscorbutic herbs (because scorbutic medicines should always be added with others when there may be some suspicion of scurvy) were put in her broth:[4] scurvy-grass, brooklime, watercress, bugloss and other stuff of the same sort. **[p. 3]** I prescribed antiscorbutic beer of this sort:

℞: scurvy-grass 4 handfuls, watercress, brooklime each 2 handfuls, wormwood 1 handful, agrimony, betony, fumitory, germander each 1 handful, fennel, borage, chicory roots each 1oz, elecampane ½oz, liquorice 1oz, borage, bugloss, rosemary flowers each 2 pinches.

---

1 Ranzau, *De conservanda*, pp. 63–64.
2 Clocks were becoming a feature of well-to-do households in Hall's lifetime, so this way of expressing time is not anachronistic.
3 A medicine mixed with honey or other sweetener.
4 A similar idea, though not in the same words, is found in Matthaeus Martini, 'De scorbuto', in Sennert, *De scorbuto tractatus*, p. 708.

Boil in 5 gallons beer, with the following in a bag: sarsaparilla, sweet flag, cinnamon, mace, aniseed, fennel each ½oz, juniper berries 8oz. After boiling remove the bag and suspend in the beer brewer's yeast previously discharged from a barrel.

After fifteen days the beer will be wholesome for drinking, so I wished her to drink it alone, forbidding all other drink for the whole of April. Until the beer was ready for drinking she used the following decoction:

℞: sarsaparilla 2oz, guaiacum 1oz, sassafras root 2dr. Soak overnight in 15 pints spring water. The next day add scurvy-grass 2 handfuls, brooklime, watercress each 1 handful, betony, agrimony, each ½ handful. Reduce by boiling to 10 pints. After boiling, add currants 2oz, prepared coriander seeds 1dr. When boiled, remove from the fire, add bruised cinnamon 1dr. Strain through a sleeve. Take **[p. 4]** 6oz hot, in bed. *Prepare the body for a light sweat, with the head and neck covered, wrapped in hot smooth sheets. The body should be wiped dry of sweat with dry clean cloths, not too soft but slightly rough.*[1]

Her usual drink was the second decoction. On the days on which she does not sweat, take properly prepared scurvy-grass juice, 6 spoonfuls in the above drink, and salt of scurvy-grass in broth. By these remedies, praise almighty God most high, she was properly cured beyond the expectation of the Earl and her friends at Ludlow.

[Case 2]

Concerning the most illustrious hero and Lord, William [1st] *Earl of Northampton,*[2] *most worthy President of His Majesty's Royal Council of Wales, suffering from burning urine.* 4 April 1622.[3]

---

1 Solenander, *Consiliorum* [...] *Solenandri*, p. 258.
2 William Compton, 1st Earl of Northampton. The Compton family seat was Castle Ashby. In 1599 he married Elizabeth Spencer, an heiress. Queen Elizabeth I was godmother to their first son. William was often at Ludlow Castle, and in 1617 became Lord President of Wales. Hall visited them at Ludlow. Compton died in London in 1630, aged 62.
3 Bruele, *Praxis medicinae*, f. 2r.

℞: newly extracted cassia flowers 1oz, washed turpentine 1dr, rhubarb 1sc, liquorice ½sc. Mix with sugar. Make a bolus.

℞: mallows 1 handful, liquorice 1oz. Boil in 2 pints cow's milk. To the
strained liquid **[p. 5]** add Fernel's marsh-mallow syrup 6oz. Take
4 or 5oz every morning and at bedtime swallow Cyprus turpentine,
in the form of a pill cooked in an apple under ashes.

Thus he was quickly and rightly cured. At Ludlow.

[Case 3]
Mrs Smith of Stratford-upon-Avon:[1] pious and respected. Age: 54.
She was wretchedly tormented by a hot rheum trickling from her
eyes, so that she could not open them in the morning.

℞: Crato's amber pills ½dr. Make 3 pills. Take them at bedtime.

Continue for four nights: four to six stools each day, without pain.
For external use:

℞: houseleek juice 1 spoonful, white wine 2 spoonfuls. Instil one or
two drops in the eyes, then place a cloth soaked in it over the eyes,
all night.

She felt great relief when the heat was alleviated. I instructed her
to instil the following water into the eyes:

℞: *preserved sarcocol 3dr, prepared tutty 2dr, aloes 1dr, sugar candy 1½dr,*
camphor 4gr, saffron 3gr, rose water 4oz. Mix. Soak a long while, stirring
frequently.[2]

One or two drops were dripped into her eyes three times daily.
Cured.

---

1 Anne Smith, born 1580, youngest daughter of a prosperous wool merchant.
Married in 1596, four children. Hall treated her in 1634, a year before her death.
Her brother, July Shaw, was an alderman, and a witness to the will of his neighbour William Shakespeare.
2 Platter, *Praxeos* [...] *de doloribus*, p. 310.

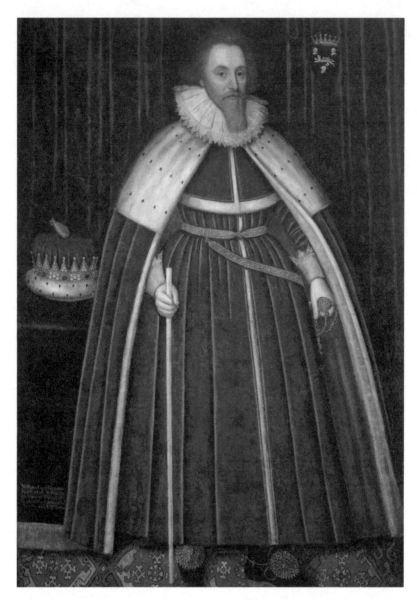

22 Portrait of William Compton, 1st Earl of Northampton. He became
Lord President of Wales from November 1617, and Hall travelled to Ludlow
to treat him for 'burning urine' (Cases 2 and 68), a swollen face caused by
catarrh (Case 79), and loss of appetite and catarrh (Case 83). Hall records
his treatment of the Countess for fainting in Case 1, which presumably
coincided with his visit to Ludlow to treat the Earl.

[Case 4]

[p. 6] Mr Wilson, vicar of Stratford-upon-Avon:[1] wretchedly troubled by a flux from the eye, as if weeping. Age: 40.

℞: pills – amber 1dr, aureae ½dr, trochiscated agaric 1sc. Make 10 pills with betony syrup. Take 5 at bedtime: the next day, six stools.

Repeat again at bedtime. For external use:

℞: *bole Armeniac ½oz, gypsum 3dr, dragon's blood, acacia each 2dr, pomegranate rind, galls each 1dr. Make a plaster for the temples and forehead using egg white and a little red vinegar as excipients.*[2]

℞: bole Armeniac, gypsum each. Make a plaster with vinegar and egg white.

I wished it applied behind the ears. Over the eye:

℞*: beaten egg white, add the same amount of rose water and a little woman's milk.*[3] Apply to the eye. Instil 1 or 2 drops of our ophthalmic water as for Mrs Smith, page 5, three times daily.

It happened that after a space of ten minutes of an hour he tasted a strong bitterness on his palate. Then I enquired and investigated. I consider the taste to be the very same sarcocol which came from the eye, through all the intervening parts, all the way to the palate.[4] He was cured by these remedies. Blessed be the Lord.

[Case 5]

[p. 7] Mrs Bettes of Ludlow:[5] weighed down by severe cough and difficulty of breathing, with pain in the side. Age: 50.

---

1 Thomas Wilson, vicar of Stratford-upon-Avon, 1619–38. Graduated MA from Oxford. His appointment as vicar as 1619 was supported by John Hall, but his Puritan attitudes offended many. The Corporation once suspended him for three months. He witnessed Hall's will in 1635. Died in 1638 (Lane 1996: 9–11).
2 Platter, *Praxeos* […] *de doloribus*, p. 300.
3 Platter, *Praxeos* […] *de doloribus*, p. 305.
4 Dunus, *De curandi ratione per venae sectionem*, p. 44.
5 Hall treated her while staying at Ludlow. She may have been an upper servant in the Compton household.

℞: Conserve of red roses 2oz, raisins without seeds 1oz, sugar candy 1oz, oils of vitriol and sulphur enough of each for tartness. Make an electuary. Dose: morning and evening, as much as a nutmeg.

℞: *frankincense, mastic, each 1½dr, sulphur 2½dr, juniper wood 2scs, styrax 1sc, sufficient turpentine. Make a lump for fumigation. At the time of use, put one or two pieces on glowing coals, and lead the smoke to the mouth by a suitable tube. The skin of the head should be fumigated. This gently dries up the superfluous humour of the brain.*[1]

For stomach pain:

℞: labdanum 1 part, wax 2 parts, sufficient Gabrieli's aromatic rose powder and a little caranna. Make a plaster.

For pain in the side:

℞: *marsh-mallow ointment 2oz, sweet almond oil 2dr. Spread it warm on the affected side, and afterwards put a hot cloth smeared with butter on the anointed part.*[2]

She became much better, then afterwards used the following for a long time:

℞: distilled waters of coltsfoot, ground-ivy, mullein, speedwell, elecampane, knapweed **[p. 8]** (i.e., herb trinity), figwort (i.e., scrophularia major), scabious, hyssop, the cordial flowers, horehound, maidenhair ferns, either orris root, roots of angelica or soapwort.

℞: 12 pints of this water, inner guaiacum 12oz, sarsaparilla ½lb, orris root 2oz, china cut in small pieces 3oz, elecampane root 3dr, maiden-hair, speedwell each 1 handful, liquorice 2oz, anise 1oz, stoned raisins 6oz. Boil in a double vessel, strain. Clarify the decoction. Dose: a good draught in a bowl, two or three times daily.

Each night: conserve of red roses to the amount of a walnut with a bolus of the electuary, from 1sc. to 1oz of the conserve. She should often drink a julep of the following distillation during the day:

---

1 Bruele, *Praxis medicinae*, p. 182.
2 Ruland the Elder, 'Centuria VII', *Curationum* [...] *centuriae*, p. 540.

℞: prepared snails 1lb, good white breadcrumbs ½lb, 30 egg whites, cream of milk 4 pints, cinnamon 2oz, choice sugar 2lb, muscadel wine 2 pints. Make a distillation of everything in a double vessel.

She should take a draught of this water often with pearled manus Christi, and finally the following lohoch:[1]

℞: lohoch sanum et expertum 2oz, barley sugar 2oz, syrups of maiden-hair fern, hyssop, liquorice, coltsfoot each 1oz, angelica and preserved elecampane roots each ½oz, orris root 1dr. Add flowers of sulphur 2dr, to 4oz of this linctus.

She was cured by these within five weeks. Later she died. I do not know what the illness was.

[Case 6]

[p. 9] Cure of yellow jaundice with tertian fever: for Mr Nash's serving maid,[2] who was staying at the Sign of the Bear. Age: 28.

℞: Wine of squills ½oz, oxymel of squills 1oz, our chymical cup ½oz. Seven vomits.[3]

℞: powdered rhubarb 1oz, diaphoenicon electuary 3oz, laxative senna powder ½dr, syrup of rose juice 1oz, celandine water 3oz. Mix. Eight stools.

After her body was properly purged on four mornings, she took 1oz of the following powder on an empty stomach, with a soft-boiled egg:

℞: inner bark of barberry, turmeric, shavings of ivory and hartshorn each 1 pinch, saffron ½ pinch. Make a powder.

1 A soft-formed medicine administered by licking.
2 The Latin makes it clear that this was a female servant, but Cooke's translation made the gender male. Lane identified the patient as Joseph Jelphes, which cannot be correct. She was probably a maid to the publican Anthony Nash, at the Sign of the Bear in Bridge Street. The patient is now unidentified. The consultation remains undated.
3 Ruland the Elder, 'Centuria V', *Curationum* […] *centuriae: poculum nostrum chymicum* is described on pp. 281 and 303–304.

She was very well cured, even though her whole body was spotted with jaundice.

[Case 7]

Mr Powell, a gentleman of Ludlow:[1] suffering from a disease of the eyes with an incessant flow of rheum that excoriated his face. He could see neither light nor lamp. *He was about 50 years old.*[2]

℞: amber pills ½dr. Make 3 pills: five stools the next day, and continue the course for four days.

℞: *mastic, frankincense, myrrh each 1½dr, dragon's blood 1dr, bole Armeniac, bean flour each 1dr, saffron 1sc. Make a paste for the forehead with egg white, rose oil and a little vinegar. Take them up with wool or woven cloth, or soak them in a softer cloth. Apply to the forehead.*

[p. 10] ℞: *prepared tutty, very finely powdered so that it can easily pass through muslin, 1½dr, camphor, saffron each 12gr. Soak them together enclosed in clean muslin, in rose water and white wine, 3oz. Make a collyrium, instill two or three drops in the eyes.*[3]

The patient should lie on his back in bed, and 1 or 2 eye drops should be placed in the eyes, introduced with a feather of a black hen. The patient should close and open their eyes so that the instilled water is diffused throughout the eye cavities, two or three times daily. He was cured.[4] With this water he used the decoction of sarsaparilla and guaiacum as above for the Countess on page 3, omitting the herbs. He was rightly cured within twenty days, beyond the expectation of his friends and servants.

---

1 Hall treated him while staying with the Compton family at Ludlow. No other information.

2 Ruland the Elder, 'Centuria III', *Curationum* [...] *centuriae*, p. 169: vir hic fuit annorum circiter 60.

3 Bruele, *Praxis medicinae*, p. 127.

4 Croll, *Basilica chymica*, p. 197.

[Case 8]

Mrs Chandler of Stratford-upon-Avon, age 34:[1] wasting away after a long illness and unbridled flux of the reds.

℞: senna decoction as for the Countess, pages 1 and 2, for five days. She was cured of the unbridled red flux by venesection, as if by magic.

Three years later she was weakened by the red flux after childbirth, so that she expects death at the door. She was cured by venesection.

[Case 9]

[p. 11] Christiana Basse of Southam:[2] age 29, wretchedly attacked by wind and phlegm in the stomach. She was relieved for a time by a drink of distilled spirits. Her complaint soon returned with very severe stomach ache, so that she was almost suffocated, then tormented by colic.

℞: the chymical cup 5dr, wine of squills ½oz. She was rightly purged, *upwards and downwards.*[3]

Next day:

℞: prepared laurel powder with vinegar, the weight of sixpence,[4] with syrup of violets and sufficient posset ale. Seven stools.

When the body was very well purged:

℞: *London treacle,*[5] Mithridate each 1dr, wormwood conserve 3oz, for three mornings.

---

1 Second wife of William Chandler, a prosperous merchant. She had eight children, seven of whom survived. She was 34 at the time of this illness, and Hall treated her again two years later after childbirth.

2 She may have been Christian Bate, baptised at Southam in 1601, who later married Thomas Judkin. Hall treated that family. She died in 1657.

3 A phrase commonly found in Ruland the Elder, *Curationum* [...] *centuriae*, but rarely elsewhere; for example, 'Centuria I', pp. 21, 37, 43; 'Centuria II', pp. 89, 90, 141; 'Centuria III', p. 181; 'Centuria IV', p. 241; 'Centuria V', p. 346; 'Centuria X', pp. 716, 717.

4 weight of a sixpence] Approximately 3 grams, or 2 scruples and 6 grains.

5 *Pharmacopoeia Londinensis*, p. 90.

Her drink was a decoction of lemon balm and mint in steeled water. She was rightly cured by these, and returned me great thanks and declared herself never afterwards tortured by these torments. Praise God.

[Case 10]

Mrs Wincoll,[1] a gentlewoman, companion to the [1st] Countess of Northampton, about 48 years old: tortured by anal prolapse and tenesmus.

> R: *camomile 1 handful, malmsey wine 1½ pints. Soak for one to two hours over glowing coals on a slow fire. Keep the anus warm with cloths soaked in this, as hot as can be borne, then replace it in the proper place with a finger,* **[p. 12]** *and then with a sponge soaked in the same warm wine and the fluid squeezed out. The patient should sit on the warm sponge and squeeze it tightly when sitting.*[2]

NOTE: these did free her from the tenesmus and prolapse, but chamomile flowers are much better and of higher quality.[3] Mr Broad's tutor was cured in the same way.

[Case 11]

Mrs Hanbury, a gentlewoman:[4] to preserve the face from pimples. She was disfigured as if by leprosy with itchy excoriation.

> R: amber pills 1dr at bedtime, and her body was purged thus three times. She took *Penot's mercury water* made with emulsions of white poppies, borax and candy sugar.[5]

Using this cleared her face.

---

1 Companion to the Countess of Northampton. She had some status in the household, and a regular annuity of £5.

2 Penot, *De denario medico*, p. 64.

3 As recommended by Penot.

4 Her father was an alderman, who left her £500 when he died in 1643. Anne then married John Thornborough, a great-nephew of the Bishop of Worcester, and had one son. Her husband died in 1648, aged 26. Anne died in the same year, aged 34.

5 Penot, *De denario medico*, p. 61: a lengthy recipe contains the ingredients mentioned.

[Case 12]
Ann Gibbs, a gentlewoman aged 19:[1] cure of a ruptured stomach abscess.

℞: hyssop and coltsfoot syrups each 1oz, oxymel of squills 3dr, vinegar of squills 1dr. Make a linctus, which she licked often.

Then she was purged thus:

℞: newly extracted cassia with endive water 1oz, powdered rhubarb 1dr, scabious water 4oz, chicory syrup with rhubarb 1oz. Make a draught: 8 stools.

℞: sufficient wormwood, roses, bugloss. Make a plaster for the stomach with oils of roses, mastic, violets. Apply hot.

[p. 13] Finally:

℞: roots of our iris, lilies, each 1oz. Boil in 1 pint white wine, reduce to half. Drink 4oz in the morning.

She was very well cured, with a good colour.

[Case 13]
John Emes, aged 15:[2] urinating in bed.

Take the gullet of a rooster roasted, with crocus Martis in a soft-boiled egg. Freed.

[Case 14]
Francisca Reyland of Quinton:[3] caught a cold while menstruating and fell into a swelling of the hands and feet, so that she could not move.

---

1 Hall describes her as *Generosa*, with some social status, but there is not enough detail to identify her accurately.
2 Son of John Emes, gentleman (1573–1655) and Elizabeth Bellers (died 1627). Their monument, described by Dugdale, is in St Nicholas' Church, Alcester. Hall's patient grew up and became a mercer.
3 Probably the wife of the churchwarden, who had many children. Not described as *Generosa*, so of low social status.

R: caryocostinum electuary 3dr, tartar crystals 1sc. Make a bolus with sugar, from which six large foul-smelling stools.

Then venesection freed her. She relapsed after twenty days and was again purged with prepared laurel, and afterwards used the following potion:

R: guaiacum ½lb, green shoots of agrimony, brooklime, watercress, sage, betony, rosemary each 1 handful. Boil in 8 pints spring water, reduce to 4 pints. Immediately after boiling, add cinnamon 2dr, aniseed 2dr. *At dawn sip 8oz by weight, which will provoke sweating.*[1]

At bedtime she took a bath:

R: oak leaves 20 handfuls, chamomile, sage, rue each 2 handfuls, salt 2lbs, alum 1lb, rock sulphur 4oz. Boil in sufficient water for a bath.

After the bath the limbs were anointed with this ointment:

R: Martiatum ointment 1oz, oil of worms and turpentine 1oz. Mix.

She was completely cured.

[Case 15]

[p. 14] Mrs Hunt,[2] a gentlewoman aged 46 of Stock Green: suffering from scabs and itch.

R: *fumitory, borage, bugloss, scabious, wormwood, each as much as you wish. Extract juice to make 2lbs, heat with whey until the whey is consumed,* skim constantly. At the end let the residue settle. During the day *drink it as you please, a good draught really cold with sugar.*[3]

---

1 Amatus Lusitanus, *Curationum medicinalium centuriae quatuor*, p. 67.
2 Mary Hunt. Her father was Richard Russell of Flyford Flavell. She married Henry Hunt, a farmer, in 1612. Widowed in 1635. In 1647 she made a will, which lists her possessions and also income owed to her in bills and bonds.
3 John of Gaddesden, *Praxis medica*, p. 1122.

This is John of Gaddesden's scabious syrup, and it is one of the secrets[1] with which he cured many of scabs. I have freed many from disfiguring scabs in the same way.

[Case 16]

Mr Dyson:[2] weighed down by heartburn on an empty stomach in the morning, with faintness and illness of the stomach.

> ℞: pills – Ruffus's, amber, stomachic, hiera simplex each 1sc. Make 7 to 9 pills.

He was rightly purged. Afterwards:

> ℞: best Mithridate ½oz, rose conserve 1oz, wormwood conserve 3oz, *London treacle* 6dr.[3] Mix. Give 1½dr in the morning.

He was completely freed. *This griping (according to Giovanni Battista de Monte, Centuria prima, consultation 72, page 389) appears around the end of digestion and it feels like this, that he appears to weaken unless he takes food. This is by reason of the acid biting humour which causes griping so that he falls* **[p. 15]** *into such a weakness, from which he is calmed by the taking of food. The reason he feels the weakness before food, is because when digestion takes place, the organs become greedy. Then the veins draw on the liver, the liver on the meseraic veins, the meseraics on the stomach. When digestion is entirely completed, the stomach feels the griping. It becomes weak, because it requires much nourishment, moreover this is because of the griping humour. The acridity of the humour is blunted by the consumption of food, and the liver manages to get what it is drawing, and the veins, and then the symptoms cease.*[4]

---

1 Secrets: in this context, 'more about technical know-how, or "how to", than hidden knowledge' (Leong and Rankin 2011: 8).

2 Thomas Dyson of Morton Underhill. His family owned land in Worcestershire, acquired at the Dissolution. Thomas had a farm near Inkberrow, and kept turkeys and poultry. He married Elizabeth Manning in 1628, and had seven children. He died in 1651 and is buried in Inkberrow church porch.

3 *Pharmacopoeia Londinensis*, p. 90.

4 da Monte, *Consultationum medicinalium*, pp. 388–389, 391.

[Case 17]
Mary Heath, aged 34 of Libington:[1] wretchedly tortured by
dysentery, catarrh, backache, worms. She was tormented by the
excretion of thick, foul-smelling stuff in the urine, and pain of the
kidneys. She was previously fleshy and fat, now lean.

R: powdered rhubarb 1½dr, loosening rose syrup 1oz, borage water
3oz. Make a draught.

Then she took this enema:

R: decoction of roasted barley in water 1pt, omphacine oil of roses
3oz, 2 egg yolks, brown sugar 1½oz. Mix. Make it.

R: yellow wax ½oz, crocus Martis 1dr. Make small lumps like nutmegs by the usual method.

*I prescribed a whole apple cored, the cavity filled up with the wax, and the top
covered. Move the apple in the coals until the wax is to entirely liquefied and
has intermingled with the flesh of the apple.* **[p. 16]** *I instructed her to eat an
apple prepared in this way before every meal.*[2]

A steeled drink: make a pap from roasted barley and breadcrumbs
with steeled water and sugar. Within a few days of using these
remedies, *she was made entirely whole.*[3] I have cured many with wax
prepared in this way.

[Case 18]
Mrs Lane, a gentlewoman of Alveston:[4] weighed down by heavi-
ness of the chest and difficulty of breathing. Age: 49.

R: *trochiscated agaric 2sc. Make a bolus with rose sugar and preserved ginger
conserve.*[5] Four stools, then one vomit, afterwards three stools.

---

1 Of humble social status, possibly the wife of John Heath, a labourer's son.
2 Valleriola, *Observationum* [...] *libri sex*, p. 139.
3 Valleriola, *Observationum* [...] *libri sex*, p. 139.
4 Joan Lane (*c.* 1564–1613). A gentlewoman, born in Mitcham, Surrey. Married in
1588 to Richard Lane of Stratford, who bought Alveston Manor in 1603. She died
in 1613, soon after her husband. Hall treated her in her final illness.
5 Crato, *Consiliorum* [...] *Liber quartus*, p. 53.

The following day and for several days, she is to take the following oxymel:

> ℞: raisins ½oz, *green shoots of hyssop, oregano, horehound, penny-royal, germander speedwell, scabious,* coltsfoot, *blessed thistle,* nettles *each ½ handful, sliced orris root,* sweet flag *each 1oz, agaric 2dr, senna 2oz, ginger 2dr.* Make a decoction of these in 2 pints *good vinegar. Mix in a third part of water.* Boil until reduced by a third. *To the strained liquid add refined honey 12oz, then boil again to the thickness of an oxymel. Whenever she is threatened with difficulty in breathing, she should drink one spoonful often, sipping it a little at a time. One may add cinnamon, cloves and sweet flag. Everything is powdered and tied in a fine cloth, so that it keeps longer and has a more agreeable flavour.*[1]

She returned to full health and said the oxymel was worth gold.

[Case 19]

[p. 17] Mrs Hall, a gentlewoman, my wife:[2] wretchedly tortured by colic.

> ℞: diaphoenicon, diacatholicon each 1oz, Holland powder 2dr, oil of rue 1oz, sufficient milk. Make an enema: two stools.

The pain remained and was little relieved, so I wished at once to inject 1 pint of hot Spanish wine as an enema. She immediately produced a large amount of wind, and was freed from all pain. I applied Crato's labdanum plaster with caranna, aromatic rose powder and mace oil. With this enema alone I freed the Earl of Northampton from a most severe colicky pain.

[Case 20]

Mrs Herbert:[3] wretchedly tortured by pain in the side.

---

1 Crato, *Consiliorum* […] *liber quartus*, pp. 53, 43.
2 Hall's wife, Susanna (1583–1649), was the Shakespeares' eldest daughter. When her father died in 1616 she inherited New Place, and other houses in Stratford and London. She and Hall had one daughter, Elizabeth. Susanna was widowed in 1635. She probably hosted Queen Henrietta Maria at New Place in 1643. Died aged 66 (cf. Case 129).
3 Hall refers to her as 'Mistress', but there are no further details.

℞: *wine spirit or aqua vitae, whichever is to hand, 6oz, camphor 1dr. Boil a little until the camphor dissolves, then add powdered sandalwood while it is still hot. Soak cloths in this liquid and apply hot.*[1]

Freed.

[Case 21]
Mary Wilson:[2] weakened by a hectic fever with severe cough, obstructed menstruation. Age: about 22 years.

Foods should be boiled, because they moisten more: veal, fowls, also young chickens if they are fed on barley or fattened on pellets formed out of a paste. This is prepared from the flesh of frogs, snails and river crabs bound together with barley flour.[3] That is how I am accustomed to encourage weight gain. **[p. 18]** *Eggs are recommended, the yolk most of all, boiled with wine and sugar, as our restaurative*[4] (that is, a caudle). For a pap:

℞: *breadcrumbs soaked in milk and then almond milk, mixed with rose water and sugar. A ptisane or barley cream prepared in this way:*[5]

℞: barley 2oz, purslane, borage each ½ handful. Boil in 10 pints spring water until 4 are gone. Drink a sufficient quantity of the strained liquid.

I wished her to have frequent recourse to sugar of roses tablets.[6] An enema:

℞: well beaten broth of a small chicken 10oz. Boil in it poppy seeds, flowers of water-lilies, violets, lettuce, mallows each ½ handful, then strain. To the strained liquid add oil of violets 1½oz, white sugar 2oz, violet honey 1½oz, household salt 1½dr, egg yolk 1. Make the enema.

I wished her to drink woman's milk. *It is best when it is drunk from the breast of a woman nourished on cooling and moistening foods such as lettuces,*

---

1 Platter, *Praxeos* […] *de doloribus*, p. 442.
2 No further identification. Died aged 23 in 1636.
3 Platter, *Praxeos* […] *de doloribus*, p. 221.
4 Platter, *Praxeos* […] *de doloribus*, p. 222.
5 Platter, *Praxeos* […] *de doloribus*, p. 222.
6 Platter, *Praxeos* […] *de doloribus*, p. 225.

barley, milk of melon seeds;[1] and if possible, *best chosen from a woman who has passed four menstrual cycles after giving birth.*[2] Though used properly they were of little benefit, because after a year she rested in peace with the Lord.

[Case 22]

Mr Drayton,[3] an excellent Poet, is troubled by a tertian fever:

℞: the chymical cup 1oz, syrup of violets ½ spoonful. Mix them.

He was properly purged *both upwards and downwards,*[4] and cured.

[Case 23]

[p. 19] Goodwife Bettes, aged 40:[5] wretchedly tortured by pain in the right side of the head, once a month, sometimes two or three times, and often ending with vomiting. During an attack she could neither walk nor stand.

℞: the chymical cup 1oz: six vomits.

The next day:

℞: pills – amber 2dr, *Fernel's for headache* 1dr.[6] Make 15 pills. Take 3 before dinner.

---

1 Vettori, *Exhortatio ad medicum recte*, p. 374.

2 Platter, *Praxeos* […] *de doloribus*, p. 223.

3 Michael Drayton (1567–1631). Poet and playwright. He had been a page in the household of Anne, Lady Rainsford, who later lived at Clifford Chambers after her marriage in 1595. Drayton was a regular visitor there. Buried in Westminster Abbey.

4 See Case 9, n. 3.

5 Possibly the same woman Hall treated at Ludlow (Case 5). Possibly the wife of William Betts, a servant of the Compton family. The case report ends abruptly with the second decoction, suggesting that Hall inadvertently omitted his usual final words.

6 Crato, *Consiliorum* […] *liber quintus*, p. 338. I have not found this recipe in Fernal, nor did any seventeenth-century author. If a source is mentioned, it is Crato.

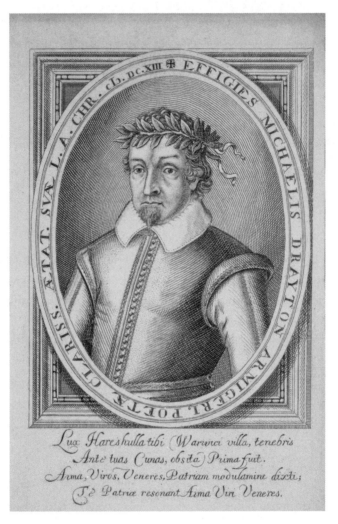

23 The poet and playwright Michael Drayton (1563–1631), a friend and possible collaborator of Shakespeare, in a print from 1796 based on the 1619 engraving by William Holle (d. 1624). Drayton regularly visited the village of Clifford Chambers, about a mile from Stratford-upon-Avon, where he stayed with the Rainsfords. Hall treated him for a tertian fever (Case 22). The Latin can be rendered as: 'A likeness of Michael Drayton esquire, renowned poet. Aged 50. 1613. 'Your first light was at Hartshill (a Warwickshire town covered in darkness before your cradle). Arms, Heroes, Loves, Albion you expressed in sweet melody; from you, Albion, Arms, Heroes, Loves, resound.' Translation by Amy Hurst.

When the pills were finished, she was bled up to 6oz. Finally she took the simple decoction of sarsaparilla, greatly praised by Johannes Crato for headache:[1]

℞: *sarsaparilla 4oz, water 10 pints. I break the sarsaparilla into small pieces, cut in small bits, then I soak them hot water for twenty four hours. I boil it, reduce to half.* Take a draught morning and at bedtime.

I make a second decoction:

℞: *the prepared sarsaparilla and water 15 pints, and without soaking, I boil them until reduced by a third. This decoction is powerful at dinner and lunch.*[2]

[Case 24]

Mrs Boughton,[3] a gentlewoman, pregnant: freed from vomiting and diarrhoea by this alone:

℞: *Malmsey wine 6oz, oil of vitriol 6 drops, dilute well. She took 1oz of this dilution on an empty stomach in the morning, daily.*[4]

℞: oils of wormwood, mace, each ½oz, Gabrieli's aromatic rose powder ½dr. Mix. Make an ointment for the stomach.

℞: poppy syrup 3oz, scabious, mint waters each 2oz, borage 1oz, a few drops of oil of vitriol.

Cured, praise God.

[Case 25]

[p. 20] Mr Randolph, a gentleman:[5] wretchedly overwhelmed by headache and catarrh and troubled by constant expectoration, so that at night he wrapped his head in a triple skullcap. Age: 35.

---

1 Crato, *Consiliorum* […] *liber sextus*, p. 663.
2 Falloppio, 'De morbo Gallico', in Luisini, *De morbo Gallico omnia*, p. 472.
3 Joyce Boughton of Cawston, Dunchurch. Born ?1593. A gentlewoman. She had five sons and four daughters. Widowed at 49 in 1642.
4 Ruland the Elder, 'Centuria I', *Curationum* […] *centuriae*, p. 10.
5 Ferrers Randolph of Wood Bevington (1584–before 1651). He inherited property but was much in debt. Married Elizabeth in 1619. William Dugdale refers to him as a Royalist in *The Antiquities of Warwickshire*.

℞: the chymical cup 1oz. Six vomits, three stools.

The next morning:

℞: pills cochiae 1dr, aureae ½dr, alhandal trochees 7gr. Make 7 pills with betony syrup.

He was rightly purged; cephalic vein bled to 6oz. Afterwards he took the following powder morning and evening. This is Martin Ruland's powder for rheum:

℞: *simple senna powder 6dr, rocket seed ½oz, long pepper 1½dr. Make a powder.*[1]

With these very few, in few days – seven to be exact – he was made entirely well.[2]

[Case 26]

Mrs Boughton,[3] a gentlewoman of Cawston aged 28: fell into a fever with excessive uterine flux three days after a miscarriage at five months, in danger of death. She was vomiting, thirsty, off her food and overwhelmed by fainting.

℞: prepared hartshorn 1oz, spring water 6 pints. Boil until 2 pints are gone, then remove from the fire. Afterwards add **[p. 21]** lemon syrup 2oz, rose water 4oz, sufficient sugar for a pleasing acidity.

In place of continuing this, she took a beverage which greatly comforted her. She took the following decoction morning and evening, *for it dispels, assails, leads away, and banishes thirst. A decoction for the chest*:

℞: *wheat barley 3 handfuls, violets 2 pinches, liquorice ½oz, jujubes 1oz, sebestens 2oz, blessed thistle 1½ handfuls. Make the decoction in enough water for 12 pints. To the strained liquid add violet sugar 4oz. Make the beverage.*[4]

---

1 Ruland the Elder, *Balnearium restauratum*, p. 142.
2 Ruland the Elder, 'Centuria III', *Curationum* […] *centuriae*, p. 221.
3 As Case 24.
4 Ruland the Elder, 'Centuria III', *Curationum* […] *centuriae*, pp. 170–171.

By these remedies alone she was made well past all expectation, praise God the one and three.

[Case 27]
Captain Basset, about 50 years old:[1] seized by a tertian fever.

R: the chymical cup 5dr, wine of squills 2dr, syrup of violets 1 spoonful. Mix.

He was rightly purged *both upwards and downwards*,[2] an hour before the attack. When the vomiting had ended:

R: electuary of cold gems 2sc, diascordium ½dr, field poppy syrup 1oz, scabious water 4oz. Mix.

He was purged in this way on the quiet days:

R: diaphoenicon, diacatholicon each 2dr, powdered rhubarb, Ruland's laxative senna powder each ½dr, Holland powder 1dr, scurvy-grass syrup 1oz, betony and blessed thistle waters each 2oz. Mix.

He was purged and cured. Three months later, he fell into a dropsy with swollen feet.

R: the chymical cup ½oz, wine of squills **[p. 22]** 2dr, barley water, syrup of violets each ½oz. Seven vomits, two stools.

The next day:

R: leaves of chicory, borage, bugloss, violet, strawberry each 1 handful, anise, caraway seeds each 1dr, roots of garden celery, bitter dock each 1oz, flowers of borage, bugloss, violet, roses each 1 pinch. Boil in enough water for 12oz. Take 4oz of the strained liquid. Infuse trochiscated agaric, rhubarb each ½dr, mechoachan ½dr, ginger

1 Probably the man who petitioned King James for a pension in 1605, 'having long served in the wars of Ireland' in 1599 and 1600. One of his fellow soldiers was the husband of another of Hall's patients, Katherine, Lady Hunks. Hall saw him in about 1620. Lane's identification of this patient as Captain Basset from Devon, who was commissioned Captain under Count Mansfeldt in 1624, does not fit with the age Basset was when he consulted Hall.
2 See Case 9, n. 3.

1½sc, spikenard 4gr, cinnamon ½sc. Strain again in the morning. To 3oz of the pressed strained liquid add loosening rose syrup 1½oz, strained manna ½oz. Mix. Make a drink. Repeat on four mornings.

When this was finished, he was purged thus:

R: aggregative pills 1sc, gamboge gum 5gr, anise oil 5 drops, sufficient chicory syrup with rhubarb. Make 2 pills per dose: seven stools.

The second day he took 1 pill: five stools, with the desired happy result because he could breathe and walk better.

A sweating potion:

R: sarsaparilla 2oz, sassafras root ½oz. Boil in 8 pints of spring water, reduce to 4 after soaking for twenty four hours. At the end add bruised cinnamon, 2dr, anise, caraway, coriander seeds each ½oz. Dose: 6oz hot, and sweating is provoked according to practice.

Afterwards he took laxative beer, prepared like this:

R: sarsaparilla 2oz, china cut in rounds 1oz, sassafras 6dr, guaiacum **[p. 23]** 2oz, senna 1½oz, rhubarb ½oz, agaric 3dr, mechoachan 1oz, shavings of ivory, hartshorn each ½oz, fennel seeds, nutmeg, cloves each 2dr, violet, rosemary, fumitory leaves each 3 handfuls. Put them in a bag for 3 gallons of beer.

These freed him from dropsy. In August he suffered from hypochondriac melancholy with headache.

R: pills of amber 2dr, powder for Galen's simple hiera picra electuary 2sc. Make 12 pills with chicory syrup with rhubarb. Take 3 at bedtime.

He was freed from the headache.

R: aggregative pills 1sc, gamboge gum 5gr. Make 2 pills with 5 drops of anise oil and apple syrup. Eight stools with great relief.

Next:

R: *origanum, wormwood, mint each ½ handful, toasted seeds of millet, anise each ½oz, camomile, lavender, rosemary leaves each 1 pinch, bayberries 1dr, nutmeg ½dr. Powder coarsely, sew into a thin red silk cloth, and make a bag sewn in the form of a stomach shield. Apply to the stomach sprinkled with some good wine and well heated.* Repeat as is beneficial.[1]

He was freed and cured of all the above symptoms by these remedies, and remained well for a long time.

[Case 28]

[p. 24] Mrs Chandler of Stratford-upon-Avon,[2] aged 36 or thereabouts: fell into an erratic fever on the fifth day after giving birth, with frequent shivering, hot spells and rigors day and night.

℞: hartshorn decoction with lemon juice, rose water and sugar for a pleasant sharpness, 3 pints.

She took it all time, always shaking it so that she drank the powder with the decoction. When this was finished:

℞: prepared hartshorn 3dr, rain water ½ pint. Reduce by boiling to 4oz. After boiling add syrup of field poppies 2oz, rose water 1oz, sufficient oil of vitriol. This is for two doses.

When these were finished, she recovered.[3]

[Case 29]

Mr Fortescue, aged 20:[4] tortured by epilepsy with consent of the stomach, hypochondriac melancholy with loss of movement and feeling of the ring and middle fingers on the right hand. When I was summoned to him, I purged him in this way. Urine: heavy, clear like spring water, in large quantity.

---

1 Feyens, *De flatibus*, pp. 144–145.
2 Cf. Case 8. This time Hall treated her for fever, five days after childbirth.
3 Ruland the Elder, 'Centuria III', *Curationum* [...] *centuriae*, p. 219.
4 William Fortescue of Cook Hill. Heir to an estate near Inkberrow. Married Jane Wylde in 1621. Fortescue was a Catholic, and the family harboured a Catholic priest. He was also a Royalist, and Charles I spent a night at his house in 1645 before the battle of Worcester.

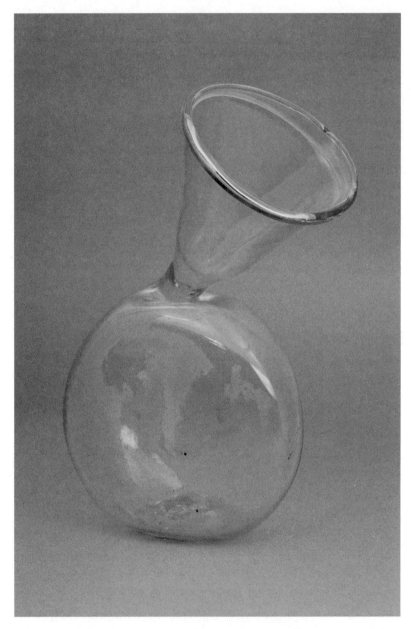

24 A seventeenth-century urine flask, rather like the one seen in Osias Dyck's *A Doctor Casting the Water* (Plate 25). The elegant bend in the jar made it easy for the patient to use. Hall took a sample of Mr Fortescue's urine and described it as 'heavy, clear, like spring water' (Case 29).

℞: pills – sine quibus 1dr, foetidae 2sc, castor 1sc, sufficient borage water. Make 7 pills: seven large stools.

After purgation, movement and feeling returned to the fingers. 5 June 1623. 6th: Section of the cephalic vein to 6oz **[p. 25]** and the same day 3 amber pills at bedtime. The following day three stools from these. 8th:

℞: best castor, assafoetida each ½dr, peony root finely powdered 1dr, aromatic rose [powder] 2dr. Mix with mint syrup. Make 7 pills from the mass. Take one when going to bed.

In the morning take this opiate, the amount of a walnut:

℞: conserves of bugloss, borage, rosemary each 1½oz, alkermes confection 2dr, electuaries – Galen's laetificans, of gems each ½dr, peony root powder, aristolochia each 1sc, shavings of ivory, hartshorn, coral each 2sc. Make the opiate with hyssop syrup by the usual method.

At the time of an attack:

℞: *benzoin gum, mummy, naval pitch each 1sc. Combine them with rue juice. Make a fumigant for the nostrils or after dissolving it, anoint the inside of the nose.*[1]

NOTE: he used this sneezing powder in the morning, before the opiate:

℞: *Spanish pellitory, peony root powder each 2sc, nutmeg 1sc, powdered black hellebore ½sc. Make a powder to be blown into the nose.*[2]

These, through God's mercy, freed him in a short time and he is now alive and well ten years later.

[Case 30]
Mrs Nash, a gentlewoman aged 62:[3] suffered from phthisis for a long time, now with wind in the stomach and very marked hot

---

1 Houllier, *De morbis internis*, p. 122.

2 Houllier, *De morbis internis*, p. 125.

3 Mary Nash of Stratford-upon-Avon. Born 1565, one of ten children. One of her brothers died with Drake off the West Indies. Married Anthony Nash, who owned

spells **[p. 26]** and sweating from the mouth of the stomach to the top of the head, with great pain especially after food.

> ℞: *white sugar 4oz, cubebs, grains of paradise, galangal, ginger each 1dr, long pepper ½dr, cinnamon 3dr, white wine 2 pints.* Stand to infuse for twenty four hours, *then strain through a sleeve. Make the potion commonly called hippocras.*[1] Take 3oz in the morning.

She used an enema of linseed oil with great effect. Finally take 3oz of the following syrup:

> ℞: *cinnamon roughly crushed 4oz, sweet flag 1oz. Soak in malmsey wine 2 pints for three days, in a glass vessel near the heat of a low fire. Strain. To the strained liquid add 1½lbs sugar. Boil it all slowly and make syrup according to practice.*[2]

These freed her from the wind and she could again take food. She said she was very much better and freed from wind. This has been proved.

[Case 31]

Mr Kempson, a gentleman aged 60:[3] overwhelmed by melancholy and tormented by fever with the very highest heat. He was likewise continuously overcome *by deeper sleep than* **[p. 27]** *he was accustomed to,*[4] without any sense of illness, as if unconscious. I cured him with the following:

> ℞: *leaves of mallow, beet, violet, mercury, hops each 1½ handfuls, borage 2 handfuls, dodder ½oz,* penny-royal, rue, wormwood, chamomile each ½ handful, seeds of anise, caraway, cumin, rue, fennel, nettle, bayberry each *½oz, polypody of the oak each 1½oz,* senna 1oz, *black hellebore*

the Bear in Bridge Street, and had four children. Her elder son Thomas married Elizabeth, John Hall's only daughter.

1 Feyens, *De flatibus*, p. 142.

2 Du Chesne, *Pharmacopoea dogmaticorum*, p. 101.

3 Leonard Kempson of Stratford-upon-Avon (*c.* 1550–1625). Son of wealthy parents. Leonard and his brother were interrogated by the Star Chamber in 1601 for taking money from local men who wished to avoid muster duty. Kempson became Constable in 1620.

4 Echoing Cicero, 'Somnium Scipionis, Book VI', *De re publica*.

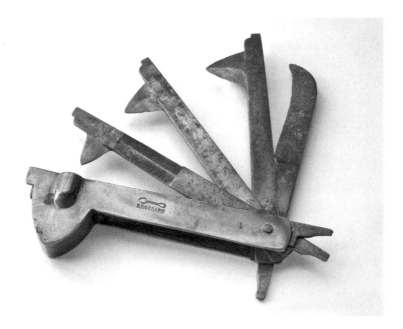

25 A seventeenth-century fleam used for blood-letting. The triangular blade was held over the vein and then struck to make the incision with minimal damage to the tissue. Hall drew eight ounces of blood from Mr Kempson (Case 31).

> *bark 1dr. Boil in milk whey, reduce to 1½ pints.*[1] Take 10oz of the strained liquid, Hamech confection, diaphoenicon each 5dr, salt 1dr.

Make an enema: two stools with a large amount of wind. Give in the morning and repeat at night. *Bind finely sliced radishes to the soles of the feet, sprinkled with vinegar and salt, renewed every third hour. The attack of the corrupt vapours should be hindered by this, the soot being attracted downwards.*[2] The next night was more restful, without the terrible dreams as before. The usual drink:

> ℞: spring water 4 pints, lemon syrup 10z, rose julep 1½oz, prepared hartshorn 4sc, spirit of vitriol as many drops as needed for a pleasing acidity.

---

1 Bruele, *Praxis medicinae*, p. 27.
2 Ruland the Younger, *De morbo Ungarico*, p. 178.

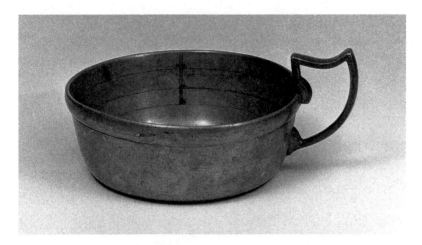

26 A late seventeenth/early eighteenth-century pewter bleeding bowl. The markings on the inside allowed the physician to measure the amount of blood that was being taken.

Then leeches were applied to the haemorrhoidal veins: **[p. 28]** 8oz of blood were taken.

℞: bezoar stone 5gr, tincture of coral 4 drops, in posset ale.

Urine: frothy with much sediment. He became much better. The enema was renewed along with the above drink which he very much enjoyed, and the bezoar stone powder and coral tincture were repeated with the desired result. He used a sneezing powder of tobacco only, to dispel sleep. He had Du Chesne's restaurative, page 187 of *Diaeteticon polyhistoricon*, section 3, chapter 9.[1] He was still worried about his stomach, so an emetic was given:

℞: our emetic 6dr, syrup of violets 2oz, oxymel of squills 1dr. Four vomits, nine stools.

He was well for five days, then relapsed in a cold and shivering fever. He recovered after an enema was given, and said farewell to his physicians. He was cured thus beyond all expectation, and

---

1 Du Chesne, *Diaeteticon polyshistoricon*, p. 187.

lived very well for many years. *It was these (by divinely declared mercy) which restored a desperate patient to good health.*[1]

[Case 32]
Mrs Garner, a gentlewoman of Shipston aged 22:[2] wretchedly weakened by a flux of the whites.

> ℞: newly extracted cassia 6dr in parsley water, turpentine washed in the same 2dr, guaiacum gum 2dr. Make a bolus with sugar.

[p. 29] The next day, I instructed her to apply the following plaster:

> ℞: comitissa ointment 1oz, gypsum, bole Armeniac each ½oz. Make a plaster with egg white.

Finally she used Jean Liébault's astringent trochees, Book 2 of *Maladies des femmes*, page 391: *take prepared coriander, sorrel seeds, plantain and chaste tree, each 1dr, sealed earth and bole Armeniac each ½dr, powder for cold diatragacanth electuary 1dr. Powder everything finely and, with sugar dissolved in plantain water, make a confection in the form of rolls or tablets* (add fish glue), *two drachms in weight. Chew one before dinner and supper and immediately afterwards swallow two or three spoonfuls of sour red wine. I am certain from experience that this confection is infinitely profitable on every occasion that the womb is affected.*[3] These controlled the discharge, and she very quickly recovered.

[Case 33]
Browne, a Romish priest:[4] suffered from Ungaric fever; in danger of death.

> ℞: the chymical cup 6dr, syrup of violets 2dr, **[p. 30]** oxymel of squills 1dr. Seven vomits, four stools.

---

1 Ruland the Elder, 'Centuria III', *Curationum* [...] *centuriae*, p. 209.
2 Probably Elizabeth Gardner (b. 1593). No further information.
3 Liébault, *Thresor des remedes secrets*, pp. 391–392.
4 No reliable information. Might be an alias, for protection. Possibly attached to a wealthy household, who would pay for his expensive medication.

He was bled the next day to 6oz. The day after venesection, a drink:

℞: *spring water 3 pints, pomegranate syrup, julep of roses each 1½oz, prepared hartshorn 3oz, enough oil of vitriol for a pleasing tartness. Then from the straining, make a julep.*[1]

He received tincture of coral 1sc in broth, and at bedtime an enema of the aperient herbs with laxative senna powder and unrefined sugar: three stools.

Take the amount of a walnut, day and night, often:[2]

℞: *blackcurrant juice, rose conserve, citron flesh conserve each 1oz, preserved citron skin ½oz, preserved oranges, liberans powder each 2dr, prepared hartshorn 4sc, prepared emerald, ruby, sapphire stones, each 6gr, flowers of sulphur 1dr, prepared red coral 1sc, pomegranate juice ½oz, enough syrup of sour citrons. Make a liquid electuary.*[3]

He also used it successfully without the gems. *The heart was also strengthened:*[4]

℞: rose conserve 1oz, coral tincture 2sc, prepared hartshorn 1dr, diascordium ½dr, prepared flowers of sulphur 2sc. Mix. Use for three days.

To quench thirst:

℞: barley 2oz, liquorice ½oz, borage, chicory each ½ handful. **[p. 31]** Boil in 3 pints water, reduce to 2 pints, add saltpetre ½dr, prepared hartshorn 3dr. Boil briefly. Take 3 draughts daily.

He also sprinkled his food with this heart-fortifying and poison-resisting powder:

℞: *prepared pearls, prepared red coral, prepared hartshorn, prepared garnet each 8gr, gold foil 1 leaf. Mix. Make the powder.*[5]

---

1 Ruland the Younger, *De morbo Ungarico*, p. 265.
2 Ruland the Younger, *De morbo Ungarico*, p. 168.
3 Ruland the Younger, *De morbo Ungarico*, p. 267.
4 Ruland the Younger, *De morbo Ungarico*, p. 168.
5 Ruland the Younger, *De morbo Ungarico*, p. 267.

When the julep was finished he used the following:

℞: *spring water 2 pints, prepared hartshorn, raw hartshorn each 3dr, liberans powder 4sc. Boil, reduce by ½ pint. Add enough lemon juice for a pleasant acidity. Boil again, skim, purify with egg white. Make a julep, of which he is to take three draughts each day, two in the morning, the third in the afternoon.*[1]

The priest recovered beyond all hope, and returned to full health. With these remedies, especially the hartshorn decoction, I have in a short time cured an infinite number tortured by this disease and other fevers, *by the power of almighty God most high, to whom alone be expressions of thanks, blessing and praise unfailingly, in endless ages. Amen.*[2]

[Case 34]

[p. 32] Captain Basset, aged 50:[3] with hypochondriac melancholy and tremor, pricking of the heart with swelling around the ankles, and headache.

℞: *leaves of chicory, borage, bugloss, violets, wild strawberries each 1 handful, black hellebore root 2dr, liquorice, polypody of the oak each 2oz, citron seeds 1½oz, anise and caraway seeds each ½oz, all the myrobalans each 2dr. Pound them coarsely and rub with the hands with sweet almond oil. Afterwards infuse for a day and a night in 10 pints fumitory water,* roots of parsley, bugloss each 1oz, borage, bugloss, violet and rose flowers each 1 handful. *Boil in 5 pints spring water until 3 pints remain. Strain, then add senna, dodder, tamarisk each 2oz. Boil again, reduce to 2 pints, and strain and squeeze out the decoction.*[4] Infuse in this agaric trochees, rhubarb each 2dr, mechoachan 2oz, ginger 4sc, spikenard ½dr, cinnamon 1dr overnight. Strain again, boil with sugar and make a perfectly concocted syrup. Add to this loosening rose syrup **[p. 33]** 4oz, manna 2oz, and keep for 4 doses.

He was very well purged with the desired result. After purging, *take one sweetmeat at a time, morning and evening, two hours before meals for a whole week*:

---

1 Ruland the Younger, *De morbo Ungarico*, p. 271.
2 Ruland the Elder, 'Centuria III', *Curationum [...] centuriae*, p. 213.
3 Cf. Case 27.
4 da Monte, *Consultationum medicinalium*, p. 336.

℞: *powders – Galen's laetificans, sweet diamoschum, aromatic rose each 1dr, cinnamon ½dr, clean pistachios ½oz,* alkermes confection, saffron, stag's heart bone, red coral, pearls each 1sc, prepared steel 2dr, sufficient sugar. *Dissolve the sugar in cinnamon water, make a sweetmeat in bite-sized pieces weighing about 2dr.*[1]

He should wear a stomach salve:

℞: labdanum 2dr, wax ½oz, mace oil 2dr, Gabrieli's aromatic rose powder 2sc. Make a stomach plaster. He used an enema with emollients and carminatives with sugar.

After meals:

℞: *prepared coriander seed 2dr, fennel, anise each 1dr, caraway ½dr, liquorice ½oz, ginger 2dr, galangal root, nutmeg, cinnamon, cloves each 1dr. Cut small, add sugar. Make a powder to be taken after meals, or make tablets with sugar dissolved in rose water.*[2]

With these he recovered rightly and properly, and thanked me.

[Case 35]

[p. 34] Cure of epilepsy by consent, for the six-month-old son of the Reverend Walker of Ilmington.[3]

Slices of peony root were hung round his neck. *I prescribed rue juice mixed with strong vinegar applied to his nostrils when the fit molested him. Using this brought him immediately to himself, but he quickly suffered a recurrence. The fits were shortened though, when it was applied to the nostrils. I instructed them to apply this plaster to the area of the heart:*

℞: *Venice treacle 1dr, powdered peony root ½dr. Mix.*

Peony root powder was also sprinkled on his hair.[4] These freed him from all the attacks.

---

1 Crato, *Consiliorum* [...] *liber secundus*, p. 151.
2 Platter, *Observationum* [...] *libri tres*, pp. 60–61.
3 John Walker of Ilmington. Born 1633. Infant son of the curate, grandson of the rector of Ilmington.
4 Platter, *Observationum* [...] *libri tres*, pp. 26–27.

[Case 36]

Elizabeth Hall, my only daughter:[1] disfigured by spasm of the mouth. See the signs in the Chapter 'De Tortura', Book 1 of Valesco de Taranta, page 88.[2] She was successfully cured in this way:

R: pills – cochiae, aureae each 1dr. Make 10 pills. Take 5: Seven stools the first day, five on the second.

The parts were fomented with aqua vitae and Venice treacle. She used the following ointment on her neck:

R: Martiatum magnum ointment 1oz, oils of laurel, petroleum, castor, oil of turpentine each ½dr, of bricks ½dr. **[p. 35]**

Using this gave much profit. Her periods were obstructed, so she was purged thus:

R: pills – foetidae 1dr, castor 1dr, of amber, rhubarb, agaric 1½sc.

She took 5 pills the size of a pea early in the morning. Eight stools, one vomit. The next day her period flowed.

For suffering from inflammation of the eye:

R: prepared tutty 1dr, for its composition see page 5 of this book.

One or two drops were instilled in the eye. When her periods stopped, I prescribed the following sweating decoction:

R: guaiacum 2oz, sassafras ½oz, sarsaparilla 1oz, china 6dr. Soak for 24 hours, then boil in 8 pints spring water, reduce to 4.

Using this day by day restored the former appearance of her mouth and face. The use of sassafras oil was not omitted, because

---

1 Elizabeth Hall, Shakespeare's granddaughter. Married 1628, aged 18, to Thomas Nash. No children. Nash died in 1647. Elizabeth remarried a year later to Sir John Barnard of Abington, a 'Royalist Northamptonshire gentleman', became Elizabeth, Lady Barnard, and stepmother to five children. She stayed at Abington until her death.
2 Valesco de Taranta, *Epitome operis*, pp. 88–90.

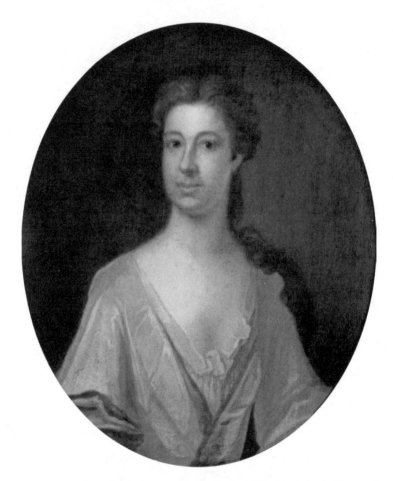

27 A presumed posthumous portrait (*c.* 1690) of Elizabeth, Lady Barnard (1608–70), née Hall, John and Susanna's daughter. Oil on canvas, 915 × 760mm (36 × 30 in). The portrait was in the possession of Thomas Hart, fifth in descent from Shakespeare's sister, Joan.

it is the equal of anything for relieving dryness of the nerves. Her neck was anointed and so she was healed. 5 January 1624.

At the beginning of April she went to London. Returning home on the 22nd, she caught cold on the way. Once more she fell into spasm of the mouth on the other side, previously on the left, now wretchedly affected on the right. Again, praise God, she was cured with the following. See Jacques Houllier, *De morbis internis Book 1*, Chapter 11, pages 96, 97, 98;[1] Felix Platter, *Book 1*, 'in Motus Impotentia', page 375;[2] see page 102, Guillaume Rondelet, chapter 38, *Methodus curandorum morbos*;[3] see page 394, cure 87, Amatus Lusitanus, *Centuria 4*.[4] I did indeed cure her again within sixteen days:

R: pills – amber ½dr, aureae 1sc. Make 5 pills, take at bedtime.

I instructed her to anoint her neck and the top of her head with oil of sassafras the same night. **[p. 36]** I gave 1½dr Ruffus's pills in the morning, and she also used oil with aqua vitae. I instructed her to drip the above eyedrops into the eye. As I was out of sassafras oil, in its place:

R: powders of castor, myrrh, nutmeg, saffron each 1sc, oils of rue, laurel, petroleum, turpentine each 2dr, Martiatum ointment ½oz, oils of costus, peppers each 1dr.

The top of the head was washed with aqua vitae in which nutmeg, cinnamon, cloves and pepper were soaked. *Nutmegs also should be chewed frequently*, as Platter strongly recommends.[5] She used amber oil to the nostrils and the top of the head. *Chew pellitory of Spain on the healthy side*.[6] She was purged often, with the following pills:

R: pills foetidae 1sc, powdered castor ½sc, pills Ruffus's, amber each 1sc. Make 5 pills.

These, correctly used, cured her rightly and properly, praise almighty God most high.

In the same year, 24 May, she was vexed with an erratic fever, now hot, soon sweating, then cold, often troubled within half an hour.

---

1 Houllier, *De morbis internis*, pp. 96–99.
2 Platter, *Praxeos* […] *de functionem laesionibus*, p. 375.
3 Rondelet, *Methodus curandorum*, ff. 101v–102v.
4 Amatus Lusitanus, *Curationum medicinaliun centuriae quatuor*, pp. 394–396.
5 Platter, *Praxeos* […] *de functionum laesionibus*, p. 375.
6 Rondelet, *Methodus curandorum*, f. 102r.

She was purged in this way:

℞: fennel, parsley roots each ½ handful, bark of elder root 2 handfuls, common iris root, tincture of madder 1 handful, asparagus
roots 2 handfuls. Boil in sufficient water to 6 pints. To the strained
liquid add rhubarb, agaric each ½oz, senna 6oz, mechoachan 2oz,
sweet flag 1oz, anise seeds 1oz, cinnamon ½oz. Soak in a closed
vessel by the usual method, then strain. Add sufficient sugar to the
strained liquid, make a well boiled syrup. Take 4oz of this, rhubarb
2dr, soak **[p. 37]** in 5oz chicory water. Mix. Give 7 spoonfuls on an
empty stomach: seven or eight stools without discomfort in one day.

℞: sarsaparilla 1oz, sassafras 2dr, guaiacum 1oz, liquorice ½oz,
leaves of chicory, sage, rosemary each ½ handful. Boil in 10 pints
water, reduce to 5 pints. Take a draught hot, in the morning.

The following balsam was used to anoint the spine, prepared in this way:

℞: *galbanum and bdellium gums. Dissolve ½oz each in spirits, benzoin 1oz,
liquid styrax 1dr, rue and ground pine leaves, French lavender and ordinary lavender flowers each 2dr, costus root ½oz, castor 1sc. Infuse, sliced and pounded,
in aqua vitae, stand to soak in the heat for a few days before use. Rub the spine
with it.*[1]

An hour after using it, *all symptoms diminished, and daily over a few days
she reached complete health, freed from death and deadly illness*[2] and has
remained well for many years.

[Case 37]
Lady Sandys,[3] after her purification:[4] wretchedly attacked by
swelling and pain of the haemorrhoids. I prescribed populeon
ointment to be anointed on the swollen haemorrhoids.

---

1 Platter, *Observationum* [...] *libri tres*, p. 220.
2 Ruland the Elder, 'Centuria III', *Curationum* [...] *centuriae*, p. 217.
3 Penelope, Lady Sandys of Ombersley (1587–1680). Came of a titled family, married Edwin Sandys, heir to Ombersley. She had four children, the youngest born
after Edwin's early death. One son died at Edgehill. Penelope lived on, through
the Civil War and Restoration, and died aged 93.
4 Purification: see 'The Thanksgiving of Women after Childbirth' in *The Book of
Common Prayer*.

R: *one egg yolk, beat well with rose oil in summer, sweet almond oil in winter, and add a little powdered saffron and rub on the spot.*[1]

This is well tested. It softens hard haemorrhoids and removes pain. Cured.

[Case 38]

[p. 38] Mr Quiney:[2] weakened by a bad cough with a large amount of phlegm, vomiting food, a slow fever. Urine: red, without sediment.

R: *trochiscated agaric 1½dr, frankincense, mastic each ½dr, sufficient turpentine. Make 5 pills from 1dr. Take 5 on going to bed. Saffron in seasonings*[3] *because it benefits the chest, and mustard with honey stimulates expectoration very well.*[4]

R: *simple hydromel freshly prepared, with choice honey 1½lb. Add fat stoned raisins 1oz, 10 fat figs, orris root, sweet flag each 1dr. Boil everything together several times, and strain. To the strained liquid add sugar candy, barley sugar each 3oz, choice broken cinnamon ½dr (it strengthens all the organs with its fragrance). Make hydromel, of which I instructed him to drink 8 or 9oz morning and evening. Large quantities of this medicine must be given, so that the power reaches the lungs.*[5]

A plaster should be applied to the shaved head, worn day and night:

R: *roots of iris, galangal, cypress, angelica each 2dr, roots of pellitory of Spain, agaric, rhubarb, squills each 1dr, senna 2dr, marjoram 1dr, coriander seeds, bayberries, cloves, nutmeg, mace each 1dr, nigella* **[p. 39]** *and mustard seeds each ½dr, benzoin, styrax each 3dr, white calcanso, calamine, alum 1dr. Make a plaster by adding old nut oil, some drops of distilled marjoram and sage oil, and sufficient larch gum and wax. Make a plaster.*[6]

---

1 Castro, *De universa mulierum medicina*, p. 198.
2 Probably George Quiney of Stratford-upon-Avon, one of eleven children of a wealthy mercer. Took a degree at Balliol, then became curate at Holy Trinity. His brother Thomas married Shakespeare's daughter Judith. George died aged 24, probably of tuberculosis.
3 Valleriola, *Observationum* [...] *libri sex*, p. 151.
4 Platter, *Praxeos* [...] *de functionum laesionibus*, p. 454.
5 Valleriola, *Observationum* [...] *libri sex*, p. 151.
6 Platter, *Observationum* [...] *libri tres*, p. 164.

On the quiet days, in the morning:

℞: saffron 1sc, musk 1gr. Give it in white wine. *Saffron is the soul of the lungs.*[1]

For hoarseness:

℞: *liquorice juice 1dr, myrrh ½dr, tragacanth gum 1sc, sugar candy and barley sugar each ½dr. Make bite-sized pieces. He should hold one inside the cheek when going to bed and allow it to dissolve on its own, while he lies on his back.*[2] *Saffron in seasonings benefits the chest, and mustard with honey stimulates expectoration very well.*[3] *Emulsion or milk of sweet almonds, with some added pine nuts, and freshly bruised gourd seeds, squeeze out 4oz. Dissolve in it rose sugar tablets 2dr.*

He drank this lukewarm, fasting on alternate mornings, and continued it for two weeks.[4] He was not completely freed, and the following year fell into the same illness. After trying many treatments in vain, he sleeps peacefully with the Lord. He was of good character, expert at languages, and for his young age learned in everything.

[Case 39]

[p. 40] Joan Judkin of Southam, aged 50:[5] with trembling and weakness of the arms and legs. She then feels a vapour rising to the heart, then the throat, until she thinks she is going to be suffocated. Age: 40.

℞: mercurius vitae 5gr, diaphoenicon 1dr. Mix.

---

1 Cardano, *Ars curandi parva*, p. 385.
2 Platter, *Observationum* […] *libri tres*, pp. 201–202.
3 Saffron … very well] Platter, *Praxeos* […] *de functionum laesionibus*, p. 454. See also Case 38, n. 3.
4 Platter, *Observationum* […] *libri tres*, p. 318.
5 Born *c.* 1584 as Joan Twigge. Married 1609 to Robert Judkin, one daughter. Note the two different ages. The second has been added in a different ink, which I see as a correction, which Hall then failed to follow through by deleting the age he wrote first. The patient's identity is unchanged but the consultation moves to 1624.

Two stools; she passed two worms. Then Venice treacle 1dr, in posset ale. She was purged again:

℞: mercurius vitae 6gr, diaphoenicon 1dr. Mix: four stools.

Finally, Venice treacle with hartshorn shavings. By these few, within four days, *with the favour and help of almighty God most high, all her symptoms vanished as if miraculously.*[1] The bell sounded for her twice.

[Case 40]
Mr Winter, aged 4:[2] attacked by worms and fever.

℞: *a honey suppository.*[3]

To drink: a decoction of prepared and raw hartshorn; ointment for worms on the umbilicus. His body was purged with ½oz manna in broth which expelled many dead worms with foul-smelling excreta. He took the following powder in broth and food:

℞: prepared coral, prepared pearls, prepared hartshorn, prepared garnets each 8gr, pieces of zircon, emerald, ruby each 3gr, gold leaf 1 piece. He used poppy syrup, to be drunk slowly, with maidenhair syrup for the cough.

I cured him with God's help, in three days.

---

1 Ruland the Elder, 'Centuria III', *Curationum* [...] *centuriae*, p. 199.
2 This patient is misidentified by Lane as John Winter of Huddington, Worcestershire, because she follows Cooke's misreading of Hall's manuscript as reading aged 44 here. Hall wrote '*et.4.*' (with a raised dot after the 4), which is different from the dashes he used to indicate an incomplete date (as, for example, in Case 156). Hall frequently used the raised dot to indicate spaces between words. Winter suffered from worms, and his treatment, with a mild purge and an umbilical plaster, is similar to that Hall used for other children rather than for adults. The young Mr Winter may have been one of John Winter's three children, born before 1622, when the mother died (there is no record of their dates of birth). The patient's identity changes, and the consultation can be approximately dated to the early or mid-1620s.
3 Platter, *Praxeos* [...] *de vitiis*, p. 985.

[Case 41]

[p. 41] Mrs Fortescue, a gentlewoman:[1] attacked by a most violent cough and worms. Age: 12.

A honey suppository;[2] a plaster against worms on the umbilicus. For cough:

> R: *flowers of sulphur ½oz, benzoin (i.e. assa odorata) ½sc. Mix. Render into a very fine powder.*[3] Divide into 12 parts, give 1 part each day in the morning and with hartshorn in the evening.

She was freed by these, and cured.

[Case 42]

Lady Throckmorton, aged 35:[4] heartburn, and melancholy with an affection of the womb.

> R: rhubarb 1dr, agaric 2sc, senna ½oz, a little cinnamon. Soak in ½ pint wormwood wine, to 6oz. Take 6 spoonfuls of the strained liquid, chicory syrup with rhubarb 2 spoonfuls, and continue the course for 3 days.

She evacuated six times a day. She told me that on the third night her period flowed more abundantly than for many years, and so for a time she discontinued the medicines. 2 March.

When I returned on 1 April, I purged her:

> R: pills – sine quibus, Ruffus's each 1dr. Make 9 pills, give 3 at bedtime.

---

1 Martha Fortescue, born *c.* 1611. Her father was the recusant Nicholas Fortescue (cf. Case 168). She married Nicholas Lewis in 1630, and Hall treated her again later (Case 153).

2 Platter, *Praxeos* [...] *de vitiis*, p. 985. See Case 40, n. 3.

3 Ruland the Elder, 'Centuria III', *Curationum* [...] *centuriae*, p. 226.

4 Lady Mary Throckmorton of Coughton came from a wealthy Catholic family in Leicestershire. In 1615 she married Robert Throckmorton, heir to Coughton Court, the leading Catholic family in the area (who were directly involved in the Gunpowder Plot). Robert was knighted in 1642, and died in 1651. Mary remarried in 1659 and moved to Walton, Warwickshire.

After her body was purged, she used the following steeled wine, about 2 spoonfuls, then 4 then 6, gradually increasing what she took:

℞: prepared steel 1oz, middle bark of ash and tamarisk, caper roots each ½oz, sassafras, juniper wood each 6dr, roots of elecampane, angelica, galangal, sweet flag each 2dr, **[p. 42]** shavings of ivory, hartshorn, yellow sandalwood each 3dr, leaves of wormwood, ground-pine, spleenwort, dodder, lemon balm, germander each 2 pinches, flowers of borage, bugloss, scabious, broom each 1 pinch, cinnamon ½oz, cloves, ginger, mace, nutmeg each 2dr. *Crush everything coarsely and blend in turn, infuse in best wine 4 pints. After steeping place in a warm bain-Marie, in a well-closed vessel, for three or four days. Afterwards strain several times through a Hippocratic sleeve.*[1]

Give as above, and she is to take exercise. Take the following powder after meals:

℞: prepared coriander seeds 1dr, fennel, anise each ½dr, caraway 1sc, the cordial flowers each 1dr, marjoram ½dr, liquorice and elecampane root each 1dr, ginger 1dr, galangal root, nutmeg, cloves each ½dr. Pound coarsely, add sugar. Make a powder.

Anoint the stomach and hypochondrium with the following oil, three times weekly:

℞: *Oils of dill, nard, capers each ½oz, vinegar of squills 1oz. Boil until the vinegar is gone, add gum ammoniac dissolved in vinegar 2dr, asarabacca root 1dr, nigella seeds ½dr, saffron 1sc, sufficient wax. Make a liniment.*[2]

The Lady regained her health with these, within 20 days.[3]

---

1 Du Chesne, *Pharmacopoea dogmaticorum*, p. 73.

2 Platter, *Praxeos* [...] *de functionum laesionibus*, p. 140.

3 Ruland the Elder, 'Centuria III', *Curationum* [...] *centuriae*, p. 181.

[Case 43]

[p. 43] Austin, a spinster:[1] *her face was sprinkled with red spots, swollen and disfigured by red pustules around her chin,* otherwise a good-looking young woman of much talent.

> ℞: *diacatholicon 5dr, Hamech confection 2dr, fumitory water 3oz,*[2] chicory syrup with rhubarb 6dr. Make it.

She was very well purged. The next day:

> ℞: pills – foetidae, of colchicum each ½dr, aureae 2sc. Make it.

She was abundantly evacuated. After being rightly purged, *she should anoint her face with this liquid*:

> ℞: *powdered litharge of gold 1oz, alum 1dr, borax 3dr, ceruse ½oz, vinegar 2oz, rose and plantain waters each 3oz. Boil on a low fire, reduce by a third, then strain. Add lemon syrup ½oz.*[3] Make it.

NOTE: I prescribed venesection before the use of this water. *On my advice, she opened, broke and expressed the pustules morning and evening. She washed daily with the above water, which afterwards dried by itself. After she had continued with this lotion for a few days, her face was entirely healed in every part, and she was well coloured.*[4]

[Case 44]

Elizabeth Kington of Honington, aged 50:[5] with a flux of blood from the mouth.

> ℞: wild poppy syrup 2oz, scabious water 3oz, a few roses. Take 1 part in the morning, another in the evening.

---

1 Alice Austin. Hall treated this young girl, and noted her good looks and wit. She married Thomas Sheffield in 1627, and had four daughters. All of the children, and the parents, died of plague within ten days in 1638.

2 Platter, *Observationum* […] *libri tres*, p. 588.

3 Platter, *Observationum* […] *libri tres*, p. 588.

4 Ruland the Elder, 'Centuria III', *Curationum* […] *centuriae*, p. 158

5 Elizabeth Warde married John Kington, a day-labourer, in 1612. One daughter. Widowed in 1619.

R: conserve of red roses 1oz, bole Armeniac, haematite, red coral, sealed earth each 1sc. Make a mixture with poppy syrup. Take as much as a bean after the julep.

Cured.

[Case 45]
[p. 44] Symons of Knowle:[1] cure of a ruptured vein in the lung, vomiting blood. Age: 40.

R: powdered rhubarb 2dr, maidenhair syrup 1oz, chicory water 4oz. Mix.

R: philonium Persicum 1dr (highly praised by Valleriola for stopping blood) syrup of bilberries 1oz, plantain water 4oz.[2] Mix. Take goat's milk with sugar, and at bedtime, conserve of red roses.

He was cured quickly, safely, pleasantly by these few.

[Case 46]
Cooper, a married woman of Pebworth, aged 48:[3] feels a breath or wind rising from her feet to the stomach. She feels ill at once and almost faints.

R: pills – foetidae, Ruffus's each 4sc. Make 9 pills. Take 3 at bedtime.

Next she took the following powder after meals:

R: shavings of ivory, hartshorn each 1dr, Gabrieli's aromatic rose powder ½dr, seeds of coriander, fennel, anise each 1dr, caraway ½dr, cordial flowers 1dr, marjoram ½dr, liquorice and elecampane root each 1dr, ginger, galangal, nutmeg, cloves each ½dr, saffron 1sc. Pound coarsely, and add an equal weight of rose sugar tablets: after meals, ½ spoonful.

1 John Symons of Knowle, born *c.* 1580. Non-gentry. Knowle is a hamlet near Oversley. Four children baptised at Arrow before 1612.
2 Valleriola, *Observationum* [...] *libri sex*, p. 220.
3 Mary Cooper of Pebworth. A married woman, probably Mary Martin who married Thomas Cooper in 1611. Three children. Died in 1641.

She said this powder was worth gold. For the stomach: plaster of laudanum, wax, caranna, the aromatic powder and mace oil. She was freed and cured of all symptoms by these alone.

[Case 47]

[p. 45] Proven cure of scurvy, hypochondriac melancholy, heart palpitations, pain in the head and joints, inflammation of the eye, giddiness, skin rash.[1] Mrs Wagstaffe, a gentlewoman of Warwick, 46 years:[2] *almost wasted away by these long-standing illnesses.*[3] She passed changeable urine, one day clear like spring water, then thick and turbid. From the frequent change of the urine I judged that she suffered from scurvy. Nor did my judgement deceive me, for her arms were polluted with livid, purple spots, with many other symptoms which it would take too long to describe now.

I was summoned for consultation, and restored her health with the following:

> R: chicory, bugloss roots each 1oz, fennel, iris, tamarisk bark each ½oz, elecampane, wormwood leaves each 3dr, marjoram, ground-pine, germander, fumitory each 2dr, cordial flowers each 1dr, seeds of anise, fennel, parsley each 1½dr, senna leaves 1½oz, bruised safflower 1oz. Pound and soak in 2 pints white wine. Boil, reduce to 1 pint, strain. Add Foreest's scheletyrbic syrup 3oz.

She used it for five days. Dose: 4dr, from which six or seven stools, sometimes eight, every day. She was almost freed from the heart palpitations by this purge.

---

1 Note the change of heading style from mentioning the patient first to mentioning the illness.

2 Elizabeth Wagstaffe of Warwick (?–1637). Daughter of a Puritan barrister. Married aged 20 to Timothy Wagstaffe, who was soon called to the bar. He died in 1625, leaving her with six children. The heir, Thomas, was made a royal ward and later entered Middle Temple. As a widow, she managed the family estates.

3 Ruland the Elder, 'Centuria III', *Curationum* [...] *centuriae*, p. 217.

Once her body was rightly purged, I advised her to use this wine next:

℞: the opening roots each ½oz, wormwood 2oz, marjoram 1½dr, **[p. 46]** cordial flowers each 1 pinch, tamarisk bark and capers each 1dr, fennel, anise seeds each 2dr, caraway 1dr, spikenard 1sc, centaury tops 1½dr, prepared steel 3dr. Make it, put in 2 pints white wine. Take three hours before food, and take prepared scurvy-grass juice in wine, 4 or 5 spoonfuls an hour before dinner, once or twice as needed.

Take a dose of the following pills, for the bowels movements should always be kept slippery:

℞: *aloes 2dr, myrrh ½dr, gum ammoniac dissolved in vinegar 1sc, agaric, rhubarb each 1½dr, wild ginger, gentian roots each ½dr, mastic 1sc, spikenard, parsley seeds each ½sc. Make a mass with wormwood juice in the form of thickened extract. Take ½dr once a week, or a little more, two hours before dinner.*[1] *If greater defaecation is required, one may add aggregative pills. Dose: 1 pill.*

A powder after meals:

℞: *cloves, galangal root, nutmeg, cinnamon each ½dr, prepared coriander seed, elecampane root each 1dr, fennel and anise seeds each ½dr, caraway 1 sc, liquorice root 2dr, ginger 1dr.*[2] Pound coarsely, add rose sugar tablets 2oz. Mix.

Then to anoint the region of the heart:

℞: *motherwort juice, nard oil each ½oz. Boil a little, add clove oil ½sc, camphor 1sc, saffron ½sc, a little white wax. Make a liniment*[3] **[p. 47]**

Then, as she was troubled with giddiness, having stopped the other tablets gradually, I decided she should use these:

---

1 aloes … dinner] Platter, *Praxeos* […] *de functionum laesionibus*, p. 139.

2 Platter, *Observationum* […] *libri tres*, p. 60. Cf. Case 34, n.2.

3 Platter, *Observationum* […] *libri tres*, p. 69.

℞: *simple diacidonium powder, nutmeg each 1dr, eyebright leaves, marjoram, lavender flowers each 1sc, red coral 2sc, ivory shavings 1sc, sugar dissolved in rose water. Make tablets. I advised her that it should be taken in the morning after broth, seasoned with marjoram and mace, or she should take it with a soft-boiled egg with added caraway seeds and salt (or better, scurvy-grass salt).*[1]

After leeches were applied to the haemorrhoidal veins she used the following to eradicate the morphew[2] disfiguring her face:

℞: white soap 2oz, live sulphur 1oz, verdigris 1dr, camphor 1sc. Make pellets with oil of tartar. Moisten a little with vinegar, anoint the face, allow to dry. Wash off with milk the next morning: and so she will quickly be freed. This has been proved a hundred times. For watering eyes, take the ophthalmic water as for Mrs Smith, page 5.

I prescribed the plaster against rupture for the temples, to control the rheum:

℞: *bole Armeniac 2dr, mastic ½dr, dragon's blood 1dr, gall powder ½dr, with egg white and vinegar as an excipient. Apply to the temples on both sides.*[3]

These restored her to her former health.

[Case 48]

[p. 48] Cure of excessive lachrymation of the right eye, dripping for a year. Mrs Simonds, a gentlewoman of Whitelady-Aston:[4] suffered from water running from the right eye without pain or redness. Because of the troublesome weeping, her vision is cut off and she sees very little. She was 15 years old. *By a happy omen I established this method of cure in order to drive off the said water.*[5]

---

1 Platter, *Observationum* […] *libri tres*, pp. 69–70.
2 A non-specific illness of the skin, associated with freckles or scaliness, but nowhere well defined.
3 Platter, *Observationum* […] *libri tres*, p. 351.
4 Isabel Simonds of White Ladies Aston (c. 1582–1645). A gentlewoman, 15 years old. Isabel Penrice married Thomas Simonds, and had seven children. Thomas was a puritan, refused to accept a knighthood and, in 1634, disclaimed his right to a coat of arms. He died in 1641. Cromwell stayed with their son George before the battle of Worcester in 1651.
5 Ruland the Elder, 'Centuria VI', *Curationum* […] *centuriae*, p. 443.

R: *fresh fumitory, cleaned senna + 3dr. Boil in milk whey for one draught, repeating often, two are appropriate for vision.*

Then she purged with pills sine quibus.[1] *I applied Horst's vesicatory plaster* to the neck:

R: *cantharides ½oz, turpentine 2oz, olibanum, myrrh, mastic, camphor each ½dr, rose oil, wax each sufficient. Make a plaster.*

I have observed the most happy use of this for a long time.[2] *Above the affected eye, I prescribed the plaster against ruptures worn continuously on the temples to restrain the flux*[3] or, in its place, the plaster for Mrs Wagstaffe on page 47. *Dip two sponges in this eye-salve, and at night apply squeezed out to the eye, fastened with a bandage or retained by a head-dress until they are dry, for then it is not a problem if they fall off. Attach them over the closed eye in the preceding way for two hours. Prepared in this way,* this is very effective and proven:

[p. 49] R: *pomegranate rind 1oz, boil in rose, plantain and nightshade waters each 3oz. Strain. Dissolve haematite 3dr, shake until the whole eye-salve becomes red, then discard the dregs. Add myrrh ½dr, sarcocol washed in milk 1dr, ceruse, tutty each 1dr, white vitriol, starch each 1sc. Powder everything for a very fine powder. Mix with eye-salve. Also prepare linseed and fenugreek mucilage, and when the eye-salve is wanted, mix in a little of this mucilage or if not available, egg white.*[4]

These cured her.

[Case 49]

Cure of red menstrual flux. Julian West:[5] *lasting 53 years, and the use of many medicines without effect. She confirms this with certain proof. A purgative:*

---

1 Platter, *Observationum* […] *libri tres*, p. 355.
2 Horst, *Observationum* […] *libri quatuor*, p. 295.
3 Platter, *Observationum* […] *libri tres*, p. 352.
4 Platter, *Observationum* […] *libri tres*, p. 354.
5 Julian West of Honington (1574–1652). Born Julian Hannes, married John West, a yeoman; eight children. Widowed in 1633.

℞: *senna leaves 1oz, agaric trochees 3dr, sugar 6dr, ginger 1dr, raisins 2dr. Reduce at a low fire in milk whey 4 pints, until ½ pint is gone.*

She took 1½oz of the decoction morning and evening for three successive days, by which her body was properly purged of the humours.[1] On the fourth day:

℞: crocus Martis in red wine 1½dr.

An hour after taking it, take a fritter made like this:

℞: *egg yolk with little ordinary oil, and mix with these herbs, viz: motherwort, flowers of all seasons, St John's wort, yarrow and celandine, and make one fritter daily. Take one, repeat for 9 days.*[2]

At bedtime, a plaster of chalk and egg white for the back. These freed her.

[Case 50]

[p. 50] Cure of long-standing cough, impaired hearing. Mrs Sheldon, a gentlewoman of Bell-End aged 55:[3] wretchedly struck down by severe cough. She was purged thus:

℞: Pills – amber ½dr, aureae 1sc, sine quibus 1sc. Make 5 pills: 3 at bedtime, 2 in the morning.

Next day give the following powder, 1sc to 1dr morning and evening for one day, with white wine, broth or other acceptable fluid. A purgative powder of this sort:

℞: *blessed thistle, charlock each 2sc, long pepper 1sc, selected senna leaves 2dr, anise ½dr, prepared diagrydium 1sc. Make a very fine powder.*[4]

Continue for 3 days. When the cough threatens severely, the following trochees may be used. Hold one in the mouth, between the teeth and cheek while it dissolves by itself. I showed her how

1 Ruland the Elder: 'Centuria IV', *Curationum* [...] *centuriae*, p. 426.

2 Solenander, *Consiliorum* [...] *Solenandri*, p. 330.

3 Elizabeth Sheldon of Bell-End [Beoley] (1560s–1630). Born to Thomas and Mary Markham, wealthy Catholics in Nottinghamshire. Married Edward Sheldon in about 1586; six children.

4 Ruland the Elder, 'Centuria VI', *Curationum* [...] *centuriae*, p. 415.

to do this at night, while sleeping comfortably. When the powder is finished:

> R: *cold diatragacanth 1 ½dr, white henbane seeds 1sc, barley sugar 1oz, opium dissolved in good wine 6gr. Make trochees with an infusion of gum tragacanth in rose water.*[1]

This freed her completely from the cough.

For impaired hearing, a *fumigation for the ears was received through a funnel in the morning, with a decoction of origanum, rue, marjoram, valerian, bayberries, juniper, seeds of fennel, caraway, cumin boiled in wine.*[2] Afterwards, place wool with musk in the ear at night. In fact, insert garlic **[p. 51]** perforated and soaked in honey all day into the ears.

I prescribed scarlet pimpernel and beet juice sniffed into the nostrils during the day, for it is altogether appropriate, nothing indeed is its equal. It draws off the flux from the ears, and the nose:

> R: *juice of pimpernel, beetroot each 1oz. Mix. Sniff this into the nostrils, or introduce with a feather dipped in it.*[3]

I restored her with these very few and with God's help, to her former complete health.[4]

[Case 51]
Cure of frequent miscarriage at two months. Mrs Sheldon, a gentlewoman,[5] the son's wife, stout, well coloured. *Every time she suspects she has conceived, she has miscarried after about a month had passed. In the aborted matter there sometimes appeared clear evidence of a foetus. She*

---

1 Platter, *Observationum* […] *libri tres*, p. 205.
2 Platter, *Observationum* […] *libri tres*, p. 107.
3 Platter, *Observationum* […] *libri tres*, p. 109.
4 Ruland the Elder, 'Centuria VI', *Curationum* […] *centuriae*, p. 415.
5 Elizabeth Sheldon of Weston (1592–1656). Daughter-in-law of the Sheldons (Case 50). Born into a wealthy Catholic family in Essex. In 1611 she married William Sheldon, heir to the Weston estates; seven children. They were forced off their land and dispossessed by Parliamentary soldiers. They remained Royalists.

suffers nothing more serious in association, remaining well and fat.[1] She asks my advice. She said her periods *flowed appropriately. Then I told her that conception was not certain. It was therefore desirable that she be cleansed and strengthened at the time of conception, so that she would be fit to conceive.*[2] She is to take sage in her drink and food. *Take a little of the following powder in a soft-boiled egg:*

> ℞: *pomegranate tincture, daisies, tormentils each 1dr, mastic ½dr.*[3] *Mix. Make a powder. Give in an egg as much as can be taken up on a groat.*[4]

An excellent plaster for retaining a foetus:

> ℞: *pure labdanum 1½oz, galls, moss from an oak, bole Armeniac, cypress nuts* **[p. 52]** *sealed earth, myrtle, red roses, dragon's blood, wild pomegranate flower each ½oz, naval pitch 2oz, turpentine 6oz. Mix everything together. Make a plaster, spread one part of it on leather and apply to the lower back and sacral bone. Apply the other, spread on leather, from the womb to the umbilicus.*[5]

She used these at the correct time, and afterwards gave birth to a lively, vigorous son, and to others later.[6]

[Case 52]
Cure of cough. Mr Parker, a gentleman aged 24:[7] tormented by a severe cough, *but by an outpouring of divine grace*[8] cured by me thus:

> ℞: Venice turpentine washed in hyssop water 1oz, with egg yolk as is the practice in 3oz hyssop water and 1oz liquorice syrup. Mix.

After complete evacuation, take the following mixture every morning:

---

1 Platter, *Observationum* […] *libri tres*, p. 698.
2 Platter, *Observationum* […] *libri tres*, p. 698.
3 Crato, *Consiliorum* […] *liber quintus*, pp. 266–267.
4 Experiments with cardboard coin replicas, flour and sugar show that this is approximately 1.5 grams, equal to 1.16 scruples or 1 scruple and 3 grains.
5 Liébault, *Thresor des remedes secrets*, pp. 806–807.
6 Platter, *Observationum* […] *libri tres*, p. 700.
7 Identification uncertain. Possibly Henry Parker (1607–70), a wealthy London mercer, whose son later bought Talton Manor and mill in 1663.
8 Ruland the Elder, 'Centuria VI', *Curationum* […] *centuriae*, p. 416.

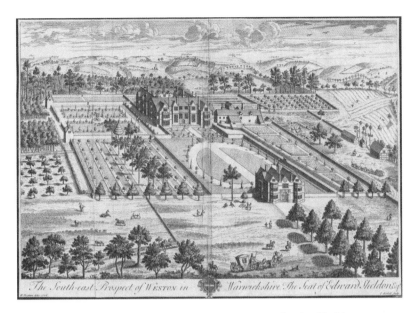

28 Weston House, Warwickshire, built in the 1580s by the Sheldons, a notable Roman Catholic recusant family, from William Dugdale, *The Antiquities of Warwickshire* (1730), p. 583. Hall would have known the house and visited it on at least two occasions (Cases 51 and 138). The gardens were laid out in the second half of the seventeenth century. This view first appeared in 1716. A new house was built on the site between 1827 and 1830, and was demolished in 1934.

> ℞: flowers of sulphur 2dr, elecampane, iris, liquorice each 1dr, sufficient honey to bind everything. Add to this oil of sulphur 10 drops. Make a linctus.

At bedtime:

> ℞: *styrax, mastic, turpentine, realgar each 4crs. Bind them with egg yolk, then smear small pieces of juniper wood with the medication, and dry. Make a fumitory with the dried pieces, received in the mouth through a funnel.*[1]

This has been proved. He was cured.

---

1 Houllier, *De morbis internis*, p. 237.

[Case 53]

[p. 53] Cure of swelling of the left testicle. Edward Rawlins, about 1½ years of age:[1] weighed down by a hard swelling of the testicle, the size of a hen's egg.

> ℞: powdered linseed and make a poultice with linseed oil. Apply hot, *then a piece of linen cloth folded double and pressed firmly.*[2]

This one remedy freed and cured him.

[Case 54]

Cure of menstrual obstruction, pain in the head and heart. Palmer of Alcester:[3] weighed down by these symptoms, and freed as follows:

> ℞: syrup of the five roots 1oz, powdered rhubarb 1sc, diacatholicon 6dr, manna ½oz, mugwort water 4oz.

Eight stools. Venesection of the foot. Then take:

> ℞: trochees of myrrh 2sc, cinnamon, castor each 1sc, mugwort syrup, white wine each 2oz. Make a draught.

This is outstanding for promoting menstrual flux. It has often been well tested.

[Case 55]

Cure of excessive menstrual flow. Mrs Barnes, a gentlewoman of Tolton:[4] with excessive red menstrual flow a month after giving birth. She was cured by this medicine alone:

---

1 This small boy was one of the Rawlins family, who owned lands in Salford Priors and Long Marston and later also Stratford. William Dugdale noted many seventeenth-century Rawlins memorials in Salford church in *The Antiquities of Warwickshire*.

2 Platter, *Observationum* [...] *libri tres*, p. 138.

3 Jane Palmer of Alcester (1608–44). Sister-in-law to Julian West (Case 49). Born in Honington, married in about 1630. Her brother John West's will left ten shillings to Jane so that she could apprentice her younger son, John.

4 Mary Barnes of Talton, in Tredington. Born about 1589. Married William Barnes in 1616, as his second wife, and had five children. Accused as a recusant in 1636 and 1640. No record of her burial.

R: hartshorn shavings ½dr with a drink in the morning. Continue the course for four days.

She immediately felt relieved, completely restored and cured.

[Case 56]

[p. 54] Cure of worms and fever. Talbot, first-born son of the Countess of Salisbury:[1] wretchedly attacked by fever and worms, so that everyone expects death at the door. About the first year of age.

An enema of milk and sugar: He passed two stools, four worms. I gave prepared hartshorn orally in the form of a julep. *I applied populeon ointment 2dr to the pulses, many spiders' webs, a little hazelnut shells. Mix.*[2] I applied it to the pulses in one arm, the following day the other. I applied Mithridate to the stomach, a plaster against worms to the umbilicus. He recovered, praise God, within three days. The Countess thanked me greatly, with a large payment.

[Case 57]

Cure of vomiting food, fever. Mrs Sheldon, a gentlewoman of Grafton aged 24:[3] wretchedly weighed down with these symptoms fourteen days after birth. She was overcome by frequent suffocation of the womb and cold sweats.

R: posset ale of hartshorn shavings and marigold flowers. For the mother she was given the white movement of a chicken (that is, the dung) 2sc, coral tincture 2½sc, bugloss water 4oz: 1 spoonful of the first, 2 spoonfuls of the latter often during the day. Apply a

1 George Talbot of Grafton (1618–42). Hall treated the infant son of the Earl and Countess of Shrewsbury (not Salisbury; Hall's mistake). The family was Catholic, with a home at Grafton Manor near Bromsgrove.
2 Platter, *Observationum* […] *libri tres*, p. 291.
3 Margaret Sheldon of Temple Grafton (?–1669). Daughter of Thomas and Letitia Kempson of Oversley, wealthy landowners. In about 1630 she married Brace Sheldon of Temple Grafton manor; eight children. Margaret and her son were accused of recusancy in 1624. Noted as a widow in 1664. Buried at Temple Grafton in 1669.

caranna plaster **[p. 55]** to the umbilicus, in the middle of which is placed 3 grains of musk.

A stomach shield:

℞: labdanum 1dr, wax 2dr, cloves, yellow sandalwood each 1sc, mastic 1dr, myrrh ½dr. Make a plaster with wormwood and mace oils.

These cured her.

[Case 58]
Cure of wind in the stomach. Mrs Davies, a gentlewoman of Quinton:[1] attacked by wind in the stomach for a long time. Age: about 63 years.

℞: Gabrieli's aromatic rose powder 2dr, elecampane root 3dr, sweet flag 2dr, liquorice ½oz, prepared turbith ½oz, senna 2oz, anise seeds ½oz, cinnamon 2dr, gentian root 1 ½oz, sufficient sugar. Make a powder. Dose: as much as can be held on twelve pennies,[2] in wine.

She was freed by this medicine alone.

[Case 59]
Cure of severe cough after smallpox. The son of Mr Bishop, a gentleman, aged 6:[3] a month after being entirely freed from smallpox, fell into a severe cough and fever with worms.

℞: *manna 2sc, diacatholicon ½dr, cassia flowers 1dr. Mix with liquorice syrup. Give it to be licked often.*[4] Give prepared hartshorn in milk. *Anoint the chest with chest ointment;*[5] our julep of poppies; an enema of milk and sugar.

---

1 Probably Frances Davies, wife of John, buried at Quinton in 1630. No children mentioned in her husband's will the following year.
2 By experiment, approximately 6 grams, equal to 4 scruples and 12 grains.
3 Might be George, the son of Anthony Bishop of Oxhill, where Hall treated other patients. Or William, born 1606, son of John Bishop of Brailes.
4 Vittori, *De aegritudinibus infantium*, p. 115.
5 Vittori, *De aegritudinibus infantium*, p. 114.

He was quickly cured.

[Case 60]

[p. 56] Cure of lower backache and white vaginal flux. Mrs Harvey, a gentlewoman, now Lady,[1] modest, devoutly pious: troubled and weakened by backache and excessive white menstrual flux, five weeks after giving birth.

> R: *good dates sliced small as you wish. Make an electuary with skimmed honey, use in the morning.*

This one remedy cured her and freed her from the pain. I have often found it to stop the white discharge, add on weight, and remove backache.[2]

[Case 61]

Cure of wind in the stomach, excessive red menstrual flux. Mrs Randolph, a gentlewoman about 27 years old:[3] discoloured by excessive red menstrual flux with torment in the stomach after food.

Apply a plaster to the back:

> R: bole Armeniac, chalk, each. Make a plaster with egg whites. To curb the flux, take one penny-weight[4] of rock alum with a sharp wine. Use the powder as for Cooper, page 44.

These cured her, within four days.

---

1 Mary, Lady Harvey of Moreton Morrell (1602–?1650; cf. Case 93). In 1620 Mary Murden (daughter of Richard and Mary Murden) married Stephen Harvey, a lawyer who had been at Balliol, then became a Knight of the Bath in 1625. Sir Stephen was on the Warwickshire bench. He died in 1630. They had eight children. His widow was a known Puritan, and loaned money to Parliament.

2 Solenander, *Consiliorum* […] *Solenandri*, p. 331.

3 Elizabeth Randolph of Wood Bevington (*c.* 1593–1657). Dates uncertain as parish records not reliable for recusants. Married Ferrers Randolph (Case 25) in about 1619. Son and heir Thomas was born 1629. Also a daughter, Elizabeth.

4 A penny weighed approximately 0.5 grams, or just under 8 grains.

[Case 62]

1617. Cure of tertian fever, thirst, sleeplessness, torment in the sides with small spots, headache. Mrs Barnes, a gentlewoman:[1] *pregnant and near to giving birth, falling into*[2] a tertian fever **[p. 57]** accompanied by thirst, sleeplessness, headache, wretched pricking pain in the left side. Age: about 28 years. *In the midst of despair, these were relieved with the help of divine grace.*[3]

> ℞: sufficient powdered white hellebore, with sliced figs. *Apply them where the arterial pulses are felt, that is to say in the region of each wrist.*[4] Renew them twice within twenty-four hours.

Her usual drink:

> ℞: *whole barley 3oz, chicory 1 handful, chicory root 3oz, rose and violet syrups each 1oz, liquorice shavings 3dr, figs 3, raisins 2oz, sugar candy 2oz. Mix together and boil in 16 pints spring water, reduce by 2 pints. Strain to make the decoction, and drink cold, as much as desired.*[5]

An ointment for pain in the side:

> ℞: *marsh-mallow ointment 2oz, sweet almond oil 3dr. Mix. Spread hot on the affected side and after anointing the area, cover with a hot cloth smeared with butter.*[6]

I alleviated the severe, troublesome headache with this ointment:

> ℞: *alabaster ointment ½oz, opium 7gr. After this was applied and rubbed to the temple, she recovered her former health*[7] and was freed from danger of imminent miscarriage.

To God be praise, honour and glory, for ever and ever.[8] She was cured within seven days. This has been proved.

---

1 Cf. Case 55. Hall treated her this time in late pregnancy.
2 Ruland the Elder, 'Centuria VII', *Curationum* [...] *centuriae*, p. 529.
3 Ruland the Elder, 'Centuria VII', *Curationum* [...] *centuriae*, p. 531.
4 Platter, *Praxeos* [...] *de doloribus*, p. 167.
5 Ruland the Elder, 'Centuria VIII', *Curationum* [...] *centuriae*, p. 563.
6 Ruland the Elder, 'Centuria VII', *Curationum* [...] *centuriae*, p. 540.
7 Ruland the Elder, 'Centuria VII', *Curationum* [...] *centuriae*, p. 479.
8 Ruland the Elder, 'Centuria VII', *Curationum* [...] *centuriae*, p. 479.

[Case 63]
Cure of nosebleed. Roberts, a tailor of Stratford-upon-Avon aged about 34 years:[1] *falls into an immoderate nosebleed, more copiously for four hours, then diminishing.*[2] *Being called to him, I restrained the blood* **[p. 58]** *as follows:*[3]

> ℞: a new piece of cloth often soaked in frog spawn in March, and dried in the sun. I made plugs with this and inserted them in the nostrils (*I squeezed tightly with the other fingers, not the little and ring finger*).[4]

Afterwards:

> ℞: *clay, burnt and powdered 2 handfuls, sharp vinegar 1 ½ pints. Mix together in the form of a plaster or poultice placed in a folded cloth. I applied it frequently, very cold, to the forehead, neck and temples. The flow ceased, and ended in less than half an hour.*[5]

[Case 64]
1617. Cure of toothache and swelling of the gums. Baron Compton, now [1st] Earl of Northampton, about 55 years of age:[6] the victim of a most unhappy toothache with very troublesome swelling of the gums, *which I took away with these few medicines:*[7]

> ℞: *amber, mastic each 2dr, aloes 5dr, agaric 2dr, true round-leaved birthwort ½dr. Make pills with betony syrup, 4 pills from 1dr.*[8] Take 1dr in the morning and another at bedtime.

He was agreeably purged. Continue so for three days.

---

1 Thomas Roberts, tailor of Stratford-upon-Avon (1579–1617). Hall notes him as Roberts Sartor (= tailor), so probably Thomas Roberts. He had one son who died in infancy.
2 Ruland the Elder, 'Centuria III', *Curationum* [...] *centuriae*, pp. 183–184.
3 Ruland the Elder, 'Centuria I', *Curationum* [...] *centuriae*, p. 35.
4 Ruland the Elder, 'Centuria III', *Curationum* [...] *centuriae*, p. 184.
5 Ruland the Elder, 'Centuria I', *Curationum* [...] *centuriae*, p. 35.
6 William Compton, 1st Earl of Northampton (cf. Case 2). Created Earl of Northampton in 1618, a year after this consultation. Hall treated him on several occasions.
7 Ruland the Elder, 'Centuria I', *Curationum* [...] *centuriae*, p. 33.
8 Aurifaber, 'Succini historia', in Crato, *Consiliorum* [...] *liber quartus*, p. 462.

A gargle:

> ℞: mulberry syrup, rose honey each 2oz, rose water 4oz, guaiacum root and barley decoctions each 4oz. Dilute with sufficient oil of vitriol to give acidity. Apply a sponge dipped in it to the painful gums often during the day, and hold it there **[p. 59]** the whole day.

These remedies freed him completely from the symptoms. On the second day he could chew food, and by the third he was perfectly cured, praise God.

[Case 65]
Cure of headache, itching all over, with a pustular rash. Anne Greene,[1] a gentlewoman, first daughter of Lawyer Greene, *has completed the first twelve years of her life. She is seized by a headache, with vivid colours all over the body, dying away and succeeded by pallor. She is vexed at the same time by itching of the whole body with a painful rash, so that at the height of the pain she could not walk.*[2]

The cure:

> ℞: sarsaparilla 2oz, colchicum 1½oz, guaiacum, liquorice each 1oz, polypody of the oak, senna each 2oz, agaric, 2dr, fennel, parsley roots 1oz, betony, sage leaves each ½ handful, rosemary 1 pinch, anise, caraway, coriander seeds each ½oz, cinnamon 1dr. Boil in 8 pints water, reduce by half. Take 2½oz, with loosening rose syrup 1oz, sufficient oil of vitriol to give acidity. Five stools. Continue the course for five successive days.

When the body was well purged, I gave a china decoction of this sort: china root sliced finely, take 3dr of it, soak in 3 pints spring water for twenty-four hours. After that time, make a decoction on

---

1 Born in New Place in 1604, where her parents, Thomas and Lettice, lodged with the Shakespeares from 1603 to 1611. Their son, William, was born in 1608, and the children's godparents were almost certainly William and Anne Shakespeare. The Greenes moved to St Mary's, a large house close by Holy Trinity Church, before moving away to Bristol in 1617. Thomas Greene liked to identify himself as Shakespeare's 'cozen', and knew Hall well.
2 Ruland the Elder, 'Centuria VII', *Curationum* [...] *centuriae*, p. 499.

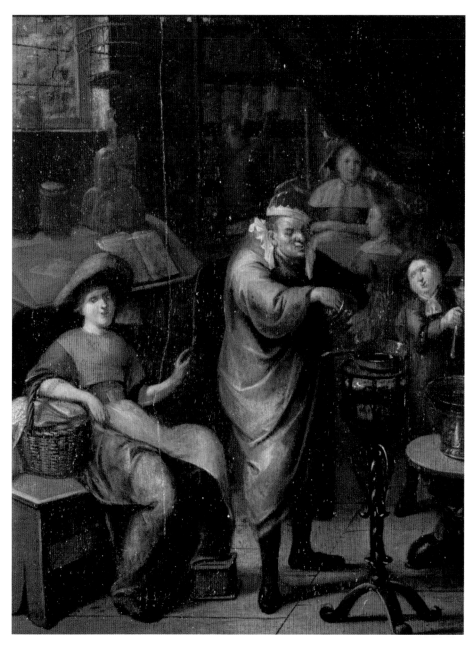

1 Richard Brackenburgh (studio of), *Interior of an apothecary's, mixing a remedy, c.* 1673, oil on panel, 31 × 24 inches. The apothecary is making a remedy in a pan on top of the brazier, and is surrounded by customers, or servants sent by physicians to collect remedies or ingredients.

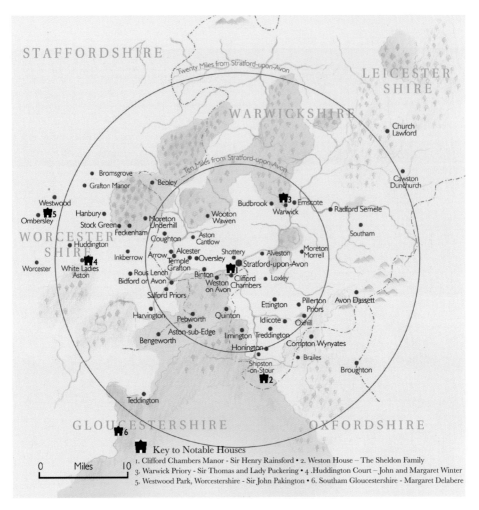

STAFFORDSHIRE

LEICESTERSHIRE

Twenty Miles from Stratford-upon-Avon

WARWICKSHIRE

Church Lawford

Ten Miles from Stratford-upon-Avon

• Bromsgrove
• Grafton Manor
• Beoley

Cawston
Dunchurch

Westwood
Ombersley Hanbury • Stock Green • Feckenham Moreton Underhill

Budbrook • █3 • Emscote
Warwick

• Radford Semele

WORCESTER
SHIRE
• Huddington

• Wooton Wawen
Aston Cantlow

Southam

• █4
Worcester White Ladies Aston

Inkberrow • Arrow • Temple Grafton
Coughton Alcester • Oversley Shottery • Alveston Moreton Morrell

• Rous Lench
Bidford on Avon • Binton • Clifford • Loxley
Weston Chambers
on Avon

█ Stratford-upon-Avon

Salford Priors /

Ettington • Pillerton Priors Avon Dassett

Harvington Pebworth Quinton Idicote • Oxhill

Aston-sub-Edge
Bengeworth Ilmington Treddington
Honington • Compton Wynyates

• Braies

Shipston -on-Stour █2 Broughton

Teddington •

GLOUCESTERSHIRE █6 OXFORDSHIRE

█ Key to Notable Houses

0   Miles   10

1. Clifford Chambers Manor - Sir Henry Rainsford • 2. Weston House – The Sheldon Family
3. Warwick Priory - Sir Thomas and Lady Puckering • 4 .Huddington Court – John and Margaret Winter
5. Westwood Park, Worcestershire - Sir John Pakington • 6. Southam Gloucestershire - Margaret Delabere

2 Travelling on horseback, carrying a portable medical chest, John Hall traversed the
county of Warwickshire, usually up to a twenty-mile radius from Stratford-upon-Avon.
He often travelled deep into Gloucestershire, Oxfordshire and Worcestershire to reach
his patients, perhaps sometimes with a servant. A visit to Sir John Pakington's residence
in Worcestershire, over twenty miles to the west, required nearly a day's ride. While main
roads were well established, the rivers in this rural landscape strongly influenced Hall's
choice of route. Travellers were reliant on landowners and borough councils carrying out
their duty to maintain vital bridges. Occasionally he travelled further afield, for example
to Ludlow to treat the Countess of Northampton. He stayed there for at least four days
(Case 1), and returned about a month later to treat the Earl (Case 2), and others while he
was there. He travelled to Worcester to treat John Thornborough, the Bishop of Worcester
(Case 164). This illustration is based on Christopher Saxton's 1576 map of Warwickshire
and Leicestershire depicting a landscape of open countryside with hills, dense woodland,
and a multitude of rivers and streams.

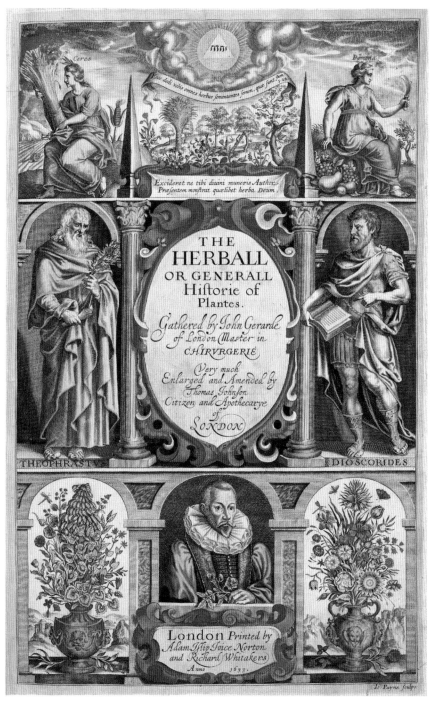

3 Title-page of the first edition of John Gerard, *The Herball or Generall Historie of Plantes* (1597). John Gerard (1545–1612) was an English botanist who had a large herb garden in London. His *Herball* became the best-known book of its kind in seventeenth-century England. It runs to 1,484 pages and includes an astonishingly detailed index which allows the reader to look up an ailment and then be directed to the plants that might aid a cure. Gerard's book translated the Dutch botanist Rembert Dodens's 1554 work, but augmented it to include North American plants.

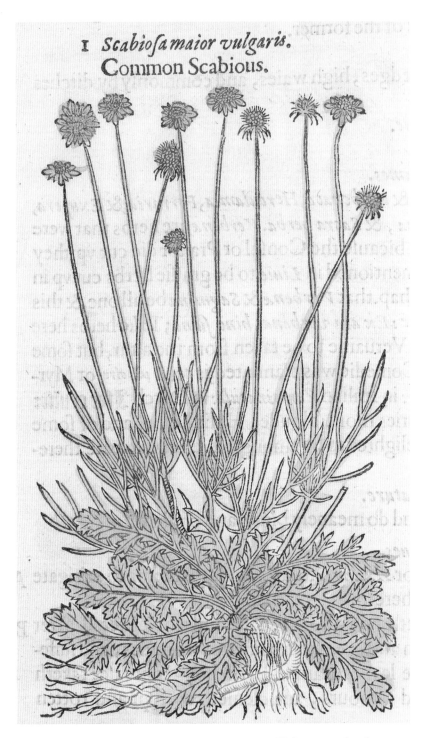

4 *Scabiosa major vulgaris*, common scabious: used by Hall to treat the chest and lungs. From John Gerard, *The Herball or Generall Historie of Plantes* (1597), p. 582.

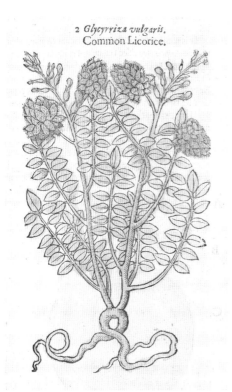

2 *Glycyrriza vulgaris.*
Common Licorice.

5 *Glycyrriza vulgaris*, common liquorice: used by Hall to treat stomach aches. From John Gerard, *The Herball or Generall Historie of Plantes* (1597), p. 1119.

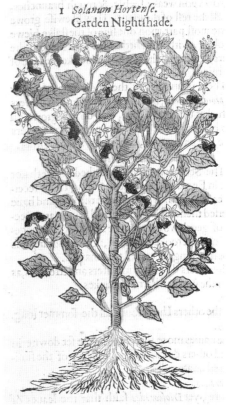

1 *Solanum Hortense.*
Garden Nightshade.

6 *Solanum hortense*, garden nightshade: used by Hall to treat stomach aches and headaches. From John Gerard, *The Herball or Generall Historie of Plantes* (1597), p. 268.

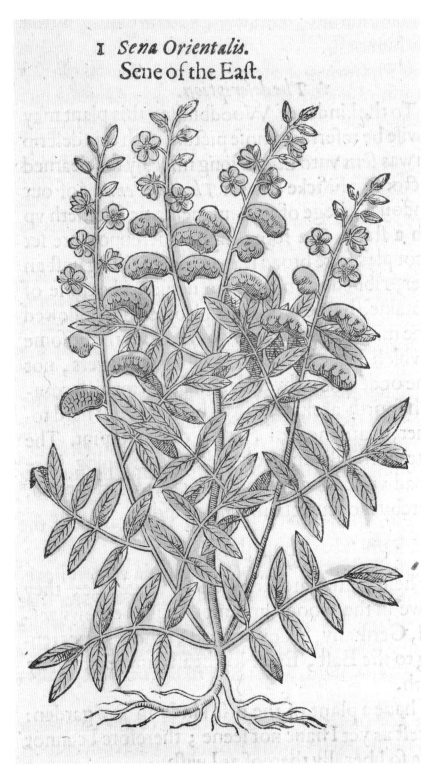

1 *Sena Orientalis.*
Sene of the East.

7 *Sena orientalis*, senna of the east: used by Hall as a laxative. From John Gerard, *The Herball or Generall Historie of Plantes* (1597), p. 1114.

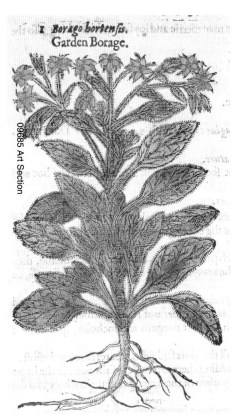

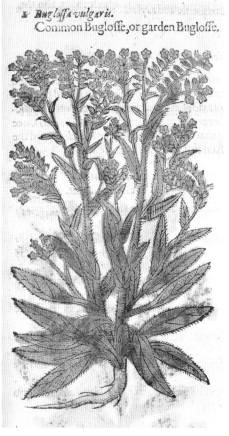

8 *Borago hortensis*, garden borage: used by Hall as a flavouring. From John Gerard, *The Herball or Generall Historie of Plantes* (1597), p. 653.

9 *Burglossa vulgaris*, common bugloss: mixed with oil by Hall to help heal wounds. From John Gerard, *The Herball or Generall Historie of Plantes* (1597), p. 655.

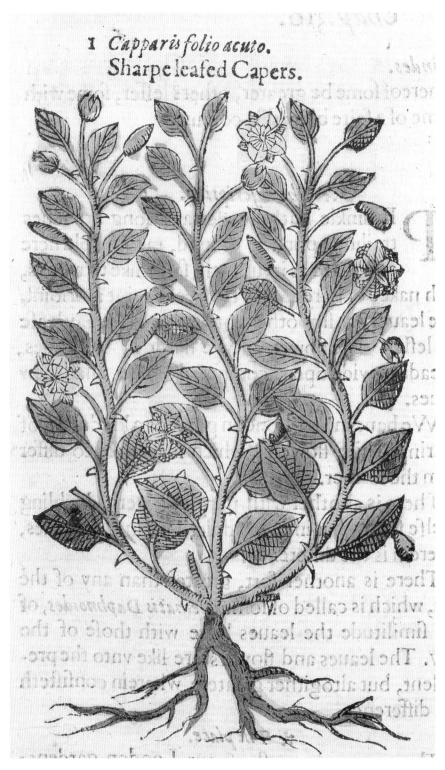

10 *Capparis folio acuto*, sharp-leaved capers: used by Hall to treat worms. From John Gerard, *The Herball or Generall Historie of Plantes* (1597), p. 748.

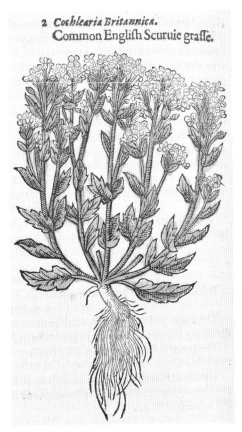

2 *Cochlearia Britannica.*
Common Englifh Scuruie graffe.

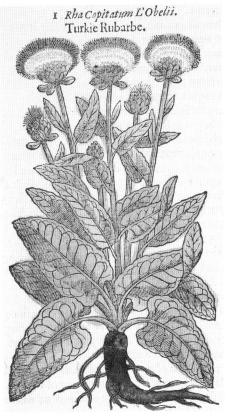

1 *Rha Capitatum L'Obelii.*
Turkie Rubarbe.

11 *Cochlearia Britannica*, common English scurvy-grass: used by Hall to treat ulcers and acne. From John Gerard, *The Herball or Generall Historie of Plantes* (1597), p. 324.

12 *Rha capitatum l'obelii*, Turkey rhubarb: used by Hall to treat wind and stomach pains. From John Gerard, *The Herball or Generall Historie of Plantes* (1597), p. 316.

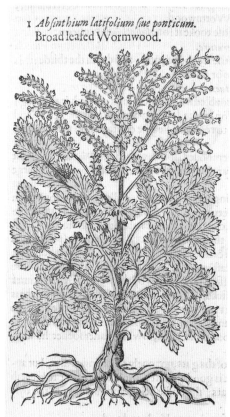

I *Abſinthium latifolium ſiue ponticum.*
Broad leafed Wormwood.

13 *Absinthium iatifolium siue ponticum*,
broad-leaved wormwood: used by Hall to
treat agues and worms and poisoning by
mistletoe and hemlock. From John Gerard,
The Herball or Generall Historie of Plantes (1597),
p. 937.

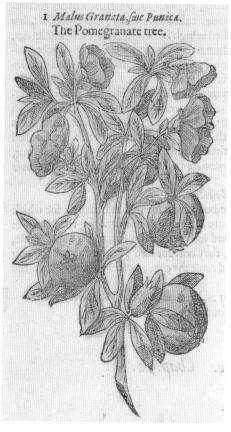

I *Malus Granata, ſiue Punica.*
The Pomegranate tree.

14 *Malus granata siue punica*, pomegranate
tree: used by Hall to strengthen teeth and
gums. From John Gerard, *The Herball or
Generall Historie of Plantes* (1597), p. 1262.

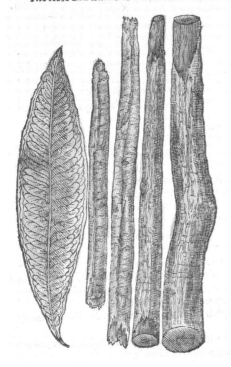

Canelle folium, & Bacillus.
The leafe and trunke of the Cinnamom tree.

15 *Canelle folium e bacillus*, cinnamon leaf
and bark: used by Hall to prevent bites
from venomous beetles. From John Gerard,
The Herball or Generall Historie of Plantes (1597),
p. 1348.

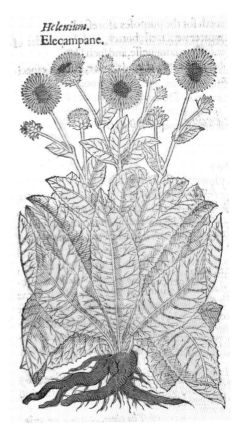

Helenium.
Elecampane.

16 *Helenium*, elecampane: used by Hall
to treat shortness of breath. From John
Gerard, *The Herball or Generall Historie of
Plantes* (1597), p. 649.

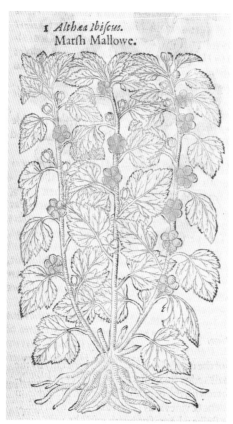

17 *Althaea ibiscus*, marsh mallow: used by Hall to treat fevers and constipation. From John Gerard, *The Herball or Generall Historie of Plantes* (1597), p. 787.

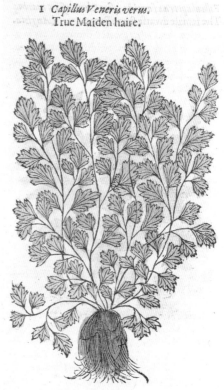

18 *Capillus veneris verus*, true maidenhair: used by Hall to treat severe coughs. From John Gerard, *The Herball or Generall Historie of Plantes* (1597), p. 982.

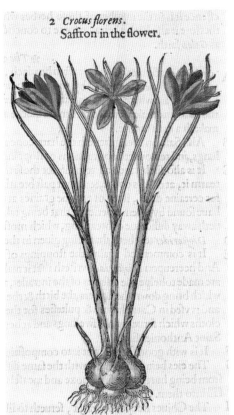

2 *Crocus florens.*
Saffron in the flower.

19 *Crocus florens*, saffron flower: used by Hall to treat headaches. From John Gerard, *The Herball or Generall Historie of Plantes* (1597), p. 123.

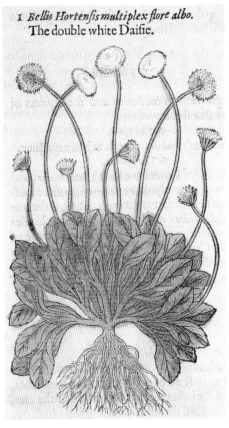

1 *Bellis Hortensis multiplex flore albo.*
The double white Daisie.

20 *Bellis hortensis multiplex flore albo*, double white daisy: Hall used the leaves in his cures for ulcers. From John Gerard, *The Herball or Generall Historie of Plantes* (1597), p. 510.

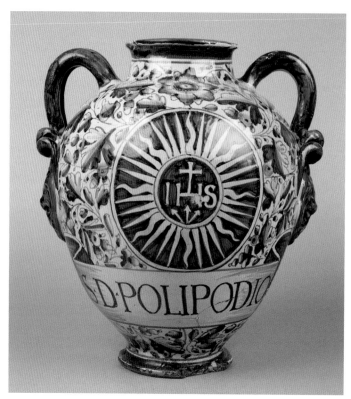

21 A seventeenth-century majolica drug jar from Venice. 'S.D.Poliopodio' stands for 'syrupus dia polypody': 'syrup of polypody', a type of fern. Hall uses 'polypody of oak' regularly (Cases 31, 34, 65, 84, 93, 97, 106, 115, 129, 141, 168 and 173).

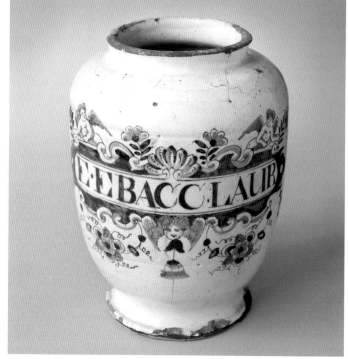

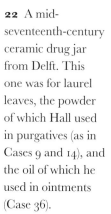

22 A mid-seventeenth-century ceramic drug jar from Delft. This one was for laurel leaves, the powder of which Hall used in purgatives (as in Cases 9 and 14), and the oil of which he used in ointments (Case 36).

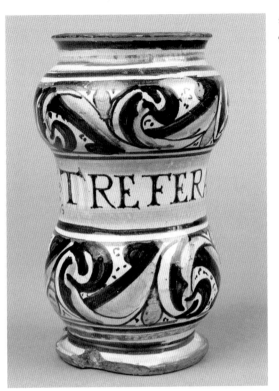

23 A sixteenth-century ceramic drug jar from Tuscany.

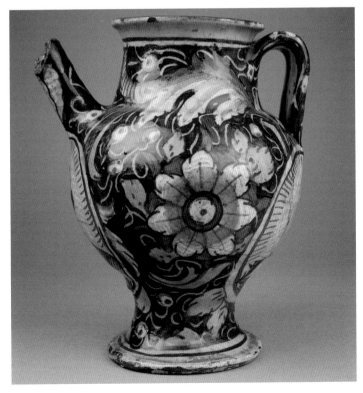

24 A late sixteenth-century majolica wet-drug jar.

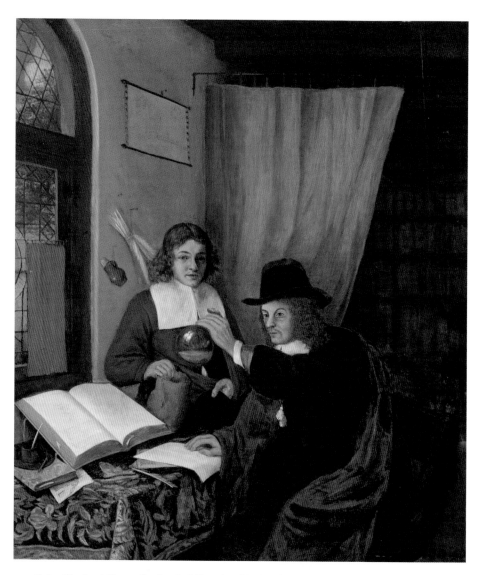

25 Osias Dyck, *A Doctor Casting the Water* (*c.* 1660s), oil on panel, 34.3 × 30.5 inches. The physician is well dressed with a lace collar, and is wearing a black travelling cloak. He is not wearing a skull-cap, so the picture depicts him while out on his travels. We are in a book-lined room in the patient's house. The tapestry-covered desk suggests someone of aspiring social status. The servant to the left has brought in the urine sample, and the physician has produced the flask in which to inspect it. Open on the table is what looks like an illustrated book: a herbal owned by the patient perhaps, or a medical textbook brought by the physician, to aid diagnosis and cure.

a slow fire until 1½ pints remain, then strain and store. Take a draught in the morning, five hours before lunch and three hours before dinner. It should be drunk hot. She should be purged every third day. **[p. 60]**

After using the prescribed sweating decoction, she used the following bath:

> ℞: oak leaves 20 handfuls, fennel 15 handfuls, sliced bryony, elecampane roots each 4 handfuls, sulphur, alum, salt each 1lb. Boil in sufficient water for a bath. On leaving the bath I ordered her to sweat in bed, and afterwards to anoint the body with an ointment of elecampane root, bryony, alum, mixed with May-butter.

These restored her looks, and made her [skin] smooth.

[Case 66]

Cure of urinary retention. John Smith aged 60, of Newnham:[1] wretchedly afflicted by urinary retention for three days. *He fell into complete suppression of urine on account of a stone, in danger of his life. Though much was tried, nothing worked to relieve it. I was finally asked for advice. I use healing medications in this way:*[2]

> ℞: winter cherries 6, parsley seeds 3dr. Boil in sufficient milk and make posset ale.

> ℞: 6oz of this, Fernel's marsh-mallow syrup 1oz, Holland powder 2dr. Make a draught.

He drank white wine in which bruised winter-cherry pips had been soaked. I prescribed an onion and sliced garlic fried in butter and vinegar to be placed hot on the pubic region and between the anus and scrotum. By these ministrations, urine began to flow **[p. 61]** *within an hour, with some stones and gravel. And so he escaped free from lamentable, long-lasting, calamitous and imminent danger, through God's grace.*[3]

---

1 John Smith of Newnham (*c.* 1560–1617). Lived in a hamlet near Aston Cantlow.
2 Ruland the Elder, 'Centuria VIII', *Curationum* [...] *centuriae*, p. 564.
3 Ruland the Elder, 'Centuria VIII', *Curationum* [...] *centuriae*, p. 564.

[Case 67]

Cure of stomach and lower back pain, yellow jaundice. John Nason, a barber of Stratford-upon-Avon, 40 years old:[1] suffering constantly from most grievous pains in the belly after food. He was wretchedly tortured by lower backache, so that he remained awake almost all night. Also yellow-tinted jaundice, urine: thin, red, the surface yellow and frothy.

R: the chymical cup 1oz: six vomits, four stools.

Next day:

R: *horehound 2oz, hops 1oz, bugloss root, elecampane root, gravel-root each ½dr, rhubarb sliced coarsely 1dr, aloes wood 1½dr. Boil everything in 3 pints strong white wine until reduced by a third, then strain without squeezing.* Add juice of goose droppings ½ pint to the strained liquid. Make it.

R: *3oz of this decoction, white sugar 2dr. Mix. Make a drink. Give it every day, in the morning at dawn.*[2]

And so within a few days, he was cured and well-coloured.

[Case 68]

Cure of burning urine. Baron Compton, about 55 years of age:[3] savagely tortured **[p. 62]** by heat of the urine. He was freed and achieved health through the following water, frequently proved by me in this illness:[4]

R: well-beaten egg whites 8, cow's milk 1 pint, red rose water ½ pint. Distil by the usual method in a common still. Take 4oz of the distilled water, Fernel's marsh-mallow syrup 1oz. Mix. Give cold on an empty stomach.

---

1 John Nason of Stratford. Dates unknown. Married Elizabeth Rogers in 1600. Was apprenticed as a barber-surgeon. Licensed in 1622 by the Bishop of Worcester to practise as a surgeon. Hall treated him in 1624. His widow died in 1653.
2 Vettori, *Exhortatio*, p. 134.
3 William Compton, 1st Earl of Northampton (cf. Cases 2, 64, 79 and 83).
4 frequently … illness] Possibly Hall's own remedy, given this comment and that it is not a borrowing.

He was properly cured and rode with King James into Scotland. Tried and proved.

[Case 69]
Cure of an impediment to swallowing with swelling of the tonsils. Mrs Boughton, a gentlewoman,[1] mother-in-law of Mr Combe, a gentleman of Lawford, good-looking, now aged about 36, of excellent and shapely figure: *harassed by the most severe illnesses and savage symptoms for two years, feeling exceedingly wretched. Although the most skilled physicians in the art were consulted nothing helped, indeed* [the symptoms] *grew worse and proved even more severe within days.*[2]

At first *she could hardly swallow or breathe.*[3] She felt something hard, the size of a dove's egg in her throat, which allowed her to swallow no food and hardly any drink. This was caused by a wind, because she felt it moving, and as it moved it caused more or less pain. Though the swelling of the tonsils was not large, she was most troubled at night by catarrh dripping from the head. *The illness and pain deprived her of sleep, and led to fear of choking.*[4] *Her head was assailed by a notable lethargy, and she was affected by an extraordinary constant sleepiness. Her body was equally oppressed by the catarrh, which caused great difficulty in walking and deprivation of the natural actions.* **[p. 63]** *From these she was seized by a long series of symptoms: a creeping discoloration in the hands at intervals, not without cold,*[5] and swollen legs like a scorbutic dropsy. All this was caused by the spleen and liver and suppression of her periods.

R: senna 2½dr, cream of tartar 2dr, best turbith, colchicum each 1dr, rhubarb, trochiscated agaric each 2sc, prepared scammony ½dr, mace, cinnamon, galangals each 3dr, violet sugar equal in weight

1 Elizabeth Boughton of Lawford (1575–1619). Daughter and heiress of Edward Catesby, the son of one of the Gunpowder Plotters. Married Edward Boughton in 1593, three children. Her tomb is in St Botolph's church, Newbold-on-Avon.
2 Potier, *Insignium Curationum*, pp. 34–35.
3 Ruland the Elder, 'Centuria II', *Curationum* [...] *centuriae*, p. 151.
4 Ruland the Elder, 'Centuria II', *Curationum* [...] *centuriae*, p. 151.
5 Potier, *Insignium curationum*, p. 35.

to everything. Make the powder. Dose: 1 to 2dr in broth boiled with herbs – penny-royal, mugwort, horehound, sage, betony.

Once that is finished, take a china decoction prepared in this way:

℞: *china root shavings 1oz, sassafras root 3dr, spring water 6 pints, lemon juice 2oz. Soak for twenty-four hours then boil, reduce by a third, then strain through a hippocras bag. She should drink 5oz of this morning and evening,*[1] with 2oz prepared scurvy-grass juice.

On the third day, although the bowel movements were not bound, I wished an enema injected: 12oz of this decoction, red sugar 2oz, rosemary honey 3oz. Make an enema.

For the mouth:

℞: *spring water 2oz, sufficient Roman oil of vitriol to give intense acidity.*

Insert a feather dipped in this water in the swollen throat, several times an hour, from which she repeatedly brought up and spat out much phlegm. After the water, by my advice white amber was put on coals, and the smoke led to the mouth through a funnel.[2] I wanted her to wear our stomach salve, page 17, all the time.

℞: simple mulberry juice 5oz, rose honey 4oz, cleavers juice 8oz, barley water 12oz, sufficient oil of sulphur to give acidity. I wished her to gargle often during the day.

These made her well, and she lived for eight years afterwards.

[Case 70]

[p. 64] Cure of fever from over-indulgence. Sir Beaufou[3] (whom I always name as a sign of honour): ate a large quantity of milk

---

1 Du Chesne, *Pharmacopoea dogmaticorum*, p. 63.

2 Ruland the Elder, 'Centuria II', *Curationum* [...] *centuriae*, pp. 151–152.

3 Sir Thomas Beaufou of Emscote (1544–1630). Owned the manor at Emscote. Married an heiress, Ursula, and had seven children. In Ursula's last years, he cohabited with her widowed sister Dorothy. When a widower, he married Dorothy's daughter, which led to his being fined by the Worcestershire consistory court in 1617. In 1626, a widower again, he received a pardon.

curds after dinner. Age: about 70 years. Soon after going to bed he felt ill, and worse each day. Coming on the second day, I found his pulse rapid. He passed a little red urine, urinating frequently. His stomach was full of phlegm and choler, for whatever he took, he freely brought up choler in large quantity, like the yolk of a bad egg. Considering this, I gave him the chymical cup 1oz. Vomits ten, and the belly returned to its duty three times. To drink: hartshorn decoction with sugar and lemon juice for a pleasing tartness.

He was properly cured, praise God, within four days.

[Case 71]
Cure of exhausted appetite. Sir Pakington:[1] suffering from distaste for food and poor appetite. He requested a medicine to restore it quickly, for which I prescribed the following senna powder, to be taken for several days:

> R: *best senna leaves 3dr, ginger, mace each 1sc, cinnamon ½dr, cream of tartar 2dr.*[2] Mix Make a powder. Dose: 1dr in broth.

This one powder restored his appetite. He thanked me greatly and asked how it was made. The following year he said he used the prepared powder often, with the desired result. This has been proved.

[Case 72]
[p. 65] Cure of sore throat, inflammation of tonsils and palate. Mr Rogers, vicar of Stratford-upon-Avon, about 40 years old:[3] the

---

1 Sir John Pakington of Westwood Park, Worcestershire (1548–1625). Queen Elizabeth met him at Worcester in 1575, and later made him a Knight of the Bath. Married Dorothy; seven children. Pakington was very wealthy, and had a great house with two deer parks.

2 This is the recipe for *pulvis senae Montagnanae*; it matches that in the 1613 *Pharmacopoeia Augustana* better than that in *Pharmacopoeia Londinensis*.

3 John Rogers, vicar of Stratford-upon-Avon, 1606–19 (Lane 1996: 139). Previously vicar of St Nicholas, Warwick. Unpopular with many townspeople. Married with six children. He would have officiated at Shakespeare's funeral in

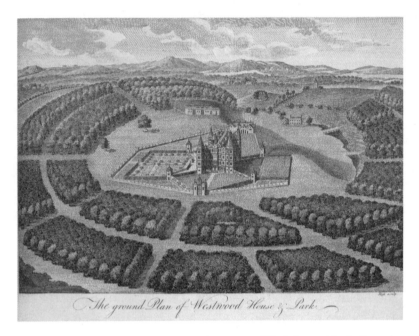

The ground Plan of Westwood House & Park

29 Westwood Park, Worcestershire, the home of Sir John and Lady Dorothy Pakington, from *The History of Worcestershire* (1781), p. 352. Sir John (1548–1625) was known as Lusty Pakington in court circles. Hall treated him for 'an exhausted appetite' (Case 71). The house depicted was built between 1614 and 1617 as a large hunting lodge, and had the diagonal wings added in 1625.

victim of pain in the throat with inflamed tonsils and uvula. He swallowed painfully, breathed with difficulty and felt almost as if choked. I rescued him quickly with the following:

℞: figs, liquorice, raisins, anise seed each 10z, spring water 4 pints. Boil by the usual method. Make an ordinary drink.

He took amber fumes often during the day.

I made this plaster to be applied to the neck and visible swelling:[1]

℞: green wormwood 2 handfuls, sufficient pork fat. Beat together and make a plaster.

1616. Dismissed in 1619 by 18 votes to 7, and replaced by Thomas Wilson (Case 4).
1 Ruland the Elder, 'Centuria IV', *Curationum* [...] *centuriae*, p. 268.

He was cured within one night, *and the ability to swallow was soon restored.*[1] This has been proved a hundred times.

[Case 73]

Cure of the Hungarian disease, with smallpox. Lady Beaufou,[2] pious, respected, held in the highest regard by everyone: Everyone was calling on God for the recovery of her lost health. Age: 28 years. 1 July 1617. She was seized by a continual malignant burning fever, with most severe headache. *She is exceedingly hot, feels pain in the belly and all organs.*[3] She was marked on the body, the arms particularly, with little spots. Urine: little and red. These revealed signs of the new fever (as it was commonly called) *which at that time prowled the streets and attacked everyone exposed to it. I was called on the* **[p. 66]** *third day of the attack,*[4] and observed the stomach stuffed full and laden with bad humours. On my advice she downed the following emetic:

> ℞: the chymical cup 1oz 1dr, which gave twelve vomits without much trouble.

The previous day she drank a lot of milk, to quench her thirst. This was her own idea, from which she threw up an amazing amount of coagulate in the vomit. She was almost choked by the first vomit, it was such a large amount and such complete ejection of the curdled milk. Afterwards she vomited much choler mixed with phlegm, then burnt black bile, with the greatest effort. With this there were 6 bowel movements, returning phlegm and green bile mingled

---

1 Ruland the Elder, 'Centuria IV', *Curationum* [...] *centuriae*, p. 271.
2 Ann, Lady Beaufou of Emscote (1589–1626). Ann Aldersey was the daughter of the first Lady Beaufou's sister Dorothy. She married the widowed Sir Thomas, who was fined for this prohibited marriage (cf. Case 70). Baptismal records indicate two sons. She died aged 37, and Sir Thomas was then pardoned. An example of the changeable nature of illnesses in this period: Lady Beaufou's illness started with a malignant fever, which after seven days changed into smallpox. See also Case 84.
3 Ruland the Younger, *De morbo Ungarico*, p. 242.
4 Ruland the Younger, *De morbo Ungarico*, p. 242.

with a large quantity of watery outpourings. Three hours after the emetic was finished, I gave Paracelsus's laudanum pills 7gr. After taking the pills she slept soundly, the headache ceasing.

Then her companion gave her a drink of milk whey without my knowing. This deception gave her three black vomits immediately, without any trouble, and two stools of the same colour. She was wretchedly tormented with hiccups, which were curbed by a drink of claret wine mulled with spices. The rest of the night was more peaceful, but she could not **[p. 67]** fall fast asleep.

In the morning I gave chicken broth with appropriate herbs, and she rested for four hours. At the end of that time I gave a draught of hot hartshorn decoction. She had her monthly period, neverthe-less I would have preferred her to drink the hartshorn decoction cold. The pocks tormented her wretchedly, with the greatest heat in the throat and tongue, so that she could swallow the drink only with the greatest difficulty. She used the following gargle:

R: simple mulberry juice 3oz, rose honey 2oz, rose water ½ pint, sufficient oil of sulphur for tartness.

Then she used the cold hartshorn decoction.

The smallpox appeared on the seventh day, notwithstanding which she used the above gargle for her throat and a draught of the cold hartshorn decoction four times a day, and so, praise God, was cured.   .

I prescribed this ointment for anointing the smallpox:

R: blessed thistle water, common salt, each. Stir them for some time.

She was cured without scars. *I healed this desperately ill lady with these few* [remedies] *and the help of God.*[1]

---

1 Ruland the Elder, 'Centuria VI', *Curationum* [...] *centuriae*, p. 450.

[Case 74]

Cure of smallpox. Mr Farnham,[1] a young gentleman of the same family, talkative, affected, witty: infected with smallpox while staying with Lady Beaufou, so that he could not return to his paternal home at Leicester. To bring out the pocks:

> ℞: diascordium 1dr, Mithridate ½dr, saffron ½sc, tarragon water 3oz, prepared hartshorn 1sc. Make a sweating draught. **[p. 68]**

Once he had drunk this, they began to spread the same day. Previously he was senseless, but seeing this *joy could not be confined*[2] and his sister reported he was freed from all danger of death. His grieving and reserved sister poured out her wide flowing joy, *holding her hands to heaven*[3] she gave everlasting thanks to God, because her brother had been freed beyond all hope from the jaws of death.

To control thirst he drank hartshorn decoction as he pleased. For his throat he used the gargle as for Lady Beaufou. To prevent disfigurement of his face, he used the following oil when the pocks started to dry:

> ℞: blessed thistle water 2oz, olive oil 1½oz. Mix. Shake together in the form of oil.

He was cured, praise God, without scars.

[Case 75]

Cure of fever after giving birth. Lady Rous of Rous Lench, devout, aged 27:[4] fell into a quotidian fever two days after giving birth.

---

1 Thomas Farnham of Leicester. Came of an old-established family at Quorndon, where there are fine tombs. It is unclear which generation of the family he belonged to. In 1617 he is described as a young man, and his sister was grateful for his cure.
2 Echoing Livy, *Historiam ab urbe condita*, Lib. XXX, Cap. XVII.
3 Echoing Virgil, 1 *Aeneid* 93.
4 Esther, Lady Rous of Rous Lench, Worcestershire (1589–1620). Daughter of Sir Thomas Temple of Stowe. Married at 16 to John Rous, heir to a Worcestershire timbered manor with a moat and large park; seven children. Her son Thomas was a noted anti-Royalist. Hall treated her on three occasions, and noted her as devout.

She was wretchedly attacked by a most violent headache at the moment of the attack, and tortured by extreme pain in her neck.

℞: diascordium ½dr, magisterium of pearls, coral tincture each 12gr, blessed thistle water 2oz. Give two hours before the attack, repeat the potion when the attack comes. Continue the course for two days.

This plaster for the sore neck:

℞: caranna 1oz. Dissolve in white hyssop wine 1oz. Make a plaster. Spread it on thin leather and apply to the neck.

She was freed from the headache and fever. Praise God.

[Case 76]

[p. 69] Cure of virulent gonorrhoea. William Clavell of Feckenham:[1] most wretchedly seized by virulent gonorrhoea with extremely hot urine for forty days. He consulted a surgeon use-lessly for a month, but did indeed recover in our hands with the following remedies, in fifteen days. In the month of October:

℞: guaiacum gum 1oz powdered, in beer. Five stools.

Afterwards:

℞: sarsaparilla decoction 4 pints.

He drank a pint morning and evening, but because he often mentioned sarsaparilla decoction, I wanted to give him these:

℞: sarsaparilla 2oz, colchicum 1½oz, guaiacum, liquorice each 1oz, senna 2oz, anise, caraway, coriander seeds each ½oz. Boil in 8 pints, reduce to four. Strain and store for use.

He took 4 pints of this. Next, the following electuary:

℞: tragacanth gum ½oz. Dissolve in sufficient plantain water. Strain. To the strained liquid add guaiacum gum powder, burnt turpentine 1dr. Dose: 1½dr.

---

1 Not further identified. Low social status.

He was suitably and correctly purged by the use of the sarsaparilla decoction, and entirely freed from lower backache and burning urine in four days. The use of the electuary completely cured his gonorrhoea.

[Case 77]

Cure of astonishing worms. Richard Wilmore of Norton, aged 14:[1] vomited black worms about one and a half inches long, with sixteen legs and small red heads. When he vomited they were almost dead, but revived after a short time had passed. They were expelled with mercurius vitae.[2] The day after they were brought up **[p. 70]** his father brought them to me wrapped in paper. They crawled slowly as if with earwig feet, but not the same colour as earwigs. Once we had seen these he continued to ask me for further advice because he judged it would benefit his son. Next I observed the state of the illness and robustness of his strength, that he was most vexed once a month, that is, at the new moon, and was wretchedly wracked by their attack (unless he gorged himself with plain food, and greedily took food by mouth, because of *frenzied hunger and immoderate greed of the stomach*).[3] He was so overwhelmed by the greatness of his suffering that those around him were wounded in spirit. *He passed urine with shining sparks the colour of amber powder, otherwise satisfactory and good.*[4] He was strong, well coloured. Two years previously I had cured him properly of the French disease, and he became well and freed from pain. Then he fell into this very painful condition, *indeed the most severe kind of affliction, which lurks in the stomach and is deeply destructive unless quickly and correctly treated. I did indeed feel pity, and started its cure with the following remedies:*[5]

---

1 Richard Wilmore of Norton Curlieu, Budbrooke (1603–49). Lived in a hamlet near Warwick. Married Joan Awry; two children.
2 They were expelled with mercurius vitae] I read as a home remedy before Hall was consulted.
3 Echoing Virgil, 6 *Aeneid* 85 and 2 *Aeneid* 357.
4 Ruland the Elder, 'Centuria X', *Curationum* […] *centuriae*, p. 718.
5 Ruland the Elder, 'Centuria X', *Curationum* […] *centuriae*, p. 728.

℞: mercurius vitae 3gr, a little rose conserve: vomits two.

He brought up six live worms, of a sort that I have never seen or read of before. On the following day:

℞: the chymical cup 5dr: vomits five, worms three.

On the third day he was purged in this way:

[p. 71] ℞: diaturbith powder with rhubarb 1dr, laxative senna powder ½dr, purslane water 3oz, solutive syrup of roses 1oz, oil of vitriol 8 drops. Mix.

He was properly purged but passed no worms. He was set free by these and gave me many thanks. I saw him in passing two years later, and asked whether he ever felt any corrosion of the stomach or passed worms. He replied that he had been free of all pain and torment since that time. Praise God.

[Case 78]

Cure of toothache. Mrs Kempson, a gentlewoman:[1] *endured grim and pitiful torture from a decayed molar tooth day and night. She contrived many things as cures but with no success. When she comes running to me, I give her the following water whose rapid application calmed the pain. She brought up much thin sputum:[2]*

℞: *field poppy water 2oz, sufficient oil of vitriol to render it sharp. Mix well. Place a cloth soaked in it over the sore tooth often.*

At last, when the fourth application had been made, all the pain suddenly left.[3] Her head was still hurting, so she used the following pills:

℞: pills – cochiae ½dr, aureae 1dr, trochiscated agaric ½sc. Make 7 pills with betony water. Ten stools and three vomits.

---

1 Margaret Kempson of Stratford-upon-Avon (1589–1643). Daughter of John Sadler, a wealthy miller. Married Leonard Kempson (cf. Case 31), becoming 'a gentlewoman'. Widowed in 1626, Margaret soon married again to John Norbury of Alcester.

2 Ruland the Elder, 'Centuria IV', *Curationum* [...] *centuriae*, p. 251.

3 Ruland the Elder, 'Centuria IV', *Curationum* [...] *centuriae*, p. 273.

She passed four large long worms at one evacuation. These alone freed her from the above symptoms.

[Case 79]

[p. 72] Cure of a swollen face. Baron Compton, President of Wales:[1] severely tortured and disfigured by swelling of the face, springing from catarrh. I visited him and prescribed the following treatment:

> ℞: marsh-mallow ointment ½oz, oils of chamomile, violet, sweet almond each 2dr, chicken fat 1dr. Make an ointment, spread it on a folded cloth. Amber pills: 1½dr at bedtime.

In the morning the swelling was entirely gone. He used the following gargle often:

> ℞: poppy syrup 1oz, poppy water 3oz, sufficient oil of vitriol to render it sharp.

He was cured of everything after two days.

[Case 80]

Cure of malignant fever, pain in the spleen, testicular swelling. 1618. Sir Rainsford, aged 35:[2] wretchedly tortured by malignant fever, thirst, wind, splenic pain, swelling of the testicles, hypochondriac melancholy. He purged himself with manna ½oz, expressed rhubarb 1dr, sufficient posset ale: five stools without any relief. Then he asked my advice. I applied this plaster to the spleen:

> ℞: labdanum 2dr, yellow wax 1oz, melilot plaster 2oz, *plaster of red lead* ½oz.[3]

---

1 William Compton, 1st Earl of Northampton (cf. Cases 2, 64, 68, 83).

2 Sir Henry Rainsford of Clifford Chambers (1575–1622). Son and heir of Hercules Rainsford, he inherited the manor in 1583. His mother then married William Barnes of Talton (cf. Case 90). Henry entered the Middle Temple in 1594. Married Anne Goodere *c.* 1595 (cf. Case 163). Received a knighthood on the occasion of James I's coronation in 1604.

3 Martini, 'De scorbuto', in Sennert, *De scorbuto tractatus*, pp. 746–747, refers to a similar plaster, but I have not found a recipe.

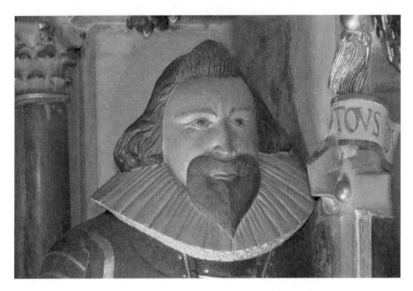

30 Effigy of Sir Henry Rainsford (1575–1622) in St Helen's Church, Clifford Chambers, about one mile away from Stratford-upon-Avon. Hall treated Sir Henry for a fever, a pain in the spleen and a testicular swelling (Case 80). Hall treated Anne, Lady Rainsford as well (Case 163).

He was rightly freed from wind. For the fluctuant swelling of the testicles:

> ℞: our lead and melilot plasters in equal amounts, but first a poultice of rue, chamomile, feverfew in **[p. 73]** in claret wine. Boil and spread this on the swelling.

When this was removed, the above plaster was applied with the desired result, for the swelling was entirely removed.

He used this softening enema:

> ℞: linseed oil 8oz or rue, chamomile oil each 1oz, diaphoenicon and diacatholicon each ½oz. Dissolve in Spanish wine. Make an enema: two stools with wind.

He was freed from the swelling and pain of the spleen. Neither the stomach nor the appetite were yet as they should be, so on the third day I gave the chymical cup 1oz, caelestis water 3 drops. Six vomits. The next day he started eating. The same day after the vomit, before sleeping:

> R: diascordium 1dr, lemon juice 1oz, sufficient posset ale. The day after the vomitory, an enema of diacatholicon, red sugar and milk. Two stools.

And so, praise God, he was restored to his former health.

[Case 81]
Cure of a canker on the leg. Mr Barnes, a gentleman aged 36:[1] limping for a long time because of a canker of the leg. His body was suitably purged with pills, then he used guaiacum decoction, then external applications. He was properly cured:

> R: *white vitriol 2oz, bole Armeniac 1oz 2dr, camphor 3dr. Make a powder. Take 1oz of this, put it in water almost boiling.* **[p. 74]** *Leave a little while to get hot and remove from the fire. The dregs will settle. Clean the canker with this warm water, without any other addition.*[2]

When he was nearly cured, I encouraged scabbing with the following plaster:

> R: white lead ½lb, chalk 4dr. Make a powder. Make a styptic plaster with pork fat by the usual method. Apply to a thickness of one finger. Leave for 9 days.

This lotion came first:

> R: sufficient white copperas. Boil in sufficient spring water, wash the ulcer with it. When the first plaster is removed, another should be applied which will stay for six days, and when that is removed a third, for three days. NOTE: the canker should always be washed with the above water.

---

1 William Barnes of Tredington (1586–?). The family had a coat of arms. One daughter by his first wife Mary, who died. Remarried *c.* 1616. Lived at Tredington manor. Inherited a large estate from his uncle, William Barnes of Clifford Chambers (cf. Case 90) in 1621.
2 Penot, *De denario medico*, p. 70.

He was perfectly cured in this way, after vainly trying many [remedies] from surgeons, to no purpose.

[Case 82]
Cure of dysentery, menstrual flux. Sheffield, a farmer's wife of Stratford Old Town,[1] 48 years old:[2] wretchedly attacked by dysentery and weakened by red menstrual flux. Her periods had previously been suppressed for the past five years. *She recovered with these, very little in quantity but of outstanding power:*[3]

℞: laudanum pills 6gr, Mithridate ½sc, conserve of roses 1½dr, crocus Martis 1sc. Mix.

She was freed from the menstrual flux and diarrhoea of the bowels, but was still troubled by thirst.

℞: corn poppy water 4oz, syrup of violets 1oz.

These freed her from thirst and flux, and she was cured.

[Case 83]
Cure of loss of appetite, catarrh. *For the most illustrious hero and Lord, William Compton, Lord President of Wales:*[4] **[p. 75]** with rheum from the head dripping into the gums, and loss of appetite. I cured and healed him by having him take the following:

℞: *senna leaves detached from the stalks ½oz, best rhubarb 2dr, choice agaric 1dr, excellent cinnamon 6dr. Infuse everything by the usual method for twelve hours, in lukewarm borage and chicory waters each 10oz. In the morning boil,*

---

1 The area around Holy Trinity Church in Stratford-upon-Avon still has this name.
2 Elinor Sheffield of Old Stratford (*c.* 1574–1624). Married *c.* 1594 to John Sheffield, a farmer; ten children. John was a churchwarden at Holy Trinity.
3 Ruland the Elder, 'Centuria VI', *Curationum* [...] *centuriae*, p. 417.
4 Bruele, *Praxis medicinae*, f. 2r. William Compton, 1st Earl of Northampton (cf. Cases 2, 64, 68, and 79). Described here as President of Wales, so probably seen in 1618 or after.

reduce by 4oz, then strain six or seven times, and sweeten with 4oz best sugar in the form of nectar.[1]

He took 2oz of this at bedtime. In the morning he had a single, large, foul-smelling stool. 21 April. 22nd: He took 5oz of the above decoction in the morning: eight stools from this. 23rd:

R: pills aureae, rhubarb each 1dr. Thirteen stools from these.

After the third stool he was a little better. After taking broth with herbs and a crust of bread (for it was Good Friday), he at once recovered. After a very good purge of the body, I gave the following decoction:

R: china sliced in pieces 2dr, sassafras root sliced in thin rounds ½oz. Boil by the usual method in 8 pints, reduce to 4 pints. Drink this at least four times a day, for eight days.

On alternate days he swallowed well made Ruffus's pills 2sc. When these were finished, praise God, he was very well and fit.

[Case 84]

Cure of indigestion of food, and liver obstruction. Lady Beaufou:[2] complained of indigestion of food and wind after eating. I prescribed the following beer for this, with the desired happy result:

R: washed dock root 4oz, agrimony leaves 5 handfuls, leaves of chicory with everything 2 handfuls. Boil in 3 gallons very new beer, reduce by ½ gallon. Strain. Add flowers of yeast. Put it away in a vessel, in which immerse the following inside a thin linen bag:

R: sarsaparilla, sassafras, **[p. 76]** ivory shavings each 1oz, senna, polypody each 5oz, colchicum 2oz, liquorice ½oz, galangals, rhubarb each ½oz, mechoachan 1oz, cinnamon, cloves each 1dr. Break them all up coarsely and mix (with a stone if that may be properly accommodated) and fasten it with a string at the top of the cask. After ten or twelve days, take a draught morning and evening.

---

1 Ranzau, *De conservanda*, pp. 63–64.
2 Ann, Lady Beaufou of Emscote (cf. Case 73).

She was rightly purged, and digested food very well. She thanked me.

[Case 85]

Cure of gout in the fingers and feet. Sir Pakington:[1] suddenly and wretchedly afflicted with gout in the fingers and feet, at an inn while travelling to London by carriage. He could neither stand nor handle anything. After asking my advice, he was restored with the following:

> ℞: *mallows with the roots cut small. Boil in equal amounts of wine and vinegar, reduce to a third part, then add coarse rye husks.*[2] After light boiling, bruise, apply hot to the painful joints.

He was well restored within the space of one day, and was freed from inflammation. He used a fomentation of *distilled frog spawn water*,[3] then I applied diachalcitys plaster. The same day I advised him to drink 2dr of Montagnana's senna powder with colchicum 15gr. These restored him, and on the third day he rode to London, and gave me many thanks.

[Case 86]

Cure of stomach ache with wind. Wilson of Stratford-upon-Avon, about 48 years old:[4] wretchedly tortured for a long time by stomach ache and indigestion of food, so that she dares not take food. After asking my advice, she was cured with this one powder:

> ℞: senna 6dr, white ginger, fennel seed, zedoary, cumin seed each 2dr, cloves, galangal, nutmeg each 1dr, rhubarb 2dr, sugar candy 6dr. Make the powder. Dose: the amount of a bean on toasted

---

1 Cf. Case 71. Died aged 77, buried at Aylesbury.
2 Solenander, *Consiliorum* [...] *Solenandri*, p. 429.
3 Croll, *Basilica chymica*, p. 277.
4 This patient was identified as male by Cooke, but the grammar of the Latin original makes it clear she was female. She is unidentifiable, and the consultation date is unknown.

bread moistened with wine in the morning; at bedtime the amount of a hazelnut, with a little wine.

Cured.

[Case 87]
[p. 77] Cure of colic and backache. Mrs Hanbury, a gentlewoman of Worcester aged 30:[1] so bent over by lower backache that she could not stand erect, and attacked by colic.

R: our caranna plaster.

R: green shoots of feverfew, rue, chamomile each 1 handful, seeds of caraway, cumin, lovage, anise, carrot each ½ handful. Boil by the usual method in sufficient claret wine, then strain without force, and keep the expressed wine. Apply the hot plaster to the lower part of the belly. When it becomes cold, heat it again in an oven with the above expressed wine, two or three times as needed. Boil red nettle seeds with their tops in white wine. Take this hot in the morning.

She was rightly and properly cured, and freed from all symptoms, praise God.

[Case 88]
Cure of red menstrual flux. The sister of neighbour Sheffield:[2] weakened by excessive menstrual flow. I cured her quickly, in this way:

R: plume alum,[3] the weight of 2 pennies in rose water.[4] Continue the course for three days. Fast for 2 hours, then take mutton broth and these herbs: yarrow, inner bark of oak, and drink steeled fluids.

She was cured, quickly and safely.

---

1 Anne Hanbury of Worcester (cf. Case 11).
2 No identifying details.
3 plume alum] A naturally occurring alum.
4 weight of 2 pennies] Approximately 5 grams, or about 15 grains.

[Case 89]

Cure of spasm of the mouth. 29 September. Lady Rous:[1] eight months pregnant, disfigured by spasm of the mouth. Age: 28 years more or less, tall in stature.

> ℞: sufficient rosemary ashes. Make a lye with white wine. Warm the affected area with a warm cloth folded in three.

> ℞: the ointment of oils, as for my daughter.

> ℞: rose water 6oz, oil of vitriol to make it sharp. Hold in the mouth.

These cured her; see page 34.

[Case 90]

Cure of bleeding from an extracted tooth. Mr Barnes, a gentleman of Clifford:[2] reduced to the feebleness of old age *by a rotten tooth, extracted*[3] without difficulty or pain. Two days after **[p. 78]** the extraction *a huge haemorrhage followed, from an artery which supplied the tooth in the gum bleeding copiously. I cured this in a short time, after he remained continuously bloodstained for twenty-four hours, not calling a physician.*[4]

Since I had no remedy to hand, I prescribed cold water held in the mouth and often spat out. He did that until other medicines were prepared, but the use of the water restrained the flow. Afterwards:

> ℞: *white vitriol* 2 pinches, bole Armeniac 1 pinch, camphor ½ pinch, sufficient hot rose water. *Make a lotion.*

On my instructions he applied a cold soaked cloth to the gum several times.[5] After five hours it stopped, *having kept him awake for much of the night.*

---

1 Cf. Cases 75 and 92. Hall treated her in 1618, late in her pregnancy.
2 William Barnes of Clifford Chambers (1547–1621). A lawyer. Married Jane Smith in 1567; no children. After Jane died, William married the widowed Elizabeth Rainsford of Clifford Chambers. Her wealthy first husband had died when their son Henry was 8, and William became his guardian. He died childless, and his nephew (also William Barnes) inherited his lands.
3 Valleriola, *Observationum* [...] *libri sex*, p. 212.
4 Valleriola, *Observationum* [...] *libri sex*, p. 212.
5 Ruland the Elder, 'Centuria V', *Curationum* [...] *centuriae*, p. 314.

Sleep took a stronger hold than usual.[1] Sleep released him after five hours had passed, and the bleeding restarted, not with much force. I could not stop it with the aid of lesser aids, so (*when other remedies have been used in vain*)[2] I had to fight with stronger ones. I prescribed a sponge wetted with crocus Martis and the above vitriolated water, wrapped round and filling up the eroded place, by which the flow was controlled, *and suppressed entirely, nor did it return in greater amount. Praise God the creator of medical practice.*[3]

This is well-proven. He was cured. 1 January 1619.

[Case 91]
Well-tested cure of giddiness. For Hudson,[4] a poor man suffering from giddiness: venesection of the cephalic vein to 10oz. He was purged with pills – aureae, cochiae 2sc each, alhandal trochees 8gr. Make 7 pills. Nine stools. Afterwards he took *peacock droppings, of a male for a male. Dry for a powder 1dr, soak overnight in white wine. Give when everything has been passed through a cloth, and continue from the new to the full moon.*[5] Cured.

[Case 92]
[p. 79] Cure of headache, suffocation of the womb. Lady Rous:[6] pregnant, wretchedly troubled by suffocation of the mother with fainting and extreme headache.

℞: fumes of burnt horse hoof.

She quickly came to herself when the smoke was drawn into her nose. Then she had a suppository of honey and holy powder,

1 Echoing Cicero, 'Somnium Scipionis, Book VI', *De re publica.*
2 Ruland the Elder, 'Centuria II', *Curationum [...] centuriae*, p. 71.
3 Ruland the Elder, 'Centuria II', *Curationum [...] centuriae*, p. 72.
4 No further identification.
5 Du Chesne, *Pharmacopoea dogmaticorum*, p. 148.
6 Cf. Cases 75 and 89. On this occasion Hall treated her in March 1620 during her seventh pregnancy. Both the child and his mother were buried on 12 August 1620.

resulting in seven stools with a large amount of wind. She had the fumes of fragrant things applied below, and stinking ones to the nostrils. I prescribed an ointment for her neck with spikenard, then Martiatum ointment, because she had suffered from facial paralysis the previous year and now feared it greatly. She took the following electuary in the morning, the quantity of a nutmeg on an empty stomach:

R: clove-gillyflower, borage conserve each 1oz, Mithridate, dia-cyminum each 2dr, prepared hartshorn 3dr.

She took the prepared hartshorn in broth. To the umbilicus: a simple caranna plaster, in the middle of which 3gr musk were placed. These freed her, and afterwards she bore a daughter at the due time. 16 March 1620.

[Case 93]
Cure of scanty menstruation, headache. Mary Murden, a gentlewoman:[1] suffers from headache, red face after eating, scanty and discoloured menstruation. Age: 17.

R: fennel, parsley roots each 2oz, asparagus, broom each 3oz, sweet flag ½oz, leaves of betony, mugwort, cure-all, watercress, hyssop, rosemary, penny-royal, nettles each ½ handful, elecampane root ½oz, liquorice 2oz, anise and fennel seeds each 3oz, stoned raisins 1 handful, senna, polypody of the oak each 4oz, colchicum 2oz, rhubarb, agaric each 2dr. Boil in 8 pints spring water, reduce to half. Squeeze out. Dissolve syrups of cyclamen, wallflower, chicory with rhubarb each 2oz. Dose: from 3 to 5oz.

The use of these quickly cured her.

[Case 94]
[p. 80] Cure of the emergence of worms from the umbilicus. Dixwell Brent of Pillerton, aged 3 years:[2] when a hard umbilical

---

1 Mary Murden of Moreton Morrell (cf. Case 60).
2 Dixwell Brent of Pillerton Priors (1617–?). This child was the youngest of ten.

swelling broke, five long worms (similar to worms appearing from the anus) [emerged] through a small hole like a fistula. His nurse removed four dead ones. The fifth worm was actually half dead, the front half motionless, the rear moved. Witnesses: the nurse, his mother and father, and servants. The hole being open and the swelling still hard (for I was an eye-witness) I prescribed only the application of an unrefined honey plaster. The same day I prescribed the administration of *a honey suppository*.[1] We did not see any worms appear, so the next day I wished a poultice of freshly bruised wormwood and boiled cattle bile applied to the umbilicus, and the honey suppository. The happy boy's colour was thus restored and the umbilicus healed. He is still alive, and now wears adult clothes. 27 April 1620.

[Case 95]
Cure of generalised dropsy. The [1st] Countess of Northampton, 6 May 1620:[2] fell into a generalised dropsy with swelling of the face and feet.

> ℞: the decoction as for Mrs Murden, page 79, with the addition of rhubarb 2dr, senna ½oz. Dose: 4oz.

Continue the course for four days: eight stools on the first day, eighteen on the second, fifteen stools on the third without loss of strength. Then take electuary of cubebs, as much as a hazelnut, on five mornings. Next she is to use guaiacum decoction prepared in this way:

> ℞: *guaiacum wood 1lb, dried snowbells 1 handful, cinnamon 2oz, raisins 2oz. Boil in 9 pints water, reduce to half.*

His mother came of a family with a coat of arms. No information about his later life.
1 Platter, *Praxeos* […] *de vitiis*, p. 985.
2 Elizabeth, Countess of Northampton (cf. Case 1). This consultation in 1620 took place two years earlier than Hall's other treatment of the Countess.

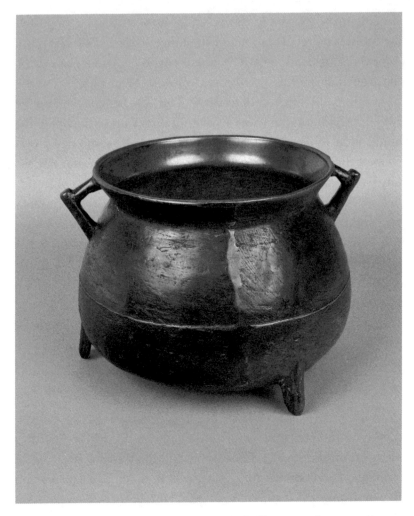

31 A seventeenth-century cauldron, used for boiling water for some of Hall's concoctions, such as Case 95.

After the boiling was completely finished I ordered it put, hot, into another glass vessel, into which I had poured three pints good wine. **[p. 81]** *I advised her to take 6oz of the hot syrup in the morning, 4oz in the evening. I advised her to cover herself completely with bed-coverings, to elicit sweat.*[1] Every morning

---

1 Valleriola, *Observationum* […] *libri sex*, p. 89.

when she sweated, she took the diacubeb electuary one hour later, and was purged every third day:

R: mechoachan 1½dr, loosening syrup of roses 1oz, wormwood water, Spanish wine each 2oz.

Two stools, then two vomits, then three stools, then one vomit; finally twelve stools with the desired result, because the swelling disappeared. She used Crato's steeled electuary. These cured her rightly and properly and restored her colour within twenty days. Praise God.

[Case 96]
Cure of stomach ache and headache. Mrs Goodman, a gentlewoman aged about 54 years:[1] oppressed by headache and stomach ache.

R: a mass of mastic pills 2sc, aloes rosata 1sc. Re-shape the pills into medium size with loosening rose syrup.

Take before meals, continue the course for three days. Finally, take this electuary on an empty stomach:

R: red rose conserve 4oz, Gabrieli's aromatic powder 1½dr, sliced cloves 1dr, ambergris 6gr. Mix with citron rind syrup. Make the electuary. Dose: as much as a chestnut.

So a little of that brought her immediate help, and she came to complete health.[2]

[Case 97]
Cure of itching hands. Mr Penell, a gentleman, son-in-law of Squire Greville of Milcot:[3] oppressed by eruptions and pustules on

---

1 Sara Goodman (?). Identification is uncertain. Might be the wife of Thomas Goodwin, a servant to Lady Hunks, who would have paid her medical expenses.
2 Ruland the Elder, 'Centuria III', *Curationum* […] *centuriae*, pp. 184 and 185.
3 Edward Pennell of Lindridge, Worcestershire (?–1657). Came of a landed family, was in the household of Sir Edward Greville at Milcote. Married Margaret Greville; five children. A Royalist, he was present at the surrender of Worcester in 1646. There are brass monuments to him and Margaret in St Lawrence's church, Lindridge.

his hands. When these ruptured, a clear poisonous water dripped out, which greatly tortured the whole of his hands with inflammation and excoriation. Many external remedies were applied in vain. His head is also overflowing with inflammation, heat and scales. Age: about 38 years. He was freed like this:

℞: agrimony, scurvy-grass, watercress each 1 handful, sage, chicory, fumitory each ½ handful, elecampane root ½oz, polypody of the oak 3oz, sassafras root ½oz. Boil in 12 pints **[p. 82]** spring water, until half is gone. Strain. To the strained liquid add rhubarb, agaric each ½oz, laxative senna 1oz, liquorice 1oz, seeds of anise, caraway, coriander each 2dr, cinnamon 1dr. Boil again until two pints are gone. To the strained liquid add loosening rose syrup 2oz, oil of vitriol 12 drops. Dose: 4oz on four consecutive days. Six or seven stools each day.

For external use:

℞: white camphor ointment mixed with juice of common houseleek as much as you like, with which anoint the hands. Venesection of the right basilic vein to 7oz.

These cured him quickly and freed him from the itch.

[Case 98]
Cure of yellow jaundice, obstructed menstruation, vomiting blood. 4 April 1621. Rogers of Stratford-upon-Avon, about 17 years old:[1] suffered from vomiting, obstructed menstruation, jaundice, bleeding.

℞: the chymical cup 7dr, syrup of violets ½ spoonful: seven vomits, five stools.

℞: sarsaparilla decoction 3oz, laxative senna powder 1½dr; very well purged.

---

1 Probably Frances Rogers of Stratford-upon-Avon (1604–?) whose father, Philip Rogers, was a town apothecary, and would have been known to Hall. Her brother went to Oxford and became a surgeon. No records of Frances's life.

On the third day:

℞: ½dr of the white droppings of fowls, in white wine with sugar.

She was cured of the jaundice on the third day.

[Case 99]
Cure of burning fever, yellow jaundice, abdominal swelling. Mrs Randolph, a gentlewoman aged 55:[1] tortured for a long time by burning fever, from which she fell into yellow jaundice. Urine: red like saffron. She suffered from abdominal pain with swelling and hardness, lower backache, splenic swelling, dropsy. She asked my advice after three weeks had passed since the beginning of the illness.

℞: the chymical cup 6dr, oxymel of squills 2dr, syrup of violets ½sp: three vomits, four stools.

The next day:

℞: electuary of rose juice 2dr, **[p. 83]** diacatholicon 1½dr, diaphoenicon 2½dr, choice rhubarb ½oz, spikenard 5gr, chicory syrup with rhubarb ½oz, chicory water 3oz. Make a draught: eighteen stools.

Her usual drink on the quiet day was hartshorn decoction. She was freed from the fever, yet the jaundice remained. To remove it:

℞: white wine 1 pint, celandine water 6oz, saffron 1dr, Venice treacle 3dr, bezoar stone 1sc, juice of goose droppings 6 spoonfuls. Make a sweating potion. Dose: 4oz on an empty stomach. Take for four days.

She used the following electuary in the evening:

℞: red and white sandalwood each 3dr, currants soaked in white

---

1 Elizabeth Randolph of Wood Bevington, Salford Priors. Dates not known. Eldest daughter of Edward Ferrers of Rowington. In about 1580 she married Thomas Randolph, son of a gentleman from Buckinghamshire; seven children. Hall also treated her son (cf. Case 25) and daughter-in-law (cf. Case 61). Thomas died in 1628.

wine then put through a sieve 4oz, rhubarb 1dr, saffron 1sc. Mix. Make the electuary. [Take] as much as a nutmeg.

For the stomach swelling:

℞: *ointments, Agrippa's 1oz, cyclamen ½oz, Martiatum 3dr, oils, of nard, rue, scorpions each 2dr, a little aqua vitae, some drops of vinegar. Make the ointment by the usual method.*[1]

She was cured, praise God, beyond her friends' expectations.

[Case 100]
Cure of sore throat, burning fever, inflammation of the tongue. Mr Broad, a gentleman of the Grange:[2] *seized by a choking sore throat. He lay incurable, despaired of,*[3] abandoned by ministers, deserted by all, with a burning fever, hot and excoriated tongue. Aged 42. *He escapes unharmed, with the aid I bring:*[4]

℞: the common decoction for enemas ½ pint, diacatholicon, diaphoenicon each 1oz. Make an enema: four stools.

Venesection beneath the tongue. A gargle:

℞: rose honey, plantain and rose waters each equal amounts, with a little oil of vitriol.

A linctus:

℞: liquorice, hyssop syrups each 3oz, oxymel of squills ½oz, rose honey 1oz. Mix. Make the linctus. Use it after the gargle.

I prescribed **[p. 84]** a plaster of wormwood wine and pork fat, to apply to the throat. Moreover, I prescribed venesection but he refused. I feared his imminent death. As venesection had been

---

1 Bruele, *Praxis medicinae*, p. 335.
2 William Broad of Bidford-on-Avon (1583–1653). He married Frances Badger, an heiress, and so in 1616 acquired the estate of Bidford Grange. In 1625 he served as Treasurer of Barlichway Hundred. He effectively declined a knighthood in 1625. Monument slab in St Laurence's church, Bidford.
3 Valleriola, *Observationum* [...] *libri sex*, pp. 259–260.
4 Ruland the Elder, 'Centuria VI', *Curationum* [...] *centuriae*, p. 439.

rejected, he fell into a continual burning fever as I foretold. His ordinary drink:

> ℞: liquorice, anise seeds, figs, raisins each 1oz. Boil in 4 pints water until 1 pint is gone.

This should be his ordinary drink. Day by day the fever increased, his strength was destroyed, and he declared that he could not survive. He sent me a messenger on a hard-ridden horse, for *in desire, swiftness is delay*.[1] After the message reached me, I found him in danger of death, unable to say anything. Immediately I cut a vein and bled to 10oz. His voice returned, and he said that he found great relief in the venesection. The same day I gave our antipyretic julep before sleeping. That night was more peaceful than others.

His ordinary drink was hartshorn decoction, and he was freed from fear of choking and fever. He recovered well, by God's will who should be blessed, and *who alone doeth great wonders*.[2]

[Case 101]
Cure of very severe cough, 1621. Mrs Sadler, a gentlewoman,[3] suffers from severe cough, difficulty in breathing and aversion to food; aged 60.

> ℞: oxymel of squills 2dr, syrup of violets ½oz, chymical cup 2dr. Mix: seven vomits, twelve stools.

She is very much relieved.

> ℞: pills – amber, cochiae, each 1sc, powdered rhubarb ½sc. Make pills with sufficient oxymel of squills. Seventeen stools.

---

1 Echoing Publilius Syrus, *Sentences*: 'celeritas in desiderio mora'.
2 Valleriola, *Observationum* [...] *libri sex*, p. 109; paraphrasing Vulgate, Ps. 135:4: 'qui facit mirabilia magna solus'.
3 Isabel Sadler of Stratford-upon-Avon (?–1636). Daughter of Peter Smart. In 1584 she married John Sadler, a miller in Stratford; five children. He acquired the status of gentleman, and served as bailiff and as alderman. He was landlord of The Bear in Bridge Street. In her will, Isabel left cash to all her grandchildren on marriage.

A linctus:

℞: lohochs – sanum et expertum, of fox lungs each 1oz, liquorice and coltsfoot syrups each 1oz, oxymel of squills 2dr. Make the linctus. *Take it with a moderately bruised liquorice root.*[1]

Before sleeping hold a pill in the mouth, made in this way:

[p. 85] ℞: *liquorice juice 2½dr, wheat flour 1½dr, saffron, myrrh each 1½sc, opium 3gr, dry styrax 3dr, sufficient syrup of violets. Make pills. Give 1sc before going to bed.*[2]

And so she recovered in a week, with God's help.

[Case 102]

Cure of loose bowels lasting for three years. Mrs Browne, a young gentlewoman,[3] endowed with very fine condition of her body: has for three years been in the grip of a watery flow of the bowels mostly at night (for she had at least six or seven stools every single night). She has been led into extreme peril with great loss of strength, and with torments and sleeplessness, though wearied by her troubles. She promises to comply with my instructions, as follows:

℞: pills – amber ½dr, best powdered rhubarb 1dr. Make 7 pills with French lavender syrup, resulting in eight stools.

℞: sarsaparilla, guaiacum bark each 2oz, sassafras 1oz, guaiacum pint, prepared coriander seed 3oz. Crush and boil in spring water 14 pints, reduce to half. At the end of the boiling add crushed cinnamon 4oz. Drink 3 draughts of this decoction each day, that is to say at dawn hot, then at 4 o'clock drink cold, and at bedtime drink cold. Make a second decoction from the dregs.

Cover the head with cloths, which are suffused with this fumigant:

---

1 Bruele, *Praxis medicinae*, p. 162.
2 Bruele, *Praxis medicinae*, p. 173.
3 Mrs Browne of Radford Semele (1602–*c.* 1633). Probably Bridget, daughter of Lady Browne of Radford. In 1623 she married Clement Throckmorton of Haseley; three sons. He was related to the family at Coughton Court, but Clement was a Parliamentarian.

℞: *Roman coriander, dry styrax, benzoin each 3oz, mace, cloves, each 1dr. Make a coarse powder for fumigation.*

℞: *flowers of sage, marjoram, French lavender each ½ handful, seeds of anise, fennel, cumin each 2oz,* **[p. 86]** bruised bayberries ½oz, millet 1lb, common salt ½lb. Parch everything in a frying pan, store in bags. *Apply them very hot to the head and neck until they cool by themselves.*[1]

After that she is to use the above fume. These *freed her from a most savage and deadly illness. To God the highest and most merciful alone be praise.*[2]

[Case 103]

1628. Cure of scurvy with associated symptoms. Mrs Mary Talbot, a gentlewoman,[3] sister to the Earl, Roman Catholic, modest and well-conducted: weighed down by these and many other symptoms: splenic swelling, erosion of the gums, livid spots on the legs, lower backache, convulsions of the jaw, tightening and paralysis of the tongue. People are ignorant of the nature of the disease, even the doctor in Salisbury, learned and experienced in other illnesses.[4] I was treating the Countess at that time. She asked me to visit her sister, taking me into a darkened room. I found the pulse uneven and small, the urine turbid and thick. While I was considering the above symptoms, the Countess asked my opinion on her life. I replied that I should not despair. I said that she suffered from long-standing, established scurvy. The gentlewoman replied that she had been cured in the Archduke's palace in the Low Countries two years previously, but now it was much worse. I described and

---

1 Fernel, *Consiliorum liber*, p. 37.
2 Ruland the Elder, 'Centuria III', *Curationum* [...] *centuriae*, p. 226.
3 Mary Talbot of Grafton, Worcestershire. Dates unknown. Daughter of Sir John Talbot, and sister to the Earl of Shrewsbury. This wealthy Catholic family was linked by marriage to many recusant families in the Midlands. Mary's eldest sister Gertrude was married to one of the Gunpowder Plotters. Mary remained unmarried.
4 Dr Nathaniel Wright MD practised in Shrewsbury (not Salisbury; Hall's mistake) about this time (Raach 1962: 95, 113).

enumerated the many signs and the nature *of the disease, which sends out shoots from deep roots*[1] in the following year. Nor is the treatment difficult but it is prolonged, requiring other medicines. I willingly gave the following advice. *First it is essential to establish* **[p. 87]** *that perseverance and fortitude is required, for nothing comes in a short time. Therefore, if she wishes to be cured, steadfast perseverance, faithful obedience, and unusual patience is required. If she delays or despairs, nothing will have an effect.*[2] Once she agreed to this, I undertook the happy cure in the name of God.

Her body was first purged with Ruffus's pills and vitriolated tartar. She used scurvy-grass salt in food, wormwood salt in broth. Her drink was the following, all others being forbidden:

> ℞: garden scurvy-grass 4 handfuls, watercress, brooklime each 2 handfuls, bruised juniper berries 1 handful, wormwood ½ handful. Boil in sufficient new beer, reduce to 4 gallons. Make beer by the usual method. After fourteen days it was ready for drinking.

She took a draught in the morning. She is to take exercise for an hour, then swallow electuary of scurvy-grass flowers, as much as a nutmeg. She did this for six days. She could walk a mile, for she went to the house of her relative, Winter. I was there, and she thanked me greatly, and said she had walked three miles. She digests food well, and from being weak has become strong. Praise [God], the One and Three.

[Case 104]
Cure of established scurvy in an elderly man. Mr Hanslap, a gentleman about 61 years old:[3] complained of constriction of the chest, troublesome shortness of breath, thirst, yellow jaundice, hard, livid and black swellings on the thighs, contraction of the knees (so that

---

1 Crato, *Consiliorum* [...] *liber quartus*, p. 100.
2 Burton 2001: 264.
3 Robert Hanslap of Southam (1568–1629). Third of eight children. At 35 he married Margaret Hill. The family was wealthy and held various parish offices.

he could not walk without a stick), loss of appetite, and vomiting. **[p. 88]** I found the pulse small, so that I hardly felt it move. Urine: variable, first thin, the next day yellow without sediment. He had unsettled bowels:

R: *diacatholicon electuary*, Solenander's opening electuary[1] *each 2dr, Hamech confection ½dr, senna powder, cream of tartar each ½sc. Make a bolus with sugar.*[2]

This resulted in six stools, but also with weakness so that he suffered from faintness. The next day:

R: prepared hartshorn, ivory shavings each 1dr, powder of worms 3dr (held to be very good in scurvy), sufficient conserve of barberries. Make a soft electuary. Take as much as a hazelnut. Afterwards take six spoonfuls of the following wine:

R: wormwood wine 4oz, Foreest's scheletyrbic syrup 2oz.

The thighs were swollen and livid, so I ordered them to be fomented twice a day with hot folded cloths.

R: brooklime, 2 handfuls boiled in beer (see Eugalenus, page 136).[3]

When these were finished:

R: *nine prepared worms, bruised in a mortar with 2 spoonfuls wine, strained through a cloth. Add to this a measure of wine. Take 3 spoonfuls in the morning and at midday and in the evening.*[4] *Mince earthworms marked with red bands near the collar* (or if you wish, with a single red band at the collar), *first washed together three times with wine, then each one once on its own.*[5]

When the medicine was made, I added 2 pints wine as above.

R: worm wine 3 spoonfuls.

An hour later:

---

1 The electuary is possibly that in Solenander, *Consiliorum* [...] *Solendri*, p. 222. See Case 177.
2 Sennert, *De scorbuto tractatus*, p. 159.
3 Eugalenus, *De scorbuto morbo*, p. 27.
4 nine ... evening] Horst, *Observationum* [...] *libri quatuor*, p. 350.
5 Mince ... own] Horst, *Observationum* [...] *libri quatuor*, p. 354.

℞: Foreest's scheletyrbic syrup 6oz, wormwood wine ½ pint. Mix. Give 2oz.

For the swollen thighs **[p. 89]** he used the following poultice:

℞: *powders of chamomile flowers, marsh cinquefoil, wormwood each 3dr, bryony, self-heal roots each ½oz, flours of wheat, vetch and beans each ½dr, all of which are mixed with two pounds of wheat breadcrumbs, cow's milk or better goat's, and reduced by slowly cooking into the form of a poultice.*[1]

The following ordinary drink:

℞: scurvy-grass 4 handfuls, brooklime, watercress each 2 handfuls, wormwood ½ handful, juniper berries ½lb, sweet flag 3dr, sassafras root 2oz. Boil by the usual method in 5 gallons new beer, reduce to 4. Add flowers of yeast as is the practice, and save in a small barrel. Drink without break after the fourteenth day.

For contraction of the knees:

℞: *juice expressed from scurvy-grass leaves 1oz, oils of St John's wort, mullein, elder each ½oz. Boil until the juice is used up. With the expression mix tacamahacca powder 1½dr, Indian balsam 4sc. Make on a slow fire stirring carefully, at the end add a little wax.*[2]

He had this cordial electuary:

℞: *scurvy-grass conserve 2oz, wormwood, Horst's diasereos, bugloss, clovegillyflowers,* damask roses, preserved elecampane root each ½oz, *rosewood, sweet flag, prepared arum root, diarrhodon Abbatis powder, diapleres archonticon, alkermes confection each ½dr. Make the electuary with Foreest's scheletyrbic syrup.*[3] Dose: as much as a bean.

I applied the following poultice to the hard swelling:

℞: *sufficient powdered common wormwood, which should be mixed to the consistency of a poultice with eggs freshly laid the same day, with the white, yolk* **[p. 90]** *and the shells broken and finely powdered. Apply cold to the swelling.*[4]

---

1 Martini, 'De scorbuto', in Sennert, *De scorbuto tractatus*, p. 737.
2 Martini, 'De scorbuto', in Sennert, *De scorbuto tractatus*, p. 705.
3 Martini, 'De scorbuto', in Sennert, *De scorbuto tractatus*, p. 686.
4 Eugalenus, *De scorbuto morbo*, pp. 136–137.

Its effect was marvellous and he sang its praises. When the swelling had subsided, I anointed the contraction with this ointment:

℞: marsh-mallow ointment, oils of chamomile, castor, worms each ½oz, veal marrow from the shinbone, linseed oil each 3dr, radish, scurvy-grass, watercress juices each ½oz. Make a liniment with sufficient wax and ammoniac solution.

He was very much alleviated. 1 May:

℞: ointments of marsh mallows ½oz, white lilies, chamomile, dill each 2dr, crushed juniper seeds 1sc. Make the ointment.

℞: steeled electuary 2oz, wormwood and scurvy-grass conserves each 1oz. Mix. Give 3dr on an empty stomach.

He was properly cured, could ride and walk, and declared himself entirely cured.

[Case 105]
Cure of palpitations of the heart. Lady Puckering:[1] often tortured by palpitations of the heart.

℞: diambra, sweet diamoschum, aromatic rose [powder] each 2dr, alkermes confection 1dr, diacorallion 1dr, Venice treacle, best Mithridate each 2sc, bugloss and scurvy-grass conserves (because she had scurvy) each 1oz. Mix. Make the electuary. Dose: as much as a hazelnut.

Freed.

I cured Mrs Iremonger, a gentlewoman, her companion, **[p. 91]** of palpitations and tremor of the heart with the following:

℞ castor 1dr, Cretan dittany root ½dr (because her periods were not flowing properly), diambra, sweet diamoschum, aromatic rose

---

1 Elizabeth, Lady Puckering of Warwick Priory (1598–1652). Daughter of Sir John Morley of Sussex. Married in 1616 to Sir Thomas Puckering; two daughters. One died aged 13, the other (later) in childbirth. When Sir Thomas died in 1636, Lady Puckering moved to Ladyholt. In her will, she founded a charity to support widows and orphans.

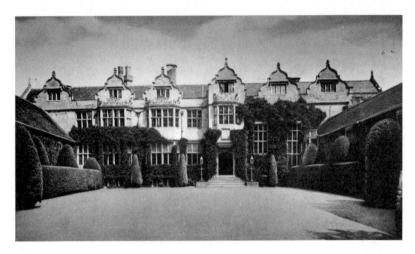

32 Warwick Priory, home of Elizabeth, Lady Puckering (1598–1652). Hall treated her for heart palpitations (Case 105). Her father-in-law, Sir John, was Speaker of the House of Commons and made Keeper of the Great Seal in 1592. He purchased the house in 1581 and remodelled it, adding the six gables seen in this photograph around 1600. The house was dismantled in 1925 and rebuilt in Richmond, Virginia.

powder each 2dr, Venice treacle, best Mithridate each 1sc, bugloss conserve 1oz. Make an opiate with sufficient mugwort syrup.

She took only half of this and was freed, although she had been weighed down with it for a long time before. She said the electuary was worth gold, and rewarded me so that I might help others as well. It cured her, and she thanked me greatly.

[Case 106]

Proven cure of scurvy. Lady Browne of Radford:[1] overcome by these scorbutic symptoms: constipation of the belly, melancholy,

---

1 Elizabeth, Lady Browne of Radford Semele (1584–1650; cf. Case 162). Married Sir William; three children. Her daughter Bridget (Case 102) died in childbirth. Sir William died in 1637. The widowed Lady Browne lived on at Radford, which her son George inherited. He and his brother-in-law were Parliamentarians. The Puritan Thomas Dugard visited Radford. Her will notes money owed by two known recusants.

sleeplessness, disturbed dreams, obstructed menstruation. She has been wretchedly tortured by these obstructions lasting a year, with windy abdominal colic and a swelling like a fist, maximally around the spleen. She was freed from the torments by passing wind. She feels a continuous palpitation at the mouth of the stomach. She feels it easily by applying a hand, in her own words, 'as theare weare some live thinge leaped in hir belly'. All this all arose from the death of her beloved, **[p. 92]** beautiful and devout daughter, whose life (a year previously) changed to death in childbirth, and she sleeps peacefully with the Lord. The remedies below cured and freed her from all symptoms:

> R: *fresh leaves of scurvy-grass, watercress, brooklime, maidenhair, spleenwort each 2 handfuls, scabious, hart's-tongue fern each ½ handful, the cordial flowers each 1 pinch, shaved liquorice root 6dr, senna leaves 1oz, polypody of the oak 6dr, rhubarb, bark of caper roots, prepared Indian myrabolans bark each 4sc, tartar crystals 2dr, stoned raisins 10dr, wheat barley 1 pinch, lemongrass 1sc.*[1] Boil in sufficient wormwood, agrimony and fumitory waters for 1 pint 4oz, after boiling stand to infuse overnight. To the strained liquid add Foreest's scheletyrbic syrup 2oz, diasereos, rhubarb syrup each 1oz. Mix with 2dr cinnamon water. Dose: 7 spoonfuls, resulting in six stools.

Afterwards, *apply Foreest's ammoniac salve to the area of the spleen, because it is very suitable for removing swelling from a painful side.*[2] This has been proved. **[p. 93]** Even though rightly purged, she was attacked by scorbutic abdominal pain. See Sennert page 95[3] and Eugalenus page 62 for the cause of this.[4] You will find the differences from colicky pain on pages 93 and 94 of Sennert,[5] and pages 603 and 638 in the same book.[6] After purging *the urine was confused, and the*

---

1 Martini, 'De scorbuto', in Sennert, *De scorbuto tractatus*, pp. 667–668.
2 Martini, 'De scorbuto', in Sennert, *De scorbuto tractatus*, p. 700.
3 Sennert, *De scorbuto tractatus*, p. 95.
4 Eugalenus, *De scorbuto morbo*, pp. 62–66.
5 Sennert, *De scorbuto tractatus*, pp. 93–94.
6 Martini, 'De scorbuto', in Sennert, *De scorbuto tractatus*, pp. 603, 638.

varieties of sediment were separated, with continuing disturbance in the urine above. These, with the greasy surface, were a warning of scurvy.[1]

Add 2 handfuls of fumitory to the beer, otherwise as for Mr Hanslap. ALSO: the haemorrhoids will be removed with leeches. After that she is to use the electuary as for Mr Hanslap, page 88. *She was freed* from scurvy by using these *and returned, by divine power, to complete health.*[2]

[Case 107]
Cure of giddiness, headache and deafness. Mrs Murden, a gentlewoman about 59 years old:[3] complained of slight giddiness, headache and deafness. I cured her quickly in this way:

R: *aloes rosatae 1dr, powdered rhubarb sprinkled with cinnamon water 2sc, freshly trochiscated agaric 1sc, mastic, myrrh each ½sc. Make 25 pills with betony syrup. Dose: 5 pills an hour before dinner.*[4]

27 April 1626. She used these pills successfully, and *did not cease extolling them with great praise, and by her urging gave me occasion to make a record of that.*[5] She also asked to have them for prevention.

[Case 108]
[p. 94] Cure of loose bowels and wind. Mr George Underhill, a gentleman about 64 years old:[6] weakened by unrestrained loose bowels and wretchedly attacked by wind due to eating gruel.

---

1 Eugalenus, *De scorbuto morbo*, p. 213.
2 Ruland the Elder, 'Centuria III', *Curationum* [...] *centuriae*, p. 185.
3 Mary Murden of Moreton Morrell, the mother of Mary Harvey (cf. Cases 60 and 93). Her monument in Moreton Morrell church shows Mary and her husband Richard kneeling.
4 Crato, *Consiliorum* [...] *liber*, p. 85.
5 Platter, *Observationum* [...] *libri tres*, p. 481.
6 George Underhill of Oxhill (1567–1650). Youngest son of Thomas Underhill of Ettington, in a gentry family. Went to Oxford, matriculated in 1583. Moved to Oxhill when he inherited the estate from his brother in 1613. Never married. Bequeathed Oxhill to his nephew, Thomas Underhill (cf. Case 132). According to William Dugdale in *The Antiquities of Warwickshire* he was politically neutral.

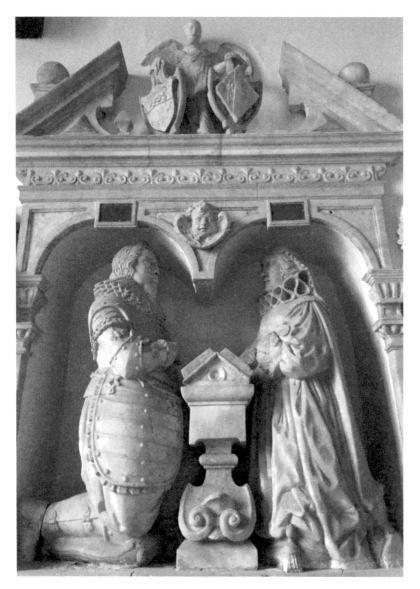

33 Effigy of Mary Murden with her husband, Richard, in the Church of the Holy Cross, Moreton Morrell. Hall treated her for giddiness, headache, and deafness (Case 107).

℞: ventrifluus electuary 6dr, cream of tartar 1sc, powdered rhubarb 2sc. Make a bolus with sugar: nine stools with relief.

At bedtime:

℞: diascordium 1dr, scabious water 3oz, lemon syrup 1oz, poppy syrup ½oz. Mix. Take hartshorn shavings twice daily on the quiet days.

For the stomach:

℞: red rose conserve 2oz, Gabrieli's aromatic rose powder 1dr, sliced cloves ½dr, ambergris 3gr. Mix with citron peel. Take as much as a chestnut in the morning.

After food, the following sweetmeat:

℞: prepared coriander, seeds of fennel, anise, caraway each 2sc, prepared hartshorn, prepared red coral, cinnamon, nutmeg each 1sc, powders, aromatic rose, Galen's laetificans each ½sc, rose sugar tablets to the weight of everything. He should wear our stomach shield.

He was thus properly cured.

[Case 109]
Cure of seminal discharge, nocturnal emission. The above gentleman[1] had been weakened by nocturnal seminal emissions the previous year, but *soon returned to health when I applied the following cure*:[2]

℞: cassia pulp 6dr, tamarind pulp 2dr, red coral, mastic each 1½sc.

Make a bolus with sugar: rightly purged. Afterwards:

---

1 Hall writes 'the above gentleman', so this refers to George Underhill (Case 108). Hall wrote 'Geneross psanno seq.' which Cooke contracted to Mr P. Joan Lane compared this with Hall's original and read 'psanno' as Psamire (an easy error with Hall's italic), and took this to be Hall's method of anonymising the patient. I translate the phrase as 'The above gentleman in the following year'. This identifies the patient as the George Underhill of the previous case, and the date of the consultation as 1631/2.
2 Ruland the Elder, 'Centuria VIII', *Curationum* [...] *centuriae*, p. 566.

R: *gum Arabic, tragacanth, carabe, mummy, bole Armeniac, pike's jaw each 2sc. Powder and make pills weighing 1sc with syrup of dried roses or myrtle. Take for the first dose* **[p. 95]** *three pills, then one pill in the morning for several days*[1] and use steeled milk. He is to wear very thin broad lead sheets on his back, over the renal area.

These cured him quickly and completely.

[Case 110]

Flux of the whites, gonorrhoea. Mrs Kenton, a gentlewoman of Northampton aged 48:[2] weakened and discoloured by a flux of the whites.

R: *clear Venice treacle ½oz. Dissolve in egg yolk by the rule of practice. Add the most refined honey 1oz, rose sugar tablets 2oz, good wine 7oz. Mix. Drink up to 1oz of the milky liquid every day. The effect of this is detected reaching up to and beyond the bladder by the smell of violets in the urine.*[3]

Her ordinary drink while taking the above potion should be the following:

R: barley water with mallows and liquorice.

Take the following bolus: *Make a bolus with olibanum ½dr, also bole Armeniac and sealed earth. Powder everything finely and mix with the white of two fresh eggs. This is something admirable and secret if used for a few days, six hours before eating.*[4]

Her drink should be of this sort:

R: *shavings of guaiacum wood 1lb, bruised bark of the same 4oz. Soak for eight days in 8 pints spring water with 2dr oil of sulphur. Clarify with horse droppings in a capacious glass vessel, well stopped earlier with wax and sulphur. Strain. Put new wood in the strained liquid as in the vessel, soak with the droppings for three days. Purify the strained liquid as you wish* **[p. 96]** *by double distillation, also sweeten and flavour as necessity and the nature of the illness*

---

1 Castro, *De universa mulierum medicina*, p. 66.
2 Of genteel status, but no identifying details.
3 Platter, *Observationum* […] *libri tres*, p. 770.
4 Liébault, *Thresor des remedes secrets*, p. 392.

demand. Give the simple strained liquid, neither purified nor sweetened nor flavoured, 2 or 3 or 4oz depending on the strength of the patient. This decoction has so much strength and efficacy in 2oz that it is equal to 1 pint of any other. It is entirely proved in yellow choler and splenic jaundice, cures dropsy and the French disease quickly, and helps with apoplexy and other very severe illnesses in the head. From the dregs a second decoction can be prepared by adding sufficient quantity of water. It was used at table in place of drink.[1]

For the back: the plaster against ruptures, that for the womb each 10z, comitissa ointment 20z, mastic powder, dragon's blood and white coral each 2dr, red roses 1 pinch, snakeweed root, oak moss each 2dr, sealed earth ½dr. Soften everything together with myrtle oil. Make a plaster. Spread one part on a piece of leather to the lower back and sacrum, the rest though on the lower belly. Wear it from one menstrual period to another, then remove it.[2]

She was properly cured.

[Case 111]

Cure of scorbutic collapse. Mrs Delabere, a gentlewoman of Southam near Gloucester:[3] ill for a long time, with aversion to food. **[p. 97]** Sometimes she takes the greatest delight in food, at other times spits it out. The urine changes frequently and while she is well when in bed, she suffers a collapse when she gets up. She was cured with the following:

> ℞: pills of hiera with agaric, Ruffus's each 2sc, amber, aggregative, cream of tartar each 1½sc, sufficient oxymel of squills. Make 15 pills, gild them. Take 2 in the evening, 3 in the morning, every third day.

She was rightly purged. For the spleen: Foreest's ammoniac salve 10z, melilot plaster ½oz. Make a plaster for the spleen, and cover it with fine red cloth.

---

1 Potier, *Pharmacopoea spagirica*, pp. 22–23.
2 Liébault, *Thresor des remedes secrets*, p. 398.
3 Margaret Delabere of Southam, Gloucestershire. Dates unknown. Married 1608 to Richard Delabere. He paid £25 effectively to decline a knighthood in 1625 at the coronation of Charles I. Margaret travelled to Bath for hydrotherapy. Hall does not record where he treated her.

On the quiet days:

> ℞: conserve of damask roses 1oz, bugloss conserve 2dr, pleres archonticon powder ½dr, cream of tartar, prepared steel powder each 2sc, prepared arum root 1sc, alkermes confection 1dr. Make a soft electuary with sufficient ginger syrup. Dose: the amount of a bean in the evening, of a nutmeg in the morning before rising. Continue so for two days. On the third day she should be purged with the prepared pills.

She was much better, so that she could walk and ride on horseback. Then she went to Bath. There she used the following decoction when she left the bath, and sweated in bed:

> ℞: *guaiacum wood chips 3oz, the same bark 2oz, sassafras 1oz, china cut into thin disks ½oz, ivory shavings 3dr,* liquorice 1oz, agrimony, *blessed thistle,* scurvy-grass, watercress, brooklime *each ½ handful, tops of fumitory, flowers of bugloss, French lavender, rosemary each 1 pinch, nutmeg, cinnamon each 2dr. Soak by the fire for twelve hours in 12 pints spring water.*[1]
> **[p. 98]** In the morning boil, reduce to half, then strain. *Sweeten the strained liquid with sugar. Dose: 4oz. This decoction should be used in the morning.*[2]

She was purged with these pills every fourth day:

> ℞: pills – of hiera with agaric, Ruffus's each 2sc, from which she was rightly purged.

She used no other medicines, and returned home well. She was freed, praise God, from all pains and symptoms, of which *to this day, glory be to God, there remain not a trace.*[3]

---

1 This is the recipe prescribed in Bath, not by Hall, so is an example of the use of a Latin source by another physician.
2 Du Chesne, *Pharmacopoea dogmaticorum*, p. 53. A combination of two recipes on that page, with the addition of antiscorbutic herbs.
3 Ruland, 'Centuria VI', *Curationum […] centuriae*, p. 460.

[Case 112]

[Cure of] dysentery of three months' duration. James Ballard aged 60:[1] attacked by a bloody and frothy flux, sometimes chylous, for three months, and tenesmus.

> R: *barley with husks 1 pinch, broken linseed, fenugreek seeds each 1oz, chamomile, melilot flowers each 1 pinch, rye bran 2 pinches. Make a decoction of everything to 1½ pints. In the strained liquid dissolve 2 egg yolks, rose honey 3oz, brown sugar 3oz. Mix. Make an enema.*[2]

> R: *philonium Persicum 2sc, plantain water 3oz, quince syrup 1oz. Make a potion, which I ordered to be given at nightfall when the patient was going to sleep.*[3]

The night was peaceful. *He said he was helped amazingly by the potion. He was settled, for the pain and flux ceased, and sweet sleep crept up.*[4]

Then he is to use an astringent enema. *It stops the belly's flux and closes an ulcer.*

> **[p. 99]** R: *tops of briars, plantains, purslane, prepared coriander, cumin dried a little and broken each 1oz, dried starch ½oz, galls, coarsely crushed cypress nuts two, both of adequate size, rye 2 pinches. Make a decoction with everything in steeled water to 1 pint. To the strained liquid add liquefied fat of goat's kidneys 1oz, prepared bole Armeniac 2dr, plantain juice 4oz, tragacanth mucilage 1oz, rose honey 2oz. Mix. Prepare the enema.*[5]

I applied a plaster on the belly:

> R: *a mass of plaster against ruptures 3oz, diaphoenicon 2oz, mastic, olibanum, prepared coriander, prepared bole Armeniac, dragon's blood each 4sc, haematite stone 2dr, plantain juice 4oz, rough red wine 3oz, myrtle oil, quince oil each 2oz. Mix with wax and turpentine. Make a roll with hands wetted with rough red wine, from which make a plaster spread on thin leather, and apply to the belly.*[6]

---

1 No identifying details. Low status. Yeomen named Ballard were recorded in Inkberrow and Ilmington. Possibly James Ballard of Ombersley, married 25 May 1576.
2 Valleriola, *Observationum* [...] *libri sex*, p. 137.
3 Valleriola, *Observationum* [...] *libri sex*, p. 437.
4 Valleriola, *Observationum* [...] *libri sex*, p. 138.
5 Valleriola, *Observationum* [...] *libri sex*, p. 138.
6 Valleriola, *Observationum* [...] *libri sex*, p. 138.

For the tenesmus:

R: *choice myrrh, saffron, dried styrax each 1dr, opium 1sc, bdellium, aloes each 18gr, sufficient liquefied yellow wax. Make suppositories. Place one in the anus.*[1]

He had one of these a day. The philonium drink was repeated as above, and the astringent electuary:

R: *prepared bole Armeniac powder 4sc, selected pearls, red coral washed 2sc, new rose powder, diarrhodon Abbatis powder each ½dr, comfrey conserve, preserved citron peel each 1dr.* [**p. 100**] *Expand with sugar dissolved in rose water. Make the electuary in small cubes weighing 2dr. I prescribed one to be eaten at dawn, the other before supper. I prescribed some grains of clear olibanum to be taken now and then, before food.*[2]

I prescribed thin food, restrained and drying[3] and with these, by the will of God, he recovered beyond his friends' expectations.

NOTE: *If there is good digestion but not separation, then dysentery is present. If there is separation and not digestion, then it is a lyentery. If neither separation nor digestion, then diarrhoea is present. If putrefaction of the stomach contents is present, then there is a flux of the belly with various colours.*[4]

[Case 113]

Cure of scorbutic epilepsy. Mrs Layton, a gentlewoman born of a noble line:[5] suffered for a long time from scorbutic epilepsy. In the first place, convulsive movements with fever always indicate it. For other signs see Eugalenus page 86 and Sennert page 620.[6] The attack starts by wretchedly troubling her with a chill, shivering and

---

1 Valleriola, *Observationum* [...] *libri sex*, p. 139.
2 Valleriola, *Observationum* [...] *libri sex*, p. 139.
3 Ruland the Elder, 'Centuria III', *Curationum* [...] *centuriae*, p. 166.
4 Croll, *Basilica chymica*, p. 251.
5 Margaret Layton of Sledwich, County Durham (1575–?). 'Born of a noble line', lived in a manor house. Daughter of John and Elizabeth Clopton of Sledwich. Her brother William married the heiress Anne Clopton of Stratford in 1589. Margaret visited Clopton House in Stratford but never lived there. No information about Margaret's marriage or children.
6 Eugalenus, *De scorbuto morbo*, pp. 86–88; Martini, 'De scorbuto', in Sennert, *De scorbuto tractatus*, pp. 620–621.

shaking of the limbs for half an hour so that she shook the whole bed. It then persists for ten hours, during which she is unaware and insensible to pain. She suffered from the subsequent attack for six hours. The same day she came to herself beyond the hope of the bystanders **[p. 101]** after having been freed from the attack. Her mother asked her how she was. She replied straight away: 'Where have you all come from to visit me? I do not feel illness or any pain.' She was barely kept awake by the conversation among her friends, but fell asleep again, as if in a waking sleep. Eventually she came to herself for twenty-four hours, but her senses were not yet fully restored.

Being there, I asked if she felt pain in her limbs. She replied that she was so attacked by pain and weariness in her limbs that she could hardly move, and was so bewildered she could not say how she was going to be. Thus Sennert, page 109: *it sometimes happens, he says, that the unhappy shaking and disturbance of all the limbs is associated with some recovery.*[1] She was also disfigured by jaundice throughout the body, with diminution of her periods. I prescribed a cure in this way, in the name of God:

℞: loosening[2] electuary 6dr, cream of tartar 1sc, powdered rhubarb 2sc. Make a bolus: six stools.

For the jaundice:

℞: best Mithridate 1dr, prepared hartshorn 2sc, powder of worms 2dr, barberry conserve 1oz: for two mornings.

She felt better when freed from the jaundice. Next she was purged in this way:

---

1 Sennert, *De scorbuto tractatus*, p. 109.
2 loosening] In Hall's Latin, *ventrifluus* ('loosening') is an adjective, not part of the proper name of the electuary.

℞: *pills* – foetidae, alephanginae, cochiae *each 1sc,* trochiscated agaric ½sc, castor 6gr. *Make 7 pills with sufficient syrup of French lavender.*[1] Give 3 at bedtime, 4 in the morning with an attendant.[2]

Then she used this sneezing powder:

℞: *nutmeg, peony root each ½dr, black hellebore 1sc, pellitory of Spain, white pepper each 1sc. Mix. Make the sneezing powder. Blow a portion of it into the nostrils through a reed.*[3] **[p. 102]** *When it is exactly the expected time of onset in the morning, give two drachms of this opiate every day:*

℞: *scurvy-grass conserve 2oz (antiscorbutic medicines should always be given mixed with others, so that you diminish the evil of the illness)*[4] *mallows, betony conserve each 1oz, old Mithridate, Venice treacle each 1dr, moss from oak, hartshorn shavings, peony seeds, powdered unburied human skull each 4sc. Mix. Take on its own or with betony water*[5] *and a little oil of vitriol.*

These, praise God, fended off the attack and freed her from everything. *She has not fallen into this misfortune any more, but has lived very well and without constraint since then, for many years.*[6]

[Case 114]
[C]ure of hemiplegia, burning fever, worms. The teacher's daughter, Lydia Trapp, about her second year of age:[7] suffered from burning fever and hemiplegia. They expected every day from all this that she would exchange life for death. I restored her in this way, by God's will:

---

1 Bruele, *Praxis medicinae*, p. 59.
2 with an attendant] 'they must especially beware, a melancholy discontented person [...] never be left alone or idle; but as physicians prescribe physic *cum custodia*, let them not be left unto themselves, but with some company or other, lest by that means they aggravate and increase their disease' (Burton 2001: 109).
3 Bruele, *Praxis medicinae*, pp. 59–60.
4 When ... illness] Martini, 'De scorbuto', in Sennert, *De scorbuto tractatus*, p. 708.
5 mallows ... water] Fernel, *Consiliorum liber*, p. 19.
6 Ruland the Elder, 'Centuria III', *Curationum [...] centuriae*, p. 199.
7 Lydia Trapp of Stratford-upon-Avon (1629–?). One of ten children. Her father, John Trapp (Case 177), was a minister and schoolmaster. Married a local minister, William Potter, in 1646.

R: prepared hartshorn 3dr, spring water 1 pint. Boil, reduce to a half, then add a little rose water, lemon syrup 1oz, sugar ½ spoonful, sufficient oil of vitriol for a pleasant tartness in her drink, laying aside all other drinks.

This was applied to the heart:

R*: Venice treacle 1dr, peony root powder ½dr. Make a plaster.* Hang peony roots cut in thin disks on a string around her neck. *Sprinkle her head with peony powder.*[1] Anoint the neck with oil of amber, oil of sassafras each ½dr, spirit of rosemary 6 drops.[2] Mix for the neck.

[p. 103] A plaster for the umbilicus:

R: aloes ½dr, pills – sine quibus 1sc, worms 1sc, myrrh ½sc. Make a plaster for the umbilicus with ox gall.

To remove thirst and provoke a stool, take this potion:

R: loosening syrup of roses 1oz, boiled water 2oz, sufficient oil of vitriol for a pleasant tartness. For the stomach, pectoral ointment.

And so with these few, her complete health was sealed in a few days.[3]

[Case 115]
Cure of painful joints. Lady Underhill, aged 53:[4] with painful joints in her hands, when she rubs them together a flatuous swelling arises at once. She also has sudden flushing of the face. When she reads her voice almost disappears, so that bystanders cannot understand her. She feels as if there are ant bites in many parts of the body. This is due to scurvy.

R: sarsaparilla 4oz, sassafras 1oz agrimony, *scurvy-grass, watercress, brooklime each 1 handful, bark of caper root, rind of Indian myrabolans each*

---

1 Platter, *Observationum* […] *libri sex*, pp. 26–27.
2 spirit of rosemary] A standard preparation; *sp.* in the MS usually abbreviates *species*, a powder, but Hall's use of *gut.* ('drops') in the quantity indicates a liquid.
3 Ruland the Elder, 'Centuria III', *Curationum* […] *centuriae*, p. 207.
4 Catherine, Lady Underhill of Ettington (1580–1662). Catherine Uvedale married Sir Edward Underhill in 1613; they had two daughters who died young. After her husband's death in 1641, Lady Underhill continued to manage the estate.

4sc, polypody of the oak, *liquorice* each ½oz, *stoned raisins 10dr*.[1] Soak overnight in 6 pints spring water. In the morning boil, reduce by half. To the strained liquid add senna 1oz, rhubarb 1dr, one or the other. Once boiled, add Foreest's scheletyrbic syrup 4oz. Make a syrup. Dose: 6 or 8 spoonfuls.

She was rightly purged and was very well, and extolled this syrup with the highest praise. *She was protected from the misfortune*, praise God, *by this one device*.[2]

[Case 116]

[p. 104] Well-tested cure of painful joints. Squire Underhill, aged 50:[3] wretchedly tortured by wandering gout. He suffered pain in the joints of the body, the ankles, knees, arms and neck. I offered the entreating patient the following medical remedy. With God's favour it entirely banished the pains.

℞: powder of sarsaparilla bark, senna each 6dr, cream of tartar 3dr. Mix. Dose 4sc, or 3, or 2, by which he daily evacuated three or four times.

Once the body was purged, he used the following bath:

℞: salt 1lb, live sulphur 1½oz, alum ½lb, squashed bay berries 4oz.

He sat in it up to his knees every day, for an hour in the morning and evening. He was not only freed from the gout, but was also truly cured of the hard flesh beneath his toes. For prevention the following October, I prescribed:

℞: caryocostinum 2½dr, tamarind electuary ½oz, cream of tartar 1sc. Make a bolus with sugar.

Then Platter's pills against gout, dispensed in this form. Swallow 5:

---

1 Martini, 'De scorbuto', in Sennert, *De scorbuto tractatus*, pp. 667–668.
2 Ruland the Elder, 'Centuria III', *Curationum* [...] *centuriae*, p. 218.
3 Edward Underhill of Ettington (1573–1641). Magdalen College, Oxford, BA 1595. Knighted in 1613, and in that year married Catherine (Case 115), daughter of Sir William Uvedale. Sir Edward was a magistrate, and High Sheriff of Warwickshire in 1638. Buried at Ettington in 1641, intestate.

℞: *true colchicum peeled ½oz, aloes, turbith, mechoachan each 1dr, rhubarb, electuaries of myrobalans, citron, yellow myrobalans, mastic each 3sc, euphorbia 2sc, round birthwort root 1sc, St John's wort seeds, ginger, cumin seeds each ½dr, salt of gems ½sc. Make a few pills with ground-pine juice, prepared scammony ½dr.*[1] **[p. 105]** Dose: 1dr each month.

He was thus released entirely from a recurrence of the pain. I nonetheless added the above powder to a ½oz quantity of betony with rose sugar 1oz. He became very well and for several years the pain never returned, praise God. Cured.

[Case 117]
Passing blood. Mr Izod, a gentleman of Toddington, consumed by old age:[2] suffers from bloody micturition on slight movement of the body.

℞: a mass of turpentine pills with rhubarb 2dr, clear turpentine 1dr. Make 15 pills with liquorice powder. Give from a spoon with marsh-mallow syrup.

He used the following tablets:

℞: winter-cherry trochees with opium ½oz, comfrey roots, turpentine boiled hard each 1dr, sugar 2½oz. Make tablets with gum tragacanth infusion, 2sc by weight. *Drink cream of refined barley often, also milk cooked with eggs to an agreeable thickness.*[3]

Cured.

---

1 Platter, *Praxeos* [...] *de doloribus*, p. 711.
2 Henry Izod of Toddington, Gloucestershire (1568–1632). Married Ann Gunn of Saintbury; four children. Their second son Henry became rector of Stanton. Daughter Dorothy married Edward Randolph (the younger brother of Ferrers Randolph; cf. Cases 25, 61 and 99), a recusant. Henry remarried in 1626. His will, made in 1629, left bequests to the church and the poor of Toddington.
3 Horst, *Observationum* [...] *libri quatuor*, p. 282.

[Case 118]

Wind in the stomach. 9 September. Lady Smith,[1] Roman Catholic, beautiful and healthy, very much vexed by wind in the stomach. She took a strong infusion of antimony from an empiric a month ago and is now very much worse. To expel the wind she takes three or four draughts of broth at night, otherwise she can neither sleep for the pain, nor lie peacefully in bed; about 27 years of age.

> R: pills – hiera with agaric, amber, Ruffus's each 1sc. Make six pills, gild them. Give three at bedtime, in the morning take the quantity **[p. 106]** of a nutmeg.

The following electuary:

> R: Crato's steeled electuary 1½oz, opening electuary ½oz. Mix.

She is to take exercise. After meals:

> R: seeds – prepared coriander, fennel, anise, caraway each 1½dr, prepared hartshorn, prepared red coral, cinnamon, nutmeg each ½dr, aromatic rose powder, Galen's laetificans powder, sweet musk each ½sc, sugar to the weight of everything. Make a sweetmeat.

24 October. She sent to me for the above powder, on behalf of the Earl of Leicester, since she had eaten what she had. The next year I saw her in passing, and she thanked me greatly for the powder because she had been altogether freed from her very severe pains. *By the very rapid administration of these, she escaped safe and unharmed, by the will of God to whom be praise in eternity.*[2]

---

1 Elizabeth, Lady Smith of Wootton Wawen (1600–58). Came of a Catholic family in Sussex. In 1620 she married Charles Smith; nine children. Her husband (also Catholic) was knighted in 1619 and inherited the Wootton estate. In 1643 Sir Charles became Viscount Carrington. During the Protectorate he went to France. Lady Carrington moved to Oxfordshire but returned to Wootton.
2 Ruland the Elder, 'Centuria II', *Curationum* [...] *centuriae*, p. 134.

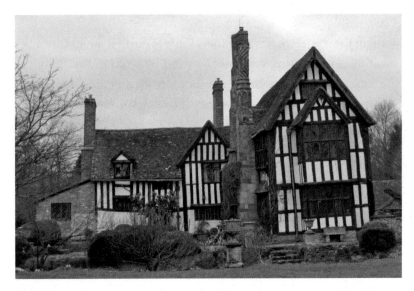

34 Huddington Court, Worcestershire, home of the Roman Catholics John and Margaret Winter. Hall treated Margaret (1595–1629) for a flux (a discharge of blood) from the belly and an excessive quantity of urine (Case 119). Robert (b. 1568) and Thomas Winter (b. 1572), both of Huddington Court, were both prominently involved in the Gunpowder Plot and executed in January 1606.

[Case 119]

[Cure] of a flux from the belly and excessive quantity of urine. Mrs Winter, a gentlewoman, a widow aged 28, Roman Catholic:[1] with a flux from the belly and inflammation of the kidneys. She passes a large amount of urine, three times more than she drinks. She is sick almost to fainting from being tortured by the stone. She has been attacked by loose bowel movements and weakened by confirmed scurvy. She was cured as follows:

℞: best Mithridate 2sc, diascordium ½dr, alkermes confection, prepared hartshorn ½sc, bezoar stone 6gr, pearled manus Christi 1dr,

---

1 Margaret Winter of Huddington, Worcestershire (1595–1629). Margaret Russell married John Winter, son of a prominent Catholic family; three sons. Her husband died in 1622. When Margaret died in 1629, the inventory of her possessions included a watch and a small striking timepiece worth £7.

magisterium of pearls 4gr, prepared coral ½sc, Galen's laetificans electuary 1dr. Mix. Make an electuary with sufficient field poppy syrup.

She swallowed half from a knife blade, which controlled the flux with great relief and **[p. 107]** cheerfulness of spirit. She took the other half at bedtime. That night was more restful than others. To drink: hartshorn decoction.

A plaster for the mouth of the stomach:

℞: Gabriel's aromatic rose powder ½dr, labdanum ½dr, best Mithridate, Venice treacle each 1dr, yellow wax 2dr. Dissolve in Crato's stomach oil. Make a plaster by the usual method.

The stomach became constipated from this: loosened by the following pills:

℞: pills – Ruffus's, of amber each 1dr. Make 10 pills. Give three at bedtime. Repeat the cordial.

Next I gave the following potion:

℞: *Dornkrell's antiscorbutic water* 4oz, *the same for the spleen*[1] 2oz, Foreest's scheletyrbic syrup. Mix. Give 8 spoonfuls in the morning.

Then she used this electuary:

℞: conserves of bugloss, clove-gillyflowers, clove pinks each 1oz, scurvy-grass conserve 2oz, preserved elecampane root 3dr, diarrhodon Abbatis powder, diapleres archonticon electuary ½oz, alkermes confection 2sc. Make an electuary with sufficient Foreest's scheletyrbic syrup. Dose: the quantity of a hazelnut on an empty stomach. Repeat the hartshorn decoction.

By these, glory to God, she was properly cured, and freed from all misfortunes.

---

1 Dornkrell, *Dispensatorium novum*, pp. 33–36.

[Case 120]

Cure of scurvy. Lady Jenkinson,[1] good-looking, devout and modest: tortured by headache, slight giddiness, heartburn, hypochondriac pain, fainting, wakefulness, heat spells briefly in the hands and feet, weakness without cause, loose flesh in the gums and often blood-stained.

℞: pills – hiera with agaric, Ruffus's each 1dr, alephanginae 2sc. Make pills with betony water, 15 pills with diatartar 2sc. Take **[p. 108]** 3 before sleeping.

Take the following decoction in the morning:

℞: the following steeled wine:

℞: orris root, bark of dwarf-elder, elder, capers, tamarisk, chicory, couch-grass, fennel, asparagus, madder each ½oz, gentian root 2dr, green shoots of wormwood ½oz, bindweed, mugwort, agrimony, white horehound each ½ handful, centaury tops 2½dr, the cordial flowers each 1½dr, sweet flag 2dr, liquorice 1oz, senna leaves 2oz, agaric ½oz, mechoachan 3dr, prepared steel filings ½oz, cream of tartar 1dr, rhubarb 3dr, ginger 1dr, cinnamon ½dr, anise seeds 2dr. Soak for three days in 4 pints white wine, in a closed vessel in a double boiler. Then boil on a slow fire for an hour, the vessel closed with a cork: [take] 4oz of this, Foreest's scheletyrbic syrup 2oz, for three mornings, as well as the antiscorbutic beer for Mrs Talbot, as on page 87. I added sassafras ½oz, sarsaparilla 2oz, betony, agrimony, fumitory each 1 handful.

℞: scurvy-grass conserve 2oz, wormwood, diaserios, bugloss, clove-gillyflowers, damask roses, elecampane root each ½oz, rhodium wood, sweet flag, prepared arum root, diarrhodon Abbatis powder, diapleres archonticon, alkermes confection each ½dr. Make an electuary with sufficient Foreest's scheletyrbic syrup, and cover with gold leaf as above.

---

1 Anne, Lady Jenkinson of Walcot, near Charlbury, Oxfordshire (1600–86). Daughter of Sir Robert Lee of Billesley, who was Sheriff in 1620. Married Sir Robert Jenkinson (of a diplomatic family); ten children. Anne's own family also had political connections. Hall may have treated her when she visited Billesley. (This was where the Halls' own daughter, Elizabeth, later married John Barnard.)

Drink the following julep:

℞: *antiscorbutic water 3oz, splenitic 2oz,*[1] *Foreest's scheletyrbic 3oz.*

For the catarrh she used the powder for the coronal suture:[2]

℞: *mastic, frankincense, amber, cloves, sandarach wood, aloes, red roses each 1dr. Sprinkle the powder on the coronal suture.*[3]

She was much better. She was purged thus, as was needed:

℞: pills – Ruffus's, alephanginae, diatartar each 1sc, pills **[p. 109]** hiera with agaric 2sc. Make six pills with sufficient antiscorbutic water. Take three at bedtime.

5 December: tortured by toothache:

℞: scurvy-grass water 6oz, red rose, plantain waters each 3oz, rose honey, simple diamoschum each 1oz, sufficient spirit of vitriol for a pleasant tartness. Dose: as much in the mouth as she can gargle.

She was freed from the toothache, and, glory to God, completely freed from all symptoms.

[Case 121]
1629. [Cure] of bloody urination, stones. Butler, of Stratford-upon-Avon:[4] produces large amounts of bloody urine on slight movement of the body, with oppressive pain in the kidneys. He has been attacked by very great heat on urinating, maximally around the prepuce. *This is* [due to] *no other material than dispersed tartar, from the coagulation of which grains of sand are afterwards produced* (see Horst, observation 39, page 284).[5] He used sarsaparilla decoction for eight days. Afterwards he used *tormentil, which when drunk with wine, cures*

---

1 Dornkrell, *Dispensatorium novum*, pp. 33–36.
2 coronal suture] The transverse suture across the top of the skull, roughly from ear to ear.
3 da Monte, *Consultationes medicae*, col. 348.
4 No positive identification. Possibly Robert Butler, a glover, whose father had been bailiff, churchwarden and alderman. But Hall does not accord him high status. Possibly Robert Butler, noted as surgeon in 1606.
5 Horst, *Observationum* […] *libri quatuor*, p. 284.

the torture of dripping urine (well-tested on Stephen Taylor of Alveston, and by John of Gaddesden, page 510).[1] *Nor is there any equal to it*, as John says in his book. *Apply thin lead sheets perforated with many holes and sprinkled with wine vinegar, to the kidney region, and change often.*[2]

The illness was in large part diminished within eight days, and he was cured by using these.

[Case 122]
Cure of scurvy, white flux, uterine wind. Mrs Richardson, a gentle-woman, Roman Catholic:[3] suffers from uterine wind (so that when she passed urine she breaks much wind from the womb, just as if from the anus), scorbutic weakness, headache, **[p. 110]** excessive red flux. When this stops she then suffers from excessive white flux. She was often attacked by lower backache with great heat in the back, very great weakness of the whole body and distress. She was oppressed by headache, worst at the back. She cannot stand light. She had a satisfactory, praiseworthy appetite, feels an aversion to medicines. A restorative of a veal joint with a rooster, and shavings of hartshorn and china were crushed every morning in our milk whey with pearled manus Christi.

To control the flux:

R: milk whey 3oz, *frog-spawn water*[4] 2 spoonfuls, pearled manus Christi 2sc, alkermes confection 2sc. *On the back: lead sheets perforated and wetted with wine vinegar.*[5]

---

1 John of Gaddesden, *Praxis medica*, p. 510
2 Bruele, *Praxis medicinae*, p. 351, and Bernard de Gordon, *Lilium medicinae*, p. 602.
3 Lane identified this patient as Elizabeth Richardson, baptised 1569, married 1607, who bore three children between 1607 and 1611. Her husband died in 1624. Cooke omitted Hall's closing remark: 'after her husband died she married and bore children six years afterwards'. It is hard to match this with Lane's patient, for whom no other marriage is recorded either before or after that to William Richardson. The identification is doubtful, and no date can be suggested for the consultation.
4 Croll, *Basilica chymica*, pp. 276, 277.
5 Bernard de Gordon, *Lilium medicinae*, p. 602.

A plaster for the womb:

> ℞: prepared hartshorn 1sc, alkermes confection ½sc, bezoar stone 3gr, scabious water 2oz, lemon syrup ½oz. Mix.

Give at the time she feels cold, because she had an erratic fever.

> ℞: snail water (my own compound), simple of frogs each 4oz, alkermes confection 2sc, pearled manus Christi ½oz, *antiscorbutic water* 6oz, *splenitic* 2oz.[1] Mix. Repeat and add 1½oz of Rodrigo de Fonseca's laetificans syrup.[2]

She recovered her lost strength wonderfully, and said this divine water far surpassed potable gold, and she wished never to be without it because, she said, it was the equal of anything. She was thus completely cured, and after the death of her husband remarried and bore an heir six years later.

[Case 123]

[**p. 111**] Cure of vomiting, swelling of the feet, quotidian fever, wasting, scurvy. Mrs Peers,[3] a gentlewoman of Alveston, Roman Catholic, beautiful, about the age of 28: oppressed by melancholy, vain attempts to vomit, swelling of the feet in the evenings, weakness of the whole body, quotidian scorbutic fever with slight shivering, splenic pain, various pains in the joints. Urine: like clear water.

> ℞: tamarind electuary ½oz, diasereos syrup 1oz, our oxymel ½oz, bugloss water 2oz, oil of vitriol 6 drops. Mix. Six stools.

The next day the urine was turbid. The following day:

---

1 Dornkrell, *Dispensatorium novum*, pp. 33–36.
2 Rodrigo ... syrup] There are several versions of laetificans syrup. I have not yet found one attributed to Rodrigo de Fonseca.
3 Clare Peers of Alveston (?–1636). Daughter of a gentleman, Andrew Benlow. Married in 1612 to Thomas Peers (of a wealthy family); six children. Both Clare and Thomas were fined for recusancy. William Dugdale notes Thomas as a Royalist in *The Antiquities of Warwickshire*. Their youngest son Philip became a physician in 1642 and died in Maryland.

℞: aromatic rose powder 1sc, tamarind electuary 2dr, with other items added as before.

At bedtime:

℞: bezoar stone 3gr, Paracelsus's laudanum 2gr, alkermes confection ½sc.

The night was restful. 14th:

℞: poppy syrup 1oz, scabious water 1oz, sufficient oil of vitriol, bezoar stone 4gr, a little rose water.

She used steeled wine as for Mrs Talbot page 87 and Lady Jenkinson page 108, to which I added Foreest's scheletyrbic syrup.

℞: wine 6oz, scheletyrbic syrup 4oz, *antiscorbutic water* 2oz, *splenitic* 2oz,[1] laetificans syrup 3oz.

℞: prepared hartshorn 1sc, alkermes confection 2sc, magisterium of pearls, tincture of coral each 6gr, pearled manus Christi ½dr, bezoar stone 6gr, sufficient scurvy-grass conserve. Make an electuary with honey. I added pleres archonticon powder.

She was freed from her symptoms. On account of sadness she fell into suffocation of the mother:

℞: castor 1dr, bryony dregs ½sc. Make 5 pills with water for the womb. Give at nightfall. To the umbilicus: caranna plaster with musk.

She inhaled assafoetida smoke through her nostrils: successfully relieved. Afterwards she was purged:

℞: pills – Ruffus's, simple hiera powder each 1½sc, castor 1sc, bryony dregs ½sc, sufficient water for the womb. Make five pills: [take] at bedtime.

She was thus properly cured.

---

1 Dornkrell, *Dispensatorium novum*, pp. 33–36.

[Case 124]

[p. 112] Cure of *motion of the womb, pain, choking.*[1] Alice Collins, Lady Puckering's companion, about 24 years old:[2] tortured by suffocation of the mother. Her periods were obstructed, when the paroxysm ends she bursts into tears. Also, the urine is like spring water. *I did indeed prescribe these medicines to root out the illness and symptoms:*[3]

> ℞: *bryony root ½oz, senna leaves ½oz, ginger ½dr, cinnamon 1dr, sugar 6dr. Infuse overnight in milk whey 1½ pints.* In the morning, boil a little and strain. Add compound mugwort syrup 2oz. *Give 5oz of this infusion to drink* hot,[4] in the morning, for a few days.

She was rightly purged and became well.

[Case 125]

Cure of worms. Hester Sylvester,[5] the daughter of Mrs Smith, gentlewoman, now married in Burford: attacked by worms last year, and cured by me with the following powder. Now she sent to me for it.

> ℞: *sea-moss, French wormwood each 1oz, white dittany, snakeweed, tormentil each ½oz. Reduce all to a powder, sprinkle with sharp vinegar and dry in shade. Take this, from ½dr to 3dr by weight* (for her, ½dr) *according to strength and the degree of the illness. It is sometimes put in wine, sometimes our purslane water, or in an apple cooked in the ashes.*[6]

She was cured again, praise God.

---

1 Ruland the Elder, 'Centuria VI', *Curationum* […] *centuriae*, p. 62.

2 Alice Collins (1602–56), waiting woman to Lady Puckering of Warwick Priory. Daughter of Francis Collins, a Warwick attorney who acted for William Shakespeare when he bought lands and tithes in 1605, and prepared Shakespeare's will. Hall treated her in 1626. Married Thomas Greene (not Shakespeare's 'cousin') in 1633. Died a widow, and buried at St Mary's in Warwick.

3 Ruland the Elder, 'Centuria VI', *Curationum* […] *centuriae*, p. 447.

4 Ruland the Elder, 'Centuria I', *Curationum* […] *centuriae*, p. 63.

5 Dates not known. This child was the daughter of Paul and Margaret Sylvester; Margaret was the daughter of Alderman Francis Smith of Stratford. Hester married Richard Cox in Burford in 1649. No record of any children.

6 Amatus Lusitanus, *Curationum medicinalium centuriae quatuor*, p. 313.

[Case 126]

[p. 113] Cure of tympany, hoarse voice. Lynes of Stratford-upon-Avon:[1] suffers from tympany. Age: 53. She has been weighed down by a huge swelling of the belly so that she could hardly get about, with hoarseness of the voice and aversion to food. Her friends despair of her as in a hopeless condition. Symptoms of dropsy also accompanied this, as they commonly do. *In order to cure and avert these most difficult of misfortunes I establish, with the help of divine grace, a method of treatment like this:*[2]

> ℞: *orris root, wild ginger, pellitory of Spain, elecampane, briar, bark of elder root each 3dr, origanum, calamint each 1 pinch, bindweed 10z, mecoachan 3dr, anise seed, bayberries each ½oz. Boil by the rule of practice in 2 pints white wine in a closed bain-Marie for four hours, then strain and sweeten with sugar. Drink 6oz morning and evening.*

Then purge her with bindweed pills in this way:[3]

> ℞: *tops of bindweed 2sc, cinnamon 1sc, aggregative pills 1dr, alhandal trochees ½sc, wild cucumber 4gr. With orris root juice, make 5 pills from 1dr. Take 3 about midnight,*[4] *repeat as needed.*

The stomach and other organs should be strengthened with this electuary:

> ℞: *orris root juice 3dr, canella, galangal each 2dr, cloves, mace each 1dr, zedoary 2sc, bindweed ½oz. Powder, mix with purified honey to form an electuary. Drink it on alternate, or every day, as much as a hazelnut.*

I also prescribed powders to be taken with meals, so that the stomach, cooled by the undigested humours, warms moderately. This promotes digestion readily and disperses wind.[5]

> ℞: prepared coriander seeds ½oz, **[p. 114]** fennel, anise seeds each 2dr, caraway 1dr, cinnamon 1dr, roots of sweet flag and galangal,

---

1 Joan Lynes of Stratford-upon-Avon (1575–?). Probably Joan Richardson, who married Humphrey Lynes in 1598; one son, also Humphrey.
2 Ruland the Elder, 'Centuria VI', *Curationum* […] *centuriae*, p. 461.
3 Feyens, *De flatibus*, p. 175.
4 Feyens, *De flatibus*, p. 176.
5 Feyens, *De flatibus*, pp. 176–177.

dried citron rind each 1dr, red roses ½dr, sugar equal to the weight of all. Take ½ spoonful after meals.

With these she began to feel much better. 4 January 1630.

[Case 127]

Cure of fits of the mother, that is, melancholy. Mrs Baker, a gentlewoman of Stratford-upon-Avon aged 38:[1] tortured by lower backache with desire to urinate. Urine: little and clear. She used the following for fear of scurvy, with the desired result.

℞: Rodericus de Fonseca's laetificans syrup 2dr, his *diartartar* 1dr, bugloss water 3oz.[2] Mix. Six stools.

℞: pills – Ruffus's 2sc, hiera with agaric 1sc, foetidae pills 1sc, castor ½sc. Make seven pills with mugwort water, gild them. Seven stools.

℞: sliced sassafras wood 1½oz, best cinnamon 1oz. Infuse in spring water 14oz, for twelve hours. Then boil, reduce to half. To the strained liquid add refined white sugar 12oz. Boil to the consistency of an electuary, add dianthos, bugloss conserve each 6oz, clove-gillyflower flowers ½oz, preserved elecampane root, preserved ginger each 2dr, aromatic rose powder 7gr, alkermes confection ½oz, ambergris, musk each 7gr. Mix. Make an electuary.

This patient started to become better within fourteen days, with ministrations for thirty days, not neglecting a rational and appropriate diet. She recovered her former strength very well. Praise God.

---

1 Katherine Baker of Stratford-upon-Avon. Dates unknown. Gentlewoman from a wealthy family. Third wife of Alderman Daniel Baker, a draper and Puritan, who already had four children. He opposed the enclosure of common land at Welcombe. Married Katherine in about 1619. In his will he left his 'well-beloved wife' well provided for.

2 Fonseca, *Consultationes*, p. 53.

[Case 128]
[Cure] of persistent cough. Smith, aged 38, of Stratford-upon-Avon:[1] tortured for a long time by persistent cough, viscous phlegm and **[p. 115]** headache.

> R: flowers of sulphur 2dr, powders of elecampane, orris, liquorice each 1dr, sufficient honey to bind everything. Make an electuary, to which add oil of sulphur 10 drops. Make a linctus.

Then:

> R: orpiment 1dr, sufficient egg yolk. Make a mass from the ingredients, dry them by the fire, then powder. Add to the powder tobacco leaves ½dr, coltsfoot 3sc, anise seed 4sc, anise oil 3 drops. Make a fumigant. Take a little through a tube in the mouth.

These cured her in a short time.

[Case 129]
Well-tested cure of scurvy. 8 February 1630. [My] wife:[2] suffered for a long time from lower backache, convulsions, diseased gums, foul-smelling breath, wind, melancholy, cardiac passion, spontaneous tiredness, difficulty in breathing, fear of choking, binding of the bowel movements, abdominal torment. She was weak and restless at night.

> R: tamarind electuary ½oz, cream of tartar 1dr. Mix.

Oxycroceum plaster was applied to the side. She was freed from the abdominal torment and lower backache. 10th: She caught a cold, relapsed wretchedly and was attacked by lower backache so that she could not lie in bed. When the attendants helped her, she cried out as if pricked by thorns. I applied this liniment for the lumbar pains:

---

1 No identification possible. Modest status.
2 Hall's wife and Shakespeare's daughter. Hall treated her in 1630, aged 44 (cf. Case 19).

℞: chicken fat, oils of sweet almonds, dill, roses, mucilage of **[p. 116]** marsh-mallow root extracted with mallow water each ½oz. Mix.

After the anointing, I prescribed oxycroceum plaster to be applied with the desired outcome, for the night was more peaceful. However, she was tortured by wind in the morning, so I used Daniel Sennert's antiscorbutic electuary, compounded in this way:

℞: *conserve of scurvy-grass buds and flowers 3oz, flowers of bugloss, clove-gillyflowers, damask roses each 1½oz, preserved coconut flesh, preserved citron peel chopped very small, juniper berry juice 3dr, alkermes confection 1½dr, cinnamon syrup 6dr. Make the electuary with sufficient scurvy-grass juice or Foreest's scheletyrbic to bind it. Add spirits of sulphuric acid for a pleasantly bitter taste.*[1] Make it.

For constipation of the belly, this suppository:

℞: honey 1oz, hiera picra powder 2sc, alhandal trochees ½sc, cumin seeds ½oz. Make a long suppository.

For the cardiac passion she used pleres archonticon electuary. She used the above electuary, ½oz on an empty stomach, and pleres archonticon electuary at any time whatever, and afterwards the steeled wine:

℞: herbs – fumitory, brooklime, watercress, scurvy-grass, betony, agrimony, harts-tongue each ½ handful, bark of capers, ash, tamarisk each ½oz, *elecampane root*, polypody of the oak each 3dr, madder, liquorice, sweet flag, *eringoes each ½oz, yellow sandalwood, red coral, ivory shavings each 6dr, cloves, mace, cinnamon, ginger each 3dr, spleenwort, broom flowers, rosemary, marigold, dodder each 1 pinch, juniper berries, steel filings* (prepared according to Crato)[2] *4oz, white wine 8 pints. Soak for eight days at least on a fire in a bain-Marie, shaking twice a day. Then strain three or four times, add saffron ½dr to the strained liquid, first extracted in sufficient scurvy-grass water, alkermes confection 2sc, with sufficient best sugar that the*

---

1 Martini, 'De scorbuto', in Sennert, *De scorbuto tractatus*, pp. 674–675.
2 *elecampane … Crato*] Crato, *Consiliorum* […] *liber secundus*, pp. 378–79.

wine tastes pleasant. Dose: one or two spoonfuls at first, thereafter increase as is needed.[1]

These cured her, praise God.

[Case 130]

[p. 117] Cure of long-established scurvy. Mrs Combe, a gentlewoman aged about 36 years:[2] seized by putrefaction of the gums, difficulty in breathing, weakness with sudden blindness. Pulse: small and unequal. Urine: thick and red, then clear, the following day full of excrement like bran. She is seized by vomiting, lower backache as if her back were broken (so that she could not move), varied pain in the parts of the body. The pain in the body and back is so severe and troublesome that she wishes rather *to die than to live* with it any longer.[3] I saw her struggle with the pain that year, even while she was pregnant. *She complains of being transfixed by something like a spike from the opening of the stomach to her mouth,*[4] and attacked by wind to a remarkable degree. A preparation for the humours, like this:

℞: our oxymel 3oz, diasereos syrup 2oz, Foreest's scheletyrbic syrup 2oz, watercress water 3oz. Give 4oz with good wine on three mornings: two or three stools each day.

Then she was purged:

℞: pills – hiera with agaric, alephanginae, Ruffus's each 2sc, oils of sage, china 6 drops. Make 10 pills with betony water, gild them. Take three at bedtime: rightly purged.

Afterwards she used steeled wine as on page 116 and the antiscorbutic electuary as for my wife. Then take our antiscorbutic water

---

1 4oz ... needed] Du Chesne, *Pharmacopoea dogmaticorum*, p. 74.
2 Katherine Combe of Old Stratford (1595–1652). A gentlewoman, daughter of Edward and Elizabeth Boughton. Married in 1612 to William Combe; one son, nine daughters. Combe was a magistrate, Parliamentary supporter and twice Sheriff. The Boughtons were firm Royalists, and there were family disputes.
3 Based on Vulgate, Tob. 3:6.
4 Eugalenus, *De scorbuto morbo*, p. 180.

as for Mrs Richardson. For the lower back: the above ointment of chicken fat and other ingredients as on the previous page. After the anointing, apply Foreest's ammoniac salve. For corruption of the gums and weaknesses in the mouth:

R: simple scurvy-grass water 6oz, *iron water* 7oz,[1] rose honey and mulberry simple each 2oz, sufficient oil of vitriol for a pleasant tartness. Make an oral rinse.

Her drink was antiscorbutic beer prepared as on page 116. A stomach plaster:

R: diambra powder, Gabrieli's aromatic rose powder each 1½sc, mastic oil 1dr, spikenard and mace oils each 1dr, cloves 5gr, liquid styrax 1dr, yellow wax 6dr, labdanum 3dr. Make a plaster. For the back, use oxycroceum plaster frequently. Take 5 pills of Cyprus turpentine and tartar before sleeping.

She was freed from this sad illness, and bore a beautiful daughter, for she was pregnant. *The use of these revived her beyond all hope, and restored her to complete health by the power of almighty God most high, to whom alone be thanks, blessing and perpetual praise, forever and ever.*[2] Amen.

[Case 131]

[p. 118] Cure of a bastard tertian fever. Lady Clark, about 44 years old:[3] seized by a bastard tertian fever. She had two attacks, with the third coming on I gave the following emetic against it:

R: the chymical cup 6dr: seven vomits, one stool.

---

1 Baudouin Ronsse, 'De scorbuto', in Sennert, *De scorbuto tractatus*, pp. 286–288. Water in which hot iron has been cooled.
2 Ruland the Elder, 'Centuria III', *Curationum [...] centuriae*, p. 213.
3 Dorothy, Lady Clark of Broom Court (1585–1669). Married twice; no children. Daughter of Thomas Hobson, a wealthy Cambridge carrier (of 'Hobson's choice' fame). Married William Hay, who died in 1617. Within the year Dorothy married Sir Simon Clark (cf. Case 136), who had five children. Continued to live at Broom Court until her death aged 84.

She had a slight attack. Then when the hot spell was coming on she had the hartshorn decoction. On the intervening day, this enema:

R: mallows, betony, spurge, origanum, calamint each ½ handful, seeds of anise, fennel each 2dr, whole barley 1 pinch, chamomile and melilot flowers each 1 pinch. Make a decoction to 100z. In the strained liquid dissolve catholicon, diaphoenicon each 10z, hiera picra powder, Holland powder each 1dr. Make an enema: rightly purged.

Before the attack:

R: alkermes confection ½sc, Paracelsus's laudanum 2gr, magisterium of pearls 3gr. Mix as one dose, which restored her.

Thanks be to God, the Lady recovered in every way.

[Case 132]
Passing blood with pain and burning urine on slight movement of the body. Age: 39. Mr Thomas Underhill, a gentleman of Lamcot, about 39 years old:[1] weakened for a long time by the above.

R: a mass of Crato's turpentine pills with rhubarb 2dr. Form 6 pills from 1dr.[2] Give 3 in the morning, coated in liquorice powder. Dose: ½dr with a few spoonfuls of Fernel's marsh-mallow syrup.

When this was finished:

R: trochees of winter cherry with opium ½oz, comfrey roots, turpentine boiled hard each 1dr, sugar 2½oz. Make tablets weighing 2sc with gum tragacanth infusion in mallow water. Take one in the evening.

---

1 Thomas Underhill of Lambcote, Ettington (1590–1669). Second son of Thomas Underhill and his heir to Loxley manor. Married Elizabeth Daston in 1616; four children. Later sold Loxley to Sir Simon Clark (Case 136). In 1650 he inherited a house in Oxhill from his uncle George (Case 108) and moved there. Buried in St Lawrence's church.
2 Crato, *Consiliorum* [...] *liber secundus*, p. 371.

In the morning:

℞: clear turpentine ½oz. Dissolve in egg yolk as is the practice, add honey 1oz, rose sugar tablets 2oz, good wine 6oz. Mix. Drink the milky **[p. 119]** liquid, up to 1oz every morning: three or four stools daily from 1oz.

He had prepared trochees at bedtime, *also a perforated lead sheet wetted with vinegar was applied to the kidneys night and day.*[1] He was cured of everything.

[Case 133]

Passing blood without pain. Katherine Sturley of Stratford-upon-Avon,[2] aged 44, stout and fat: *passing entirely bloody urine without any pain in the back*[3] or at the mouth of the bladder. *She feels nothing in the excretion, neither from a stone nor ulceration. The cause of this conditions remains to be sought in the bile-filled sharpness of the blood, and weakness of the kidneys.*[4] *I concluded from this that the over-sharp blood should be mellowed, and the retaining power of the kidneys strengthened. I therefore prescribed the following digestive potion, which was*:

℞: *liquorice shavings 6dr, wheat barley 1 pinch, jujubes 5, leaves of water-lilies, violets, roses each 1 pinch, purslane, sorrel seeds, the four greater cold seeds each 1dr, chicory root 1oz, green shoots of endive, sorrel, plantain, fumitory each 1 handful. Boil in chickpea broth. Strain. Sweeten with sugar candy 2oz. Make a potion. Drink a third on an empty stomach for eight days.*

I prescribed the following electuary to strengthen the kidneys:

℞: *burnt prepared hartshorn, prepared red coral each 1dr, old rose sugar, diacydonium without powders each 1½oz, sufficient rose juice syrup. Make a soft electuary,*[5] take ½oz two hours before meals, twice a day.

---

1 Bernard de Gordon, *Lilium medicinae*, p. 602.
2 Katherine Sturley of Stratford-upon-Avon (1585–?). Townswoman, daughter of Abraham Sturley, a Cambridge graduate who settled in Stratford. Katherine was unmarried, and 'stout and fat' when Hall treated her. No record of marriage.
3 Horst, *Observationum* [...] *libri quatuor*, p. 279.
4 Horst, *Observationum* [...] *libri quatuor*, p. 280.
5 Horst, *Observationum* [...] *libri quatuor*, p. 280.

These cured her, but chiefly the following medicine:

℞: *sanicle, lady's mantle, golden-rod, wintergreen, betony, agrimony each 1 handful, marsh mallow 2 handfuls, fern, flowers of chamomile, St John's wort, mugwort, briars, origanum, flowers and root of tormentil each 1 handful. Make a linen bag, three-quarters of a* **[p. 120]** *forearm's length long and broad. Slice the herbs finely and spread evenly so that they fill everything and are not placed too thickly. Sew the bag together wherever the herbs are not, then boil the bag in the dregs of good wine. Press the boiled bag little by little between two wooden rollers, place it on the whole lumbar region. The patient should in fact lie face down. Repeat this until the flux of blood stops. It is convenient to prepare two bags so that as one cools, the other may be applied hot.*

NOTE: *If fresh blood is thoroughly mixed with the urine but does not smell strongly, and if a stabbing pain, not really painful, appears in the back where the kidneys are, then* [the blood] *certainly stems from the kidneys. Anyone who passes blood suddenly and spontaneously, especially visibly, demonstrates a ruptured vein in the kidneys. If someone passes blood and sand, and suffers from poor urinary stream with pain in the hypogastrium – that is, the belly and peritoneum – or if it reaches the thighs, then the area around the bladder is troubled (Hippocrates Book 4, aphorism 78).*[1]

[Case 134]

Continual burning fever with abdominal constipation. Lady Hunks, aged 69:[2] attacked by a continual burning fever with torment in the sides and stomach ache, tortured by abdominal constipation for eight days. *It happened in these lamentable diseases that the urine appeared confused and heralded death. But her friends and the patient, struck by these most severe misfortunes, appealed to me. The Lady, from giving*

---

1 Willich, *Urinarum probationes*, p. 216.
2 Katherine, Lady Hunks of Arrow (1565–1646). Daughter of Sir John Conway of Ragley and granddaughter of Sir Fulke Greville. In 1587 married Thomas Hunks; ten children. Hunks was a professional soldier, who was knighted in Ireland in 1605. Her brother was Secretary of State to James I. Their five surviving sons were all soldiers. Widowed in 1631.

up hope, was healed again through almighty God the Chief Physician, and escaped in this way:[1]

R̴: green shoots of mallow, **[p. 121]** marsh mallow, good-King-Henry each 1 handful. Make a decoction.

R̴: of this 12oz, diaphoenicon, diacatholicon each 1oz, holy powder 1dr. Make an enema: two stools.

Afterwards our antipyretic julep. Apply marsh-mallow ointment with sweet almond oil to the painful side:

R̴: *marsh-mallow ointment 2oz, sweet almond oil ½oz. Dissolve, mix by the fire. For the ointment with which she anointed her side, she placed it on a folded cloth smeared with warm butter, and the pain diminished.*[2]

The next day:

R̴: ½ pint of the prepared decoction, the chymical cup 2oz. Make an enema: three stools.

An expectorant:

R̴: magisterial scabious syrup 1oz, du Chesne's raisin lohoch 2oz.

Her diet was moistening. To drink: this decoction:

R̴: *wheat barley 3oz, roses, violets each 1 pinch, liquorice shavings 3dr, raisins 2oz, figs 3, sugar candy 2oz. Boil in 16 pints water until 2 pints are gone. Drink the strained liquid.*[3]

The fever stopped, thirst diminished, appetite returned. She breathed with less difficulty, and slept well. Beyond every hope and expectation in her old age, all her symptoms improved within fourteen days, by the hand and power of God almighty. She said that she was revived from death and rejuvenated in old age. To God the all-powerful and omnipotent physician alone be praise, for ever and ever.[4]

---

1 Ruland the Elder, 'Centuria IV', *Curationum* […] *centuriae*, p. 352.
2 Ruland the Elder, 'Centuria III', *Curationum* […] *centuriae*, p. 181.
3 Ruland the Elder, 'Centuria III', *Curationum* […] *centuriae*, p. 181.
4 Ruland the Elder, 'Centuria IV', *Curationum* […] *centuriae*, p. 353.

[Case 135]
Cure of giddiness, headache, darkened vision. Baronet Puckering,
about 38 years old,[1] *a man remarkably learned, of uncommon constitution, very thin and phlegmatic,*[2] as devoted to the Muses as anyone:
he followed the best way of life and also an excellent diet. He
complained of slight giddiness, and *after meals suddenly lost strength,
accompanied now and then by headache and followed by darkness of vision and
poor appetite.*[3] Urine: well coloured but frothy. Other effects sprang
from sympathy of the vision with digestion.

[The Plan]:[4]
[1] *The weakness of the digestion should be aided;*
2. The head and nervous system **[p. 122]** *should be strengthened;*
*3. the causative fault, both when received into the head and about to be received,
should be diverted and removed.*

1. *First of all, a gentle evacuation of the main passages, with ½oz of manna
dissolved in broth.*[5] I prescribed herbs, agrimony and whole chicory,
in broth: three stools.

2. He was purged:

R: pills – of peony 1dr, amber, Ruffus's each 1sc, *Fernel's for headache*
2sc.[6] Make 15 pills with betony water. Take 3 before sleeping: three
stools in the morning.

---

1 Sir Thomas Puckering of Warwick Priory (1592–1635) (cf. Case 156). His lawyer
father, Sir John, left the priory and other estates to his young son in 1596. Thomas
travelled in Europe, and was a companion of Henry, Prince of Wales. Knighted
in 1612. Served as High Sheriff of Warwickshire in 1625. In 1630 he established
a charity for the poor of Warwick. Was a friend of the Puritan Thomas Dugard.
2 Foreest, *De febribus ephemeris et continuis,* p. 178.
3 Horst, *Observationum* [...] *libri quatuor,* p. 104. These form three subheadings in
Horst's text.
4 Plans set out and numbered like this are common in *practicae*; this one, borrowed
from Horst's *Observationum,* is the only example in Hall.
5 Horst, *Observationum* [...] *libri quatuor,* p. 104.
6 Fernel's for headache] See Case 23, n. 6.

3. When these were finished, he used the carminative powder on page 94 after meals, with added sweet diamoschum 1sc.

4. *We prescribed rolls for the head*:

℞: *powder for sweet diamoschum 1dr, pressed nutmeg oil 1sc, oil of white amber 3 drops, ambergris 4gr, sugar dissolved in lavender water 4oz. Make a confection in rolls, take two or three on an empty stomach.*[1]

With all of these God blessed him from on high, and he wrote back that his head was greatly relieved by their use.

5. Nevertheless, I wished the haemorrhoid veins to be emptied with leeches. This was happily successful. These, by the favour of almighty God the most high, perfectly cured one who deserved well of the people. He used the following for prevention, the following autumn:

℞: roots of fennel, parsley each 1oz, butcher's broom, asparagus each 1½oz, sweet flag 2oz, agrimony, betony, maidenhair each ½ handful, elecampane root 2dr, stoned raisins 1 handful, liquorice 1dr, broom flowers, rosemary each 1 pinch, anise seeds, sweet fennel each 2dr. Make a decoction in sufficient bugloss and borage waters for ½ pint. In the decoction infuse senna leaves ½oz, powdered rhubarb 2dr, cinnamon 2sc. Make an infusion in the coals overnight. Strain in the morning, add to the strained liquid chicory syrup with rhubarb 2½oz, **[p. 123]** Augsburg syrup 1oz, sufficient oil of vitriol for a pleasant acidity. Divide into 2 equal parts and pour into vials for 2 doses: four stools from the first dose, seven from the second.

After the preparation of the humour he was purged thus:

℞: pills – of peony 1dr, amber, Ruffus's each 1sc, *Fernel's for headache* 2sc,[2] oils of sage, china 5 drops. Make 15 pills with betony water. Take 3 at bedtime, in the morning 2: five stools, and continue so. Then he is to use the powder as on page 122, adding sweet diamoschum powder 3sc: in the morning 1 or 2 rolls (page 122) to which I added alkermes confection 1sc.

---

1 Horst, *Observationum* […] *libri quatuor*, p. 105.
2 Fernel's for headache] See Case 23, n. 6.

After a while, I restored him. He regained, day by day, his former health.[1]

[Case 136]
Burning tertian fever. Baronet Clark of Broom Court, about 57 years old:[2] seized by a burning tertian fever with stomach ache and headache. Urine: red, and it broke the glass at the end of the collection. *He followed my advice, so that through God's grace I rescued him within three days:*[3]

℞: the chymical cup ½oz, our oxymel 2oz: seven vomits, eight stools.

After draining this, he discharged much upwards and downwards,[4] *and in a few days everything was ejected and he was bending towards health.*[5] The next day I gave hartshorn decoction, which he took frequently during the day. He sang the highest praises of [these remedies] with which God might bless him from on high. After three days of treatment, not neglecting a prudent diet, he completely recovered his earlier strength.

[Case 137]
Cure of a desperate quinsy. The [2nd] Earl of Northampton, about 29 years of age:[6] tortured by quinsy with inflammation of the throat, with an accompanying fever. *He does not draw breath unless*

---

1 Ruland the Elder, 'Centuria III', *Curationum* […] *centuriae*, p. 217.
2 Sir Simon Clark of Broom Court (1579–1652). In 1604 he married an heir-ess, Margaret Alderford. Became a baronet in 1617, and bought the manors of Bidford and Broom. In that year his wife died at the birth of their seventh child. Remarried in 1618 (cf. Case 131). Clark was an antiquarian and scholar, friend of Dugdale. Buried at Salford Priors, in the church he had enlarged in 1633.
3 Ruland the Elder, 'Centuria III', *Curationum* […] *centuriae*, p. 198.
4 upwards and downwards] See Case 9, n. 3.
5 Ruland the Elder, 'Centuria IV', *Curationum* […] *centuriae*, p. 209.
6 Spencer Compton, 2nd Earl of Northampton (1601–43). Eldest son of William Compton (Case 2). Queen Elizabeth I was his godmother. Inherited the title at 29, but also great debts. Married Mary Beaumont (Case 144) in 1621. A firm Royalist. Spencer and three of his sons fought at Edgehill. He was killed in battle in 1643 and interred at Derby.

his neck is straight. Even speaking is painful,[1] *and he could swallow food only with difficulty.* **[p. 124]** *There is much damp and viscous stuff in his mouth.*[2] *The original disorder always comes from their flows, which are derived in this misfortune from the jugular veins and head itself.*[3] *For the disease is all the more dangerous to the degree that the character of the sore throat is more powerful, while on the contrary, as it is weaker so it is less dangerous.*[4] Most important is: *venesection immediately on the same side as the illness started,*[5] but he refused and was therefore purged in this way:

℞: senna leaves 1oz, rhubarb 3dr, agaric 2dr, cinnamon ½oz, anise and fennel seeds each 1dr, sweet flag ½oz, liquorice 3dr. Infuse for twelve hours by the usual method in spring water 3 pints, then boil on a slow fire, reduce to a third. Strain. Add chicory syrup with rhubarb, diasereos each 1oz to the strained liquid. Make it.

℞: of this (since it was to hand) 4oz, diasereos syrup, chicory with rhubarb each 6dr. Mix.

He could scarcely get it down because of the painful difficulty in swallowing. Six foul-smelling stools. *One should abstain from more powerful purges at the beginning of the illness, for the humours will be stirred up, and for this reason it gives them an opportunity to flux more freely to the affected part.*[6] Repeat the purge: eight stools.

Gargle on the first days following as I prescribed:

℞: mulberry simple, rose honey each 2oz, waters of woodbine, plantain, barley each 4oz, oil of vitriol and sulphur each sufficient for sharpness. *Hold it in the mouth hot and the amount as much as possible for a long time. It will gently wash out the inmost parts of the pharynx; and indeed it is better that the humours do not run so freely in the affected area.*[7]

---

1 He does not … painful] Bruele, *Praxis medicinae*, p. 156.
2 There … mouth] Bruele, *Praxis medicinae*, p. 157.
3 The … itself] Bruele, *Praxis medicinae*, p. 157.
4 For … dangerous] Bruele, *Praxis medicinae*, pp. 157–158.
5 Bruele, *Praxis medicinae*, p. 158.
6 Bruele, *Praxis medicinae*, p. 159.
7 Bruele, *Praxis medicinae*, p. 160.

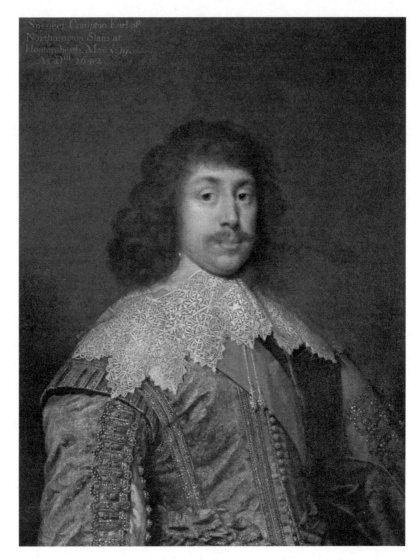

35 Portrait of Spencer Compton, 2nd Earl of Northampton, the eldest son of William (see Figure 22). He was godson of Queen Elizabeth I and became a favourite of Prince Charles. Hall treated the Earl for 'desperate quinsy' (Case 137) with a poultice and a form of lozenge (of a kind Hall said he had used on his own wife). Hall also treated the Countess (Case 144) and the Earl again for pleurisy (Case 178).

Apply a plaster of green wormwood **[p. 125]** and fat in the morning and evening; happily successful. As the night was sleepless after removal of the plaster, he requested advice from Dr Clayton of Oxford,[1] and sent [for him] at precipitate speed. Everyone feared imminent peril. He refused venesection but was instantly freed from pain and danger by the following plaster:

> R: *two whole swallows' nests, including straw, dirt, and swallows' droppings. Boil in oils of chamomile and lilies. Pound them and filter through a sieve of bristles. Add droppings from dogs which have eaten bones 1oz, flour, linseed and fenugreek seeds each 1oz, marsh-mallow ointment, chicken fat each ½oz. Make a poultice in the form of a plaster.*

I prescribed it applied hot to the place,[2] with the desired outcome. He used amber fumes, and before sleeping held a trochee of this sort in his mouth, under the tongue:

> R: liquorice juice, white sugar each 1dr, husked seeds of purslane, cucumber, melon, water-melon each 1sc, starch, tragacanth each ½dr, barley sugar 4sc. Make trochees.

I have successfully prescribed trochees like these for [my] wife and others suffering from sore throat:

> R: white poppy seeds 2sc, gums of tragacanth, Arabian each ½dr, husked seeds of purslane, melon, cucumbers, water-melons each ½dr, liquorice juice ½dr, rose sugar, barley sugar each 2dr. Make small trochees with poppy syrup.

But in fact the Earl was satisfied with [the preceding] prescriptions alone, before the doctor arrived. *He felt their present help, praise to God, Jesus Christ, our almighty and most high Saviour. His throat was opened, the swelling and inflammation of the tonsils and uvula lifted, and he breathed and swallowed easily.*[3] He gave me a large payment, and often afterwards thanked me greatly.

---

1 Dr Thomas Clayton, MD (Oxon), 1575–1647 (Raach 1962: 36).
2 Valleriola, *Observationum* [...] *libri sex*, p. 261.
3 Ruland the Elder, 'Centuria III', *Curationum* [...] *centuriae*, p. 222.

On the correct page: **[p. 126]** put in place: But I used the following (applied as a poultice which was omitted from the preceding page).[1]

A gargle:

> ℞: *plantain water 1½ pints, scabious 7oz, red rose flowers 1dr, pomegranate rind ½dr. Simmer once, boil, then strain. To the strained liquid add mulberry syrup, rose honey each 2oz. Mix.*[2]

He rinsed his mouth with this gargle frequently during the day. Then he drank half a spoonful of the following linctus:

> ℞: maidenhair syrup, liquorice syrup each ½oz, cold diatragacanth tablets 1½dr, poppy syrup to reduce saltiness ½oz. Mix. Make the eclegma.

His ordinary drink for one day:

> ℞: liquorice, anise seeds, figs, raisins each 1oz. Boil in 4 pints spring water until a pint is gone.

These, praise God, cured the Earl quickly and safely. Ruland gives *½ spoonful, equal to 3dr, of oil of hazel wood, with which he rinsed the throat and parts affected.*[3] This is a secret.

[Case 138]
Cure of yellow jaundice. Mrs Stoker,[4] a gentlewoman, aged about 44 years, companion to Mrs Sheldon of Weston: with jaundice spread over the whole body, pain and torment in the right side. Her friends judge her to be in danger of death.

---

1 Hall must have completed the case report, then decided to add a treatment missing from the previous page.
2 Foreest, *De febribus ephemeris et continuis*, p. 97.
3 Ruland the Elder, 'Centuria III', *Curationum* […] *centuriae*, p. 222.
4 Elizabeth Stoker, companion to Elizabeth Sheldon of Weston (?–*c.* 1680). Hall calls her *Generosa*, so her status was higher than that of a servant. She lived at Weston Hall, near Cherington, as companion to William Sheldon's wife after their marriage in 1611. In her will, Elizabeth Stoker left money to the English Benedictine abbey at Douai.

℞: electuary of rose juice 2dr, diacatholicon 1½dr, diaphoenicon 2½dr, rhubarb 1sc, spikenard 5gr, chicory syrup with rhubarb ½oz, chicory water 3oz. Make a draught. Two stools.

With the jaundice, she was wretchedly overwhelmed by abdominal constipation because her bowels were always bound. **[p. 127]** Venesection to 4oz (I did not wish a larger quantity, because 'blood is a restraint on choler'). The venesection freed her from the pain in the side.

℞: ammoniac 1dr, oxymel 2oz, agrimony water 1oz. Continue the course for four days. She was properly purged. I prescribed jelly of hartshorn shavings 1oz, worms 10, each one with red round the neck and washed in white wine. Boil in 1½ pints spring water, reduce to half. After boiling, add finely powdered saffron 1sc. Make jelly. Give two spoonfuls in broth with shoots of celandine, barberry bark, flowers of rosemary and marigold.

Her drink: the hartshorn decoction. A sweating drink of this sort:

℞: white wine 4oz, celandine water 3oz, saffron ½dr, Venice treacle 1½dr, bezoar stone ½sc, juice of goose droppings 3 spoonfuls. Make a sweating drink. Dose: take 4oz on four mornings.

She is to use the following electuary in the evening:

℞: red and white sandalwood 3dr, currants soaked in white wine then sieved 4oz, rhubarb 1dr, saffron 1sc. Mix. Make the electuary. Dose: the amount of a hazelnut.

These freed her from the jaundice. On my advice she used the following electuary for ten days:

℞: steeled electuary 2oz, powdered rhubarb 3sc, powdered ammoniac 4sc, tamarind electuary ½oz, diatrion santalon 3dr. Mix. Make the electuary: dose ½oz. She is to take exercise.

These, to God alone be praise, freed her from death within twenty days.

[Case 139]

Cure of an ulcer, virulent gonorrhoea. Mr Harvey,[1] gentleman of Northampton, about 65 years of age: complained of burning and dribbling urine and an ulcer at the mouth of the bladder. **[p. 128]** The previous year I gave him distilled water of milk and egg white with mallow which made him much better. He received differing opinions from many physicians. My opinion, now as before, is that he suffered from a dirty ulcer in the penile urethra, for I saw mucous pus at the bottom of the chamber-pot. As he was passing urine, I saw little pieces being excreted with the urine from the penis, and swelling under the scrotum. In addition he felt the urine dribbling and burning at the end of his penis.

I contrived the following remedies for these. A diuretic and cathartic potion: he used the turpentine potion as on page 95 for eight days. His ordinary drink: barley cream, or better, barley water with mallow and liquorice. At the same time *I prescribed lead sheet with very many perforations, to be applied to the area of the kidneys, and changed often.*[2] I prescribed the following injection for the day and night:

R: *Rhazes's white trochees without opium 1½dr, calamine stone (that is, cadmium dug up), prepared tutty each 1dr, lead burnt and washed with plantain water, the most refined bole Armeniac each 2dr. Make a very fine powder. Mix 1dr of it with the following decoction and inject, adding 1dr of gum tragacanth mucilage made with plantain water.*

R: *horse-tail fern twigs, plantain leaves each 1 handful, daisy roots 2oz, red roses 1 pinch, pomegranate rind 2dr. Beat, boil in steeled water.*[3]

When the milky-white water was finished, he used the following tablets:

---

1 Sir Francis Harvey of Hardingstone, Northamptonshire (1567–1632). Educated at Cambridge, MA in 1589. Became a lawyer. Knighted in 1626. Bought a manor for his son Stephen when he married Mary Murden (cf. Case 60).
2 Bruele, *Praxis medicinae*, p. 351.
3 Platter, *Observationum* [...] *libri tres*, pp. 781–782.

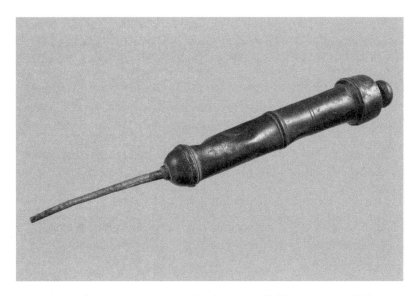

36 A sixteenth-century pewter medical syringe. Hall's treatment of Mr Harvey of Hardingstone, Northampton (about fifty miles from Stratford-upon-Avon) included injections (Case 139). Hall was treating him for an ulcer in his urethra and gonorrhoea.

R: *winter-cherry trochees with opium ½oz, comfrey roots, turpentine cooked dry each 1dr,* **[p. 129]** *sugar 2 ½oz. Make trochees with gum tragacanth, 2sc by weight.*[1] Take with milk or distilled water of eggs in the morning, for several days.

I prescribed a lead tube to be placed in the penis, to remain there as long as he could hold it, or *a wax candle, thin, flexible and long, was slowly inserted into the channel several times, covered with ointment of red lead or red camphor.*[2] For the scrotal swelling I ordered a fresh decoction of crushed sarsaparilla for several days, and he always wore a lead sheet over the kidneys. He was completely freed from the burning urine.

Now he was attacked by gonorrhoea, for which I prescribed the following powder for ten days:

---

1 Platter, *Observationum* [...] *libri tres*, p. 761.
2 Platter, *Observationum* [...] *libri tres*, p. 771.

℞: *sarsaparilla 1½oz, guaiacum bark ½oz, best cinnamon ½dr 15gr, senna 2dr, dodder, hellebore root each 1dr, best white sugar 2oz. Mix. Make the powder and divide into 1½dr per dose. Sometimes the hellebore and dodder is omitted.*[1]

These made him well, and he rode to London. It started again, by some fate unknown to me. He asked advice from the most learned Dr Harvey, and followed his counsel:

℞: Rhazes's white trochees ½oz, Gordon's trochees 1sc, best aloes 2½dr, barley sugar 1½dr, plantain water ½ pint. Make an injection.

He used an electuary, the amount of a bean at bedtime:

℞: alkekengi trochees with opium ½oz, sufficient lemon juice syrup, gum tragacanth, prepared crystal mastic, prepared coral each 1sc. Make an electuary.

These again restored him. After all of these had indeed been given, he began to pass water continuously and quickly, and was well. The next year he rode to St Vincent's Spring and took the waters. He was very well. On account of incapacity from a small growth [in the urethra], he was injured by a surgeon with an iron tube and relapsed again. He could never afterwards be cured.

[Case 140]

[p. 130] Suffocation of the womb, convulsion of the eyes and obstructed periods. 1 February 1631. Mrs Mary Combe,[2] a gentlewoman of Stratford-upon-Avon, about the age of 13: her periods started two years previously, satisfactory in quantity and every month. They started to flow plentifully from the age of 11 years, now are held back by sadness and smallpox. First she felt a slight convulsion in the right eye (in her own words, 'a twichinge as

---

1 Crato, *Consiliorum* [...] *liber secundus*, pp. 366–377.
2 Mary Combe of Stratford-upon-Avon (1619–86). She was 13 when Hall treated her. Married Thomas Wagstaffe in 1636; two children. Wagstaffe had been a royal ward after his father's early death (cf. Case 47). Sir Thomas died in 1639. Mary then married John Rous and lived at Tachbrook Mallory. Widowed in 1680. Her memorial is in St Chad's church, Bishops Tachbrook.

though hir eye was pulled inwarde, presently it would be gone')
then convulsions in both eyes with very severe headache. I prescribed *Fernel's headache pills*[1] for this, ½dr to be taken at bedtime.
This resulted in three stools, and the same the next day when
the pills were repeated. Then she was wretchedly troubled by
suffocation of the mother. The attack lasted for nine hours, with
slight intervals. Eventually, by the aid of God and the following
remedies, she was freed:

> R: fume of horse's hoof. I also gave water for the womb as described
> in the *Pharmacopoeia Londinensis*.[2]

She drank 3 spoonfuls, at intervals as she was able. I applied a
plaster for the womb below the umbilicus. Finally I prescribed the
use of the following ointment with which I ordered the womb to
be anointed from within:

> R: *musk 4gr, musk galls 1sc, lily oil sufficient, or ½oz. Mix. Make the ointment,
> by which it was aroused and restored to itself.*

Fumigants, from which the fume is sent down to the nose:

> R: *castor, galbanum dissolved in vinegar, each ½oz, sulphur 1oz, assafoetida
> 1dr. Make trochees with castor oil.*[3]

> **[p. 131]** R: pills – of peony, of ground-pine each 2sc, oil of clary
> sage 5 drops. Make 10 pills. Give three hours before sleep, add
> water for the womb 2sc. From swallowing 2 pills, five or six stools
> the next day.

The following day she was again weighed down by suffocation of
the mother, but the attack was slight, though she was in the paroxysm for a whole hour together. The above trochees, burnt and
applied to the nostrils, awakened her instantly. I also prescribed
the womb to be rubbed with the above ointment. I gave two
spoonfuls of water for the womb, though she was reluctant: the

---

1 Fernel's for headache] See Case 23, n. 6.
2 *Pharmacopoeia Londinensis*, p. 9.
3 Rueff, *De conceptu*, f. 83v.

night restful. Again I prescribed two pills to be taken at bedtime. When I came in the morning, she complained of stomach ache and headache.

11 February: She was vexed by a slight fever with a little choking. For prevention:

℞: extract for the womb 2dr. Make 10 pills with sufficient water for the womb. Give 1 pill on an empty stomach.

She became well. 28 March: She fell again into a uterine passion with convulsion of the eyes. She had convulsions of the eye for two days before being weighed down by the uterine passion.

℞: pills – of peony, ground-pine, hiera with agaric each 2sc, of amber, Ruffus's each 1dr, extract for the womb 2dr. Make a mass with water for the womb, of which make 5 pills from 1dr; cover with gold. Give 3 at bedtime.

These freed her from the uterine passion. Praise God.

[Case 141]
Cure of swelling of the lips and nasal catarrh. Lady Harington's first-born daughter:[1] after smallpox, suffers from swelling of the nose and lips and now the cheeks, with catarrh dripping from her head. About 10 years old.

℞: shoots of brooklime, watercress, scurvy-grass each 4 handfuls, juniper berries ½lb, agrimony 1 handful, wormwood, blessed thistle each ½ handful. Boil in **[p. 132]** 5 gallons new beer, reduce to 4. Take 2 pints of the strained liquid, senna 2oz, agaric ½oz, rhubarb 2dr, sarsaparilla 2oz, sassafras 1oz, colchicum 1½oz, liquorice 1oz, polypody 2oz, seeds of anise, caraway, coriander each ½oz, cinnamon 2dr. Strain. Add sufficient sugar to the strained liquid, make a syrup.

---

1 Sarah, daughter of Sir John Harington of Elmesthorpe, Leicestershire (1607–65). Came of a wealthy family. Hall treated her when she was 10. Sarah served in the household of Queen Henrietta Maria. In 1630 she married Sir John Feschville; three daughters. Sir John was raised to the peerage for his Royalist support.

℞: of this 12oz, chicory syrup with rhubarb 2oz. Dose: 3 or 4 spoonfuls.

For the lips: *Ruland's mercury water.*[1] Wear a lead sheet at night. To drink: the above beer. *When these had been continued, her lips were at once healed of everything within a few days.*[2] The following year she saw me in passing, and thanked me greatly.

Margaret Baker,[3] aged 9, was disfigured after smallpox by swelling of the nose and lips. She was properly cured as follows:

℞: amber pills ½dr. Make 3 pills. Give before sleeping, and repeat for four days.

She was rightly purged. Her lips were washed with Ruland's mercury water. She was rightly cured.

[Case 142]

Abdominal torment after birth. Lady Rainsford,[4] good-looking and of very fine structure, approaching 27 years: wretchedly attacked by abdominal torment three days after giving birth, from which I reclaimed her with the following:

℞: the white of chicken droppings in beer, with sugar to the weight of 1dr.

I also prescribed this to be applied hot to her belly:

℞: fresh milk mixed with honey each 1 pint, horehound bark 1 handful, wheat flour 3oz, saffron 1dr. Boil to the consistency of a poultice.

---

1 There is a reference to this but without a recipe in Ruland the Elder, 'Centuria III', *Curationum* […] *centuriae*, p. 158. There is also a recipe for *aqua Mercurialis Alex. Ped.* on p. 311.
2 Ruland the Elder, 'Centuria III', *Curationum* […] *centuriae*, p. 158.
3 For some reason Hall's manuscript does not treat Margaret Baker as a separate case.
4 Elinor, Lady Rainsford of Clifford Chambers (*c.* 1596–1640). Born Elinor Boswell in Combe, Hampshire. Married Sir Henry Rainsford; five children. Hall describes her as beautiful. Died six months before her husband. Their son Henry, a known Royalist, inherited the estate.

These freed her from her torments.

[Case 143]
Continual burning fever, headache, slight nosebleed. **[p. 133]**
Grace Court,[1] the apothecary's wife, aged 27: very severely
afflicted by a burning and continual fever, lower backache, slight
nosebleed, headache with slight confusion. First I prescribed opening a vein and taking 4 to 5 oz (although she was in the fourteenth
week of pregnancy). She used this for stomach problems, the same
day:

> ℞: prepared hartshorn 2sc, powder for liberans confection, red
> Pannonian powder, alkermes confection each 2sc, barberry con-
> serve 1oz. She swallowed the amount of a bean every third hour.

She drank only the following:

> ℞: *boiled spring water 3 pints, pomegranate syrup 1½oz, rose julep 2oz, spirits
> of vitriol the amount of necessary for a pleasing tartness.*[2]

I prescribed *bruised radishes sprinkled with salt and rose vinegar, applied to
the soles of the feet every fourth hour.*[3]

A gargle for inflammation of the tongue:

> ℞: *clear spring water 2 pints, rose julep 1½oz, sufficient drops of spirit of vitriol
> for a pleasing acidity,*[4] mulberry simple 6dr, rose vinegar 1oz.

*She washed her mouth often during the day and, the phlegm being thick and
also impacted, she rubbed the dried parts alternately with rose honey and butter
to cleanse and remove it.*[5] I prescribed this antipyretic to be applied on
both wrists:

---

1 Grace Court, apothecary's wife. Married John Court; five children. He died
in 1639. Two years later Grace married Christopher Pargetter. Her son John
excluded his stepfather from his will. Grace apparently left Stratford. No record
of her death.
2 Ruland the Younger, *De morbo Ungarico*, p. 194.
3 Ruland the Younger, *De morbo Ungarico*, p. 168.
4 Ruland the Younger, *De morbo Ungarico*, p. 194.
5 Ruland the Younger, *De morbo Ungarico*, p. 266

℞: *populeon ointment 1oz, lots of spiders' webs, a little walnut. Mix.*

For back pain:[1]

℞: *ointments of populeon, rose each ½oz, alabaster 2dr, oil of water lilies 6dr, camphor ½sc. Mix.*

But since this oil was not to hand, she used the following

℞: *oils of scorpions,*[2] *2dr, almonds ½oz. Make it with 1oz of rose ointment.*

For headache, this sort of oxyrrhodinum,[3] *which prevented the rising of the vapours:*

℞: *waters of roses, plantain,* **[p. 134]** *elderflowers each 3oz, rose oil, water of lettuce washed several times 1½oz, red sandalwood powder 1½dr.*[4] *Mix. Soak linen cloths and apply to the head.*

So as not to fall into a stupor, she used the following hartshorn decoction:

℞: *pure spring water 2 pints, seeds and rind of citron each 1dr, prepared hartshorn ½oz, liberans powder 2dr. Boil, reduce by ½ pint. To the strained liquid add pomegranate juice and sufficient sugar for an agreeable tartness. Boil again, skimming all the time, and purify with egg white.*

She took three draughts of this every day, one in the morning, the second two hours before lunch, and the third two hours before dinner. To strengthen the heart and more quickly subdue the malice, take a draught of the above decoction every second day fasting beforehand, after the amount of a nutmeg of the following cordial:

℞: *blackcurrant juice, conserve of citron flesh each 1oz, liberans powder, prepared pearls, prepared emeralds each 1sc. Make a soft electuary with pomegranate syrup.*

---

1 Platter, *Observationum* […] *libri tres*, p. 291.
2 Ruland the Younger, *De morbo Ungarico*, p. 142.
3 oxyrrhodinum] A generic name for a mixture of oil and water of roses, not a specific remedy.
4 Ruland the Younger, *De morbo Ungarico*, pp. 143–144.

She is to take a draught of the hartshorn decoction on the third evening, take just as much of the cordial electuary.[1]

16th: red Pannonian powder, and afterwards an enema:

> ℞: marsh-mallow root 1oz, the four emollient plants each 1 handful, barley 1½ pinches, gourds ½oz. Dissolve in it cassia 1oz, violet honey 1oz, violet oil 3oz. **[p. 135]** Make an enema with salt.

20 June: She vomited a worm with greenish bile. I then gave the following electuary, the amount of a bean every third hour:

> ℞: vitriolated rose conserve 1oz, diarrhodon Abbatis powder 1dr, red Pannonian powder 1sc, sufficient barberry conserve. Make an electuary.

With these we brought on a remission of the attacks, and returned to her possession of her mind,[2] and in a short while she regained her health. By these I set the end of her cure. *To God almighty be glory and honour for ever and ever.*[3] Amen.

[Case 144]

Bastard tertian fever, yellow jaundice, headache, lower backache, abdominal pain in pregnancy. The [2nd] Countess of Northampton,[4] a gentlewoman of noble stock, distinguished in character and education, *richly endowed with all the natural talents which adorn a well-born mother, and remarkably beautiful:*[5] she fell into a bastard tertian fever when seven months pregnant. She was also disfigured by jaundice, tortured by abdominal pains and headache, and attacked by lower backache. Age: about 26 years.

---

1 Ruland the Younger, *De morbo Ungarico*, pp. 246–247.
2 Horst, *Observationum* [...] *libri quatuor*, p. 102.
3 Ruland the Elder, 'Centuria VII', *Curationum* [...] *centuriae*, p. 555.
4 Mary, Countess of Northampton (1600–54). Daughter of Sir Francis Beaumont. Hall notes she was remarkably beautiful. In 1621 she married Spencer Compton, later 2nd Earl of Northampton (cf. Case 137); eight children. Widowed in 1643, the Dowager Countess moved to Oxford and later died in London. Buried at Compton Wynyates.
5 Valleriola, *Observationum* [...] *libri sex*, p. 67. Cf. Case 147, n. 2.

After seeking my advice, she used the following. She does not want to be purged, nor do I wish it. I prescribed this posset ale an hour before the attack:

> R: flowers – marigold, rosemary each 1 pinch, blessed thistle ½ pinch, flowers and leaves of melilot 2 pinches. Boil in sufficient posset ale for ½ pint. Take half of it hot with a little sugar an hour before the attack.

This delayed the onset of the attack for two hours. When it started to recur she drank the second half hot. She was freed from the fever, shivering **[p. 136]** and rigors. Then the jaundice appeared very strongly in her urine, the heat of the fever following on rapidly. Very severe sweating broke out but the second attack was shorter than the previous one. For the hot fever and sweating she took plenty of hartshorn decoction with lemon juice. She would not take rose water in the decoction. She swallowed the following electuary on the quiet day, the amount of a bean every third hour:

> R: barberry conserve ½oz, red Pannonian powder 2sc.

But after taking it once she loathed it, because the barberry peels were unpleasant. She took jelly of hartshorn shavings with marigold and crocus flowers.

22 July: before the attack she is to take bezoar stone 5gr, and the posset ale an hour before the attack, as before. Now, because her companion gave her nearly all the posset ale before the attack, and only a little when the fever started, she was again afflicted by shivering and rigors. But the heat and sweating quickly passed, and the attack lasted less than six hours.

23rd: at five o'clock on the quiet day:

> R: coral tincture, magisterium of pearls each 4gr, bezoar stone 5gr, red Pannonian powder 12gr: an hour before lunch and an hour before dinner.

24th: at 3 o'clock in the morning before the attack: as before, and the above posset ale. The fever was mild at the time.

25th: as on 23rd.

26th: I prescribed wormwood, rue, feverfew, nettles in equal amounts, to be applied hot to her feet. Bruise and apply to the soles of the feet; the posset ale as before. For the forehead, as the heat came on: populeon ointment with opium. For the back: **[p. 137]** oxycroceum plaster, which entirely removed the backache. The fever was so faint that it could hardly be detected.

28th:

> R: prepared hartshorn, red Pannonian powder each ½dr, water of blessed thistles 2oz, field poppy syrup ½oz, bezoar stone 4gr. Mix. Give five hours before an attack, and apply the herbs to the soles of the feet.

When the heat is returning:

> R: syrup of poppies 1oz, of lemons ½oz, scabious water 2oz, oil of vitriol 5 drops, caelestis water 7 drops Mix.

The noble Countess was completely healed by these very few remedies with twelve days,[1] and *was freed from a most savage and deadly illness. Praise be to God alone, the highest and most merciful.*[2]

1 August: she relapsed after catching cold. The herbs were applied to her feet two hours before the attack. To the pulses:

> R: *populeon ointment ½oz, a lot of spider webs, a little of a walnut tree,*[3] *which restrained the outward movement of the heat. Populeon with spider webs was definitely applied to the pulses and temples, spread on a small piece of cotton* – Gregor Horst.[4]

---

1 Hall means within twelve days.
2 Ruland the Elder, 'Centuria III', *Curationum* [...] *centuriae*, p. 226.
3 populeon ... tree] Platter, *Observationum* [...] *libri tres*, p. 291. Perhaps this means the bark or wood of the tree, rather than the nut.
4 Horst, *Observationum* [...] *libri quatuor*, p. 59.

For the rigor:

> ℞: bezoar water ½ spoonful, bezoar stone 5gr, lemon juice 2 spoon-fuls, two hours before the attack. When the heat is coming on apply to the temples populeon ointment ½oz, opium dissolved in rose water ½sc.

The noble Lady, struck a second time with this most severe fever, was quickly and entirely cured by these remedies, and attained sound good health, and rejoices. She bore a beautiful daughter afterwards and, meeting in passing, I saw her carrying her beautiful daughter in her arms. She declared that she gave thanks to God and to me for her, because she had not thought that she could survive.

[Case 145]

[p. 138] Inflammation of internal haemorrhoids. The Reverend Fawcet,[1] about 55 years old, a man distinguished for his learning: *tortured by most dangerous and intolerable pain of the haemorrhoids. To help himself he tried many different remedies in vain. He finally came to me and complained a lot about this hidden mischief. To relieve it,*[2] apply hot milk kept warm, then tepid, then the following oil:

> ℞: linseed oil 2oz, and elder oil 1oz. Mix. Apply a little with a folded cloth.

Night and day:

> ℞: sufficient tapsi valentia and rub in.

Everything was entirely curbed. An ointment:

> ℞: *populeon ointment 1oz, 1oz, dried powdered opium 1sc. Mix. Apply to the part.* Rodericus de Fonseca though, recommends box-tree oil, and

---

1 Thomas Fawcet, rector of Aston-sub-Edge, Gloucestershire (1564–1636). Born in Yorkshire, graduated from St Catherine's College, Cambridge in 1589. In 1607 married Margaret Sellers, and became rector of Aston. Died a widower, and left his books to his son-in-law, John Sellers.
2 Ruland the Elder, 'Centuria I', *Curationum* […] *centuriae*, p. 52.

says it is the equal of anything.[1] *It is a narcotic, even for toothache, which it always allays wonderfully by its strength. It alleviates both other pains and is especially good at allaying that of haemorrhoids if a drop or two is put on them with a pen wrapped in cotton wool. Also it may be mixed with linseed oil, mixing up to 1oz with 1sc of box-tree oil. Alternatively, flowers of sulphur with turpentine washed many times in rose water, and apply it in place of balsam sulphur. It has power to melt away, loosen and open internal haemorrhoids so that they drain blood, because one should be in the habit of attending to this especially in this condition.*[2]

And so he was freed from the above pain, and made healthy.

[Case 146]

[p. 139] Choking of the lungs. Anne Ward of Stratford-upon-Avon,[3] respected, good-looking, devoutly pious: passed black matter *upwards and downwards*.[4] Afterwards she felt strangled with choking of the lungs, so that everyone expected her death. She could not speak, breathed with loud gasps and continued so for an hour. Her parents called me as I was coming home. I at once applied a large cupping glass to the mouth of the stomach, and as if by a spell she was able to speak distinctly. (Twice before it was the same, with Mrs Goodyeare and Mrs Savage gentlewomen, whom everyone had forsaken in peril of death.) I prescribed our pectoral roll to be held in the mouth at night.

An enema:

℞: *Du Chesne's carminative diacolocynth oil* 2oz,[5] the carminative decoction for enemas ½ pint: two stools.

---

1 Fonseca, *Consultationes*, p. 96.
2 Fonseca, *Consultationes*, p. 97.
3 Hall did not record her status or age. Might have been Anne Cap, who married Edward Ward in 1608, or her daughter Anne born in 1610. No further records found for either.
4 upwards and downwards] See Case 9, n. 3.
5 Du Chesne, *Pharmacopoea dogmaticorum*, pp. 135–136.

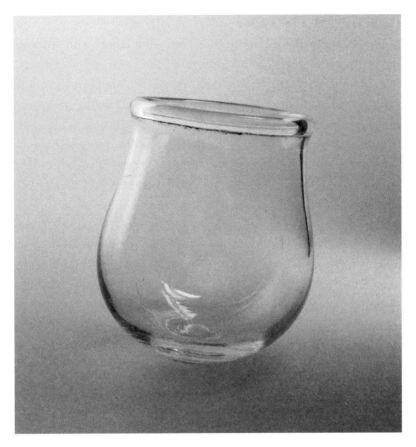

37 A seventeenth-century cupping glass. A small amount of water was placed under the glass, and a small fire lit on the top of it. As the glass heated and then cooled it created a vacuum to draw blood, or other matter, from the patient.

The next day:

R: electuaries of tamarinds ½oz, of rose juice 3oz, cream of tartar 1sc. Make a bolus with sugar: eight stools.

She was cured, *and became the greatest trumpeter of praises of the art.*[1] Praise God.

---

1 Amatus Lusitanus, *Curationum* [...] *centuriae duae*, p. 325. Cf. Case 152.

[Case 147]

Melancholy from the womb, white discharge with uterine
pains. Mrs Fiennes,[1] a gentlewoman of the noble stock of Baron
Wimbledon, 22 years, wife of the first son of Viscount Saye and
Sele, devoutly pious, good-looking, as full of remarkable inborn
qualities as anyone and *richly endowed with all the natural talents which
adorn a noble woman*:[2] has been wretchedly afflicted by these symptoms – menstrual blockage for two months. At the time they flowed
[p. 140] in laudable quantity, they had a bad watery colour, with
very severe uterine pain. In addition there is shortness of breath
with trembling of the heart, and palpitations as if her chest is going
to crack. She is unwell with abdominal pain after sleeping, and
feels a tearing sensation round the umbilicus. She was wretchedly
afflicted with these pains around the time of her menstruation. She
feels much better after passing wind. She also feels something hard
moving in her belly, like an infant, but the application of hot cloths
removes the pain with the wind. She is tortured by splenic pain,
emaciated by the white flux, weighed down by lower backache,
afflicted with slight giddiness so that she staggers as if drunk and
feels the house spinning round her.

She had also been emaciated by scurvy for a long time. *When I had
visited her, lying in bed, and studied all the symptoms*,[3] I judged that the
origin of the evil had its roots in scurvy, *of which I undertook the cure
in this way, in God's name*:[4]

℞: pills – of amber 2dr, Ruffus's 1dr. Make 5 pills from a drachm.
Take 3 at bedtime, 2 in the morning.

---

1 Frances Fiennes of Broughton Castle, Oxfordshire (1610–84). Daughter of
Edward Cecil. In 1631 she married James, heir to Viscount Saye and Sele. The
Fiennes family were Parliamentarians. Three sons, who all died young. After
James died in 1674, the title passed to his nephew. The following year Frances,
aged 64, married the Puritan writer Joshua Sprigge, twelve years her junior.
2 Valleriola, *Observationum* [...] *libri sex*, p. 67. Cf. Case 144, n. 5.
3 Ruland the Elder, 'Centuria II', *Curationum*, p. 146.
4 Ruland the Elder, 'Centuria II', *Curationum* [...] *centuriae*, p. 148. Cf. Case 153.

She grew very well again at once by the intense and happy working of these pills.[1] For wind:

> R: pleres archonticon powder 1oz, rose sugar 4oz. Mix. Take ½ spoonful after meals.

After using these, her menstruation restarted in laudable quantities. She wrote on the 16th, because she expelled large fleshy masses like liver from her womb with pain as if in labour. These would not dissolve in water.[2] She used the following pills to clean the womb:

> **[p. 141]** R: pills – hiera with agaric, amber each 1½dr, Cyprus turpentine, Ruffus's each ½dr. Make 20 pills. Give 3 at bedtime, 2 in the morning with an attendant. When these are finished take 2dr of pleres archonticon electuary, and take exercise.

5 March: Take cream of tartar 1dr in broth, for four mornings, an hour later our steeled water made in this way:

> R: *oil of sulphur 1 part, wine spirit 2 parts. Boil in a pan or newly made iron cup, evaporate on a slow fire until the moisture is gone. You are to store this powder in vials, very well closed lest air gets in, because that melts it.*[3]

> R: of this powder 2dr, place in agrimony water 4oz, and soak over hot coals.

She used:

> R: of this water ½oz in broth, and she is to take exercise.

She vomited, as it often provokes, on the first day but not on the second and third. *This is a true restorative of the liver, and it will collect all the illnesses flowing from there, such as dropsy*[4] and wasting and the green sickness. She took it for fifteen days.

---

1 Ruland the Elder, 'Centuria II', *Curationum* […] *centuriae*, p. 142.
2 would not dissolve in water] demonstrating that they were solid matter, not blood clots.
3 Béguin, *Tyrocinium chymicum*, pp. 389–390. Béguin gave du Chesne, *Pharmacopoea dogmaticorum*, p. 244 as his source, but Hall's wording is closer to Béguin's.
4 Béguin, *Tyrocinium chymicum*, p. 390.

Spread plasters – Foreest's ammoniac, oxycroceum – on yellow silk, and apply to the spleen. She took pleres archonticon with sugar every day, nor did she neglect the antiscorbutic beer as on page 3, diacubebs 2dr, in the morning. By using these *she grew well again as if by a miracle, which should be ascribed to the work of God alone, whose name be blessed through endless ages.*[1]

[Case 148]
Worms, lower backache, pain in the side, fever. Frances Finch of Stratford-upon-Avon,[2] aged 47, complained of the above. I cured her in this way, praise God, without payment: **[p. 142]**

> ℞: Dudley's powder,[3] prepared scammony each 14gr, cream of tartar 10gr, borage water 1½oz, syrup of roses ½ spoonful.

She evacuated four times with a great many small worms. It was repeated the next day. Cured.

[Case 149]
Frenzy after childbirth. Mrs Jackson,[4] a gentlewoman, devout, wife of the younger minister, about 24 years old: *after childbirth, as she was not well purged, she fell suddenly into a severe frenzy with no other illness appearing. She was enraged, chiefly with those whom previously she had most loved, though she spoke much about religion.* This happened at intervals. *An acute fever appeared, from which I judged this to be a true phrenitis.*[5] I was hampered by much business, so could not visit her. I prescribed the following with happy success:

---

1 Ruland the Elder, 'Centuria II', *Curationum* [...] *centuriae*, p. 142.
2 Frances Finch of Stratford-upon-Avon (1586–1632). Frances Jones married Thomas Finch in 1612; two sons. She died on Christmas Day.
3 A famous powder called *pulvis comitis Warwicensis*, or the Earl of Warwick's powder. Sir Robert Dudley was the illegitimate son of the 1st Earl of Leicester (*DNB*).
4 Anne Jackson of Binton (?–1634). Wife of John Jackson, the rector of Binton. Hall was too busy to visit her when she suffered a feverish illness after childbirth, but he sent her medicine and she recovered.
5 Platter, *Observationum* [...] *libri tres*, p. 86.

R: mugwort syrup 1oz, softening electuary, diacatholicon each 3dr, rhubarb, castor each ½sc, betony water 3oz. Mix.

She brought up wind when her stomach was full, then five stools without torment, as her husband wrote.

22 May: venesection to 6oz. Blood: black and watery. Yet the frenzy was not entirely removed.

23 May:

R: leaves of mallow, violets, beets, lettuce, borage each 2 handfuls, barley 1oz, cucumber, gourd seeds each ½oz. Make a decoction in sufficient water for 12oz. Strain. To the strained liquid add oil of violets 3oz, **[p. 143]** freshly extracted cassia, diacatholicon each 1oz, salt 1dr. Make an enema.

Then because of sleeplessness and restlessness I gave the following syrup:[1]

R: corn poppy syrup 1½oz, syrup of violets ½oz, scabious water 3oz, a little rose water, oil of vitriol for acidity.

I also prescribed oxyrrhodinum of this sort, applied to the forehead:[2]

R: omphacine oil of roses 3oz,[3] rose vinegar 1oz, red sandalwood powder 1½dr, waters of lettuce, plantain, roses each 1oz. Make it.

I ordered a chicken cut in half, to be placed still warm and bloody on the top of her head;[4] *on the soles of her feet radishes bruised and sprinkled with rose vinegar and salt, and changed every three hours*[5] to draw away [the humours].

25th:

R: freshly extracted cassia with betony water 1oz, loosening rose syrup ½oz, waters of bugloss, borage, violets each 1oz. Make a draught, give it at dawn.

---

1 Platter, *Observationum* […] *libri tres*, p. 86.
2 Platter, *Observationum* […] *libri tres*, p. 86.
3 roses] made from unripe fruit.
4 Platter, *Observationum* […] *libri tres*, p. 86.
5 on … hours] Ruland the Younger, *De morbo Ungarico*, p. 168. Cf. Case 143.

I also prescribed the application of scarification to the shoulders and upper arm.[1] I submit all this to the judgement of the attending physician, for they should be changed, increased or decreased, as the existing circumstances demand. She was restored by these medicinal methods alone, *and with God's help recovered from the deadly illnesses and symptoms within a week.*[2]

[Case 150]

Cure of continual and tertian scorbutic fever. 2 May. Mrs Woodward,[3] a gentlewoman of Avon Dassett, spinster of good character and greatly accomplished[4] though hump-backed, aged 28: fell into a continual burning fever six weeks ago. Then, from purging and venesection by a physician, she fell from the continual burning fever into a dangerous bastard tertian with **[p. 144]** yellow jaundice, very disfiguring spots like flea bites all over the skin, on the arms and many other parts of the body. *These at first grew red and florid, rather like the signs that remain in the skin after flea bites have faded.*[5] Seeing these, I asserted that she suffered from scurvy, for *scurvy is often joined with lasting and tertian and quartan fevers.* Nor did my opinion fail me, *for febrile and vicious material is collected in the meseraics and drying still further, finally induces the scorbutic condition.*[6] *Further (as Eugalenus says), they are not cured unless the medicines which scurvy requires are used.*[7] *Jaundice has its root, not in obstruction of the gall bladder, but from yellow humour abundantly produced in the liver from decayed scorbutic matter and diffused through the whole body.*[8]

---

1 Platter, *Observationum* [...] *libri tres*, p. 86.
2 Ruland the Elder, 'Centuria VI', *Curationum* [...] *centuriae*, p. 444.
3 Isabel Woodward of Avon Dassett (?–1668). Daughter of John Woodward and Isabella Blencowe, from a wealthy sheep-farming family. In 1643 she married her cousin's widower John Fetherston, who had seven children. They lived at Packwood Hall.
4 good ... accomplished] very witty and well-bred.
5 Alberti, 'Schorbuti historia', in Sennert, *De scorbuto tractatus*, p. 395.
6 Sennert, *De scorbuto tractatus*, p. 86.
7 scurvy ... used] Sennert, *De febribus libri IV*, p. 285.
8 Jaundice ... body] Sennert, *De scorbuto tractatus*, p. 123.

I followed the following method, in the name of God. She was without periods, and with a troublesome constipation of the bowels. When I came after an attack, I dealt with the following symptoms of fever, leaving the disease for another day.

> ℞: coral tincture 6 drops, liberans powder 1sc, manus Christi pearled 2sc, bezoar stone 5gr, with barberry conserve. I instructed her to take the hartshorn restorative with pearled manus Christi often on the same day, with these herbs chopped up in veal broth: brooklime, watercress, borage, chicory.

[p. 145] 26 May:

> ℞: diaturbith powder with rhubarb (because no other purgative was to hand) 4sc. Soak overnight in posset ale, in the morning strain and give with sugar.

While I was absent, four stools without pain. In the evening she awaited the unwelcome visitor with an anxious mind. I prescribed an antipyretic ointment to the pulses, with wormwood, rue and chamomile boiled in water for the feet, and [the same] applied hot in a bladder before the attack.

> ℞: liberans powder 2dr, barberry conserve 2oz. Take the amount of a bean often during the day. I gave our antiscorbutic water as on page 110.

For the jaundice and scurvy:

> ℞: powdered ammoniac 2sc, simple oxymel 2oz, agrimony water 1oz.

It was repeated on the quiet days as needed. She used the ammoniac plaster for the spleen, as much diacrocuma electuary as a nutmeg after meals. She was completely freed from the fever, though not yet exempt from the scurvy.

13 June:

> ℞: steeled wine (as on page 41) 6oz, scurvy-grass syrup 3oz, brooklime, watercress each 2dr. Mix. The dose should be 6 spoonfuls, and she is to take exercise, and every other day:

℞: Stomach pills, Ruffus's. Take 3 pills [made from] ½dr at bedtime.

She was rightly cured, praise God the three and one. I saw her the following year, very well coloured and fleshed out, and she gave me thanks.

[Case 151]
June 27. Cure of retained and corrupted products of conception. Mrs Hopper,[1] a gentlewoman aged 24: the products of conception are retained and corrupted after birth, so that small foul-smelling pieces are expelled. *A foul smell rises thence to the stomach, heart,* **[p. 146]** *liver, diaphragm and in consequence to the brain, so that headache, many collapses and cold sweats soon ensue, with resulting danger of death.*[2] To control these symptoms, I prescribed the following plaster to be placed on the umbilicus:

℞: *colocynth decoction in water and rue juice equal parts, with which mix myrrh, linseed, fenugreek, barley flour each a spoonful. Boil everything together. Also, place a plaster of this mixture over the whole belly from the umbilicus to the pubis.*[3]

I also prescribed anointing the womb with basilicon ointment:[4]

℞: castor 6gr, myrrh, saffron each 3gr, Mithridate ½sc. Make 3 pills. Take them about 9 o'clock or at bedtime.

These, praise God, freed her from everything within twenty-four hours.

[Case 152]
Fit of the mother, loss of speech, convulsions of the face, eyes

---

1 Cecily Hopper of Loxley (*c*. 1600–?). In 1628 she married John Hopper, of a wealthy family; two sons died in infancy. No further record of her life or death.
2 Rueff, *De conceptu*, f. 25v.
3 colocynth … pubis] Rueff, *De conceptu*, f. 26v.
4 I … ointment] Rueff, *De conceptu*, f. 26r.

and of the whole body. Archer of Stratford-upon-Avon,[1] dealer in malt: suddenly seized by a convulsion of the face and eyes, and loss of speech. *Her womb was carried off from its home.*[2] She lay there like the image of death. Sometimes she moved violently hither and thither with open eyes. Everyone expected her to die at any moment. Being present, I instructed the apothecary to prepare the following potion speedily. I prescribed:

℞: castor 1dr, rue juice 1 spoonful, sage water 2dr, mugwort syrup 1oz.

She drank this potion whether she would or not, and I wanted assafoetida applied to her nose. In the space of three minutes she recovered her speech, and recognised the bystanders. The next day:

℞: pills – hiera powder with agaric ½dr, foetidae, of peonies each 1sc, bryony dregs, diagrydium each 6dr. Make 5 pills, take in the morning with an attendant.

[p. 147] Finally:

℞: bryony root 3dr, senna leaves ½oz, ginger ½sc, cinnamon 1dr, sugar 1oz. *Infuse overnight in 1½ pints milk whey kept warm.*[3] Administer the potion from this infusion on an empty stomach for some days, 5oz.

This cure,[4] by the favour of almighty God most high and my attentive care, made her entirely and quickly well, with the above cheap and opportune medical help. Her wish was granted, and she became the greatest trumpeter [of praises] of the art and of God.[5]

---

1 Mrs Archer of Stratford-upon-Avon. No identifying information. She lived in town and dealt in malt, a major industry in Stratford in the seventeenth century.

2 Ruland the Elder, 'Centuria II', *Curationum* [...] *centuriae*, p. 133.

3 Ruland the Elder, 'Centuria IV', *Curationum* [...] *centuriae*, p. 312.

4 This ... cure] Ruland the Elder, 'Centuria II', *Curationum* [...] *centuriae*, p. 133.

5 Her ... God] Amatus Lusitanus, *Curationum* [...] *centuriae duae*, p. 325. Cf. Case 146.

[Case 153]

Puerperal fever, called milk fever. Mrs Lewis,[1] a gentlewoman, Mr Fortescue's sister: caught a cold three days after giving birth. She fell into a fever and caught a cold with abdominal pains. This sort of fever is called milk fever for when she was wretchedly obstructed with the milk, now cold then hot, again cold, she was oppressed in the danger of death. *I undertook the cure of this wretched illness in this way,*[2] with God's help:

> A drink: prepared hartshorn decoction, our antipyretic julep: 2 spoonfuls every fourth hour.

I also prescribed the injection of an enema of milk and unrefined sugar and origanum and marjoram applied to her belly, wrapped in a hot linen cloth. These quickly cured her.

[Case 154]

Confirmed scurvy, with various symptoms. 13 August 1632. Mrs Vernon,[3] a gentlewoman of Hanbury, the minister's wife, devout, very beautiful, about 30 years of age, complained of these: she feels a cold in the soles of her feet *like a vapour, and with the spreading of a colder wind into her stomach through the intervening parts,*[4] then feels wretchedly ill. Afterwards she was afflicted by hot spells, then cold sweats, and was again very well in two hours. In addition she was afflicted by melancholy, trembling of the heart and splenic pain, as if it were squeezed by a hand held over the spleen **[p. 148]**

---

1 Martha Lewis of Glamorgan, born *c.* 1611. Martha Fortescue (cf. Case 41), daughter of Nicholas Fortescue, a recusant, married Nicholas Lewis, son of the wealthy Royalist Sir Edward Lewis, in *c.* 1630. Nicholas had an income of £400 in 1645. In 1640 he was prosecuted as a recusant, as were Martha and her servants in 1642.

2 Ruland the Elder, 'Centuria II', *Curationum* [...] *centuriae*, p. 148. Cf. Case 147.

3 Susanna Vernon of Hanbury, Worcestershire (1602–81). Daughter of Thomas Holland, Regius Professor at Oxford. In 1627 she married John Vernon; ten children. Vernon was a Balliol man who was rector of Hanbury, as was his father before him. Died at Hanbury five months before her husband of fifty-four years.

4 Bruele, *Praxis medicinae*, p. 53.

with great pressure. She was attacked by toothache and pain in the gums, by lower backache and the stone. Her whole body felt exhausted. She was harassed by slight swelling of the feet in the evening. She was wretchedly attacked by torments at the time of her periods, and weakened by their excessive and irregular flux. She was often troubled by fits of the mother, not freed from them until she cried. Her thighs were at times disfigured by black spots. Her bowels sometimes did not answer to their duty once within four days, then again the flux would be let loose as if she were lifeless. Urine: various colours, now turbid at which she felt better, then clear like spring water, when [she felt] worse.

These are the symptoms with which the gentlewoman was afflicted. For the causes see Daniel Sennert, *Tractatus de scorbuto*,[1] and Eugalenus.[2] I undertake her cure in the name of God who *maketh sore and bindeth up; killeth and maketh alive; hast power of life and death.*[34] I prescribed taking an enema of this sort, because a few [items] were missing:

> ℞: mallows, mercury, marsh mallow each 1 handful. Boil in suf-ficient milk for ½ pint. In the strained liquid dissolve diaphoenicon, diacatholicon each 6dr, Holland powder 1dr. Make an enema: three stools with wind. At bedtime: *London treacle* 2dr.[5]

14th:

> ℞: brooklime, watercress each ½ handful, marigold and rosemary blossoms 1 pinch. Boil in sufficient milk whey for 1½ pints. To the strained liquid add sugar ½lb. Boil again and skim, then add saf-fron ½dr tied in thin cloth. Boil again once or twice, remove from the fire.

---

1 Sennert, *De scorbuto tractatus*, pp. 31–64.
2 Eugalenus, *De scorbuto morbo*, pp. 2–4.
3 maketh ... death] Job 5:18; 1 Sam. 2:6; Wis. 16:13.
4 Valleriola, *Observationum* […] *libri sex*, pp. 1–2. Cf. Case 155.
5 *Pharmacopoeia Londinensis*, p. 90.

[p. 149] ℞: 8 spoonfuls of this decoction, Holland powder and tartar crystals each equal parts, the amount six pennies can hold.[1] Fast for two hours, then broth with veal and herbs: borage, bugloss, brooklime, watercress and chicory. Take lunch at the usual time, dine at about five o'clock. At bedtime, take *London treacle* as before.[2]

She wrote to say she was much better. For the fits of the mother she used the *London water for the womb*.[3] For cold feet this plaster was applied:

℞: pitch 2lb, best gum powdered and sieved, best frankincense powdered each 2lb, sheep suet 1oz, saffron 2oz, mace 2oz, laudanum 4oz, cloves 1oz. Mix. Boil for the space of half an hour or longer. First put the pitch in place. Spread it on leather very thinly, so as to make plasters shaped like the soles of slippers. These are joined by sewing to a linen sock shaped to the sole of the foot. Use it on the soles for fourteen days, or for a month or for six weeks, then remove.

This is certainly powerful in any pain whatsoever. I cured old Mr Ferriman,[4] a gentleman worn out by long-standing pain in the feet, with this plaster alone.

For the swollen spleen: magisterial ointment for the spleen. For backache, our nephritic plaster:

℞: opium 15gr, wax, lead each 2oz, oils of roses, water-lilies each 2oz, nightshade juice 1oz. Boil in the form of a plaster. Make the plaster, spread some on leather and apply to the back.

For wind in the stomach:

---

1 amount … hold] approximately 7 grams, or 11 grains.
2 *Pharmacopoeia Londinensis*, p. 90.
3 *Pharmacopoeia Londinensis*, p. 9.
4 Thomas Ferriman, rector of Harvington, Worcestershire (?–1619). Matriculated from Queens' College, Cambridge in 1566. He was domestic chaplain to the Bishop of Worcester for four years, which included a visit by Queen Elizabeth I in 1575. In 1597 he married Magdalen Smalwait. He was rector of Harvington from 1579 for forty years. He left money to the poor in his will. His son Thomas succeeded him as rector.

℞: bugloss conserve 2oz, pleres archonticon powder 2dr. Dose: the amount of a nutmeg.

She also used our antiscorbutic water with clove-gillyflower syrup. She took the above antiscorbutic beer and used their steeled wine. She recovered rightly, praise God.

[Case 155]

[p. 150] Burning fever with facial convulsion and spasm of the mouth.[1] You Lord, who *hast power of life and death; thou leadest to the gates of hell, and bringest up again;*[2] I confess *neither by human work, nor help from the art, nor advice, but only by your goodness and mercy you made me whole, and recovered me beyond all hope and expectation from the most severe and deadliest signs of a lethal fever, as if rescued from the jaws of hell and restored to perfect health.*[3] For this *I give thanks to you, most merciful God and Father of our Lord Jesus Christ, who through your fatherly mercy has made me whole. Give me grace, that I may recognize and remember your blessings with a grateful mind.*[4] *It was only on account of receiving so much from almighty God the most high, that I was raised from such a severe and deadly illness. So that my friends may rejoice with me, and the divine will of God and his unbounding power be admired, I report the whole story, faithful to the truth.*[5]

About the 57th year of age, from 27 August in the year of salvation 1632 to 19 September, I had been weakened by an excessive flux from the haemorrhoids. I nevertheless had to visit patients here and there every day, riding at great speed on a hard-mouthed

---

1 Hall records his own illness in 1632, which he treated himself until he was so ill that his wife sent for two physicians. After their treatments, he prescribed for himself again, and was cured: 'God did all this.'

2 hast … again] Valleriola, *Observationum* […] *libri sex*, p. 2, based on Vulgate, 1 Sam. 2:6.

3 neither … health] Valleriola, *Observationum* […] *libri sex*, p. 1. Translation from King James Bible, Wis. 16:13.

4 I give … mind] Ruland the Elder, 'Centuria III', *Curationum* […] *centuriae*, p. 231.

5 It was … truth] Valleriola, *Observationum* […] *libri sex*, p. 2.

horse.[1] The flux of the haemorrhoids was checked for **[p. 151]**
fourteen days. Then I was wretchedly attacked by toothache, and
fell into a deadly burning fever (which was then seeking victims
everywhere, and almost all who were infected exchanged life for
death).[2] *Therefore what I used in this most severe fever as a method of driving
it away, and by the help of which alone I was protected by the aid of God's good
will, I now put forward.*[3] First I was purged in this way:

℞: rhubarb infusion 1dr, diasereos syrup 1oz, electuary of rose juice
3 dr, resulting in four stools.

Next I used hartshorn decoction with this effect. The illness was
well expelled in the urine so that at night fourteen chamber-pots
were half filled (I ordered each passage of urine to be stored in a
single vessel) and as many in the day, for I was forced to pass urine
every hour. Strange to say, I did not drink more than 2 pints of
hartshorn deocoction (all other drink being forbidden) for I feared
dropsy of the chamber pots. The flux of urine continued thus for
four days. I was emaciated, my strength exhausted, so that I could
not move in bed without the help of servants. I had spasms of the
mouth and eyes. *A breathing pigeon, dismembered, was applied to the feet,
to draw the vapours down*[4] for I was often slightly delirious. Then my
wife called in two physicians for advice. I used a softening enema
with the emollient herbs, diacatholicon, and softeners. I swallowed
the following electuary from my friends the physicians, the amount
of a nutmeg twice a day:

℞: electuary of cold gems, 2dr, pleres archonticon powder 1dr
(because scurvy was feared), pearled manus Christi 1oz, **[p. 152]**
bugloss, violet conserves each 2oz, wood-sorrel 1oz, syrup of violets
½oz, of lemons 1oz, oil of vitriol 6 drops. Make an electuary.

---

1 hard-mouthed horse] Translation following Conrad Gesner, *Historiae animalium
liber I* (Zurich: Frosch, 1551), p. 532.
2 which ... death] according to Lane (1996: xxiii), Birmingham had an outbreak
of plague at about this time, but deaths in Stratford were not unusually high.
3 Valleriola, *Observationum* [...] *libri sex*, p. 6.
4 Donne, *Devotions upon Emergent Occasions*, p. 284.

27 September: purged thus:

R: softening electuary 1½oz, wormwood water 4oz. Mix. Three stools.

At bedtime:

R: diacodium syrup and corn poppies with diascordium.

For heat in the back:

R: Galen's cooling [ointment] 1½oz, sandalwood salve ½oz, houseleek juice, wine vinegar each 1 spoonful. Make a soft ointment.

A plaster for the region of the heart:

R: labdanum 6dr, styrax calamita ½oz, aromatic rose powder 4sc, musk 4gr. Mix.

I was purged again like this:

R: diasereos syrup ½oz, electuary of rose juice 3dr, sufficient chicory water.

NOTE: Before the physicians attended me, I took 10oz of blood from the hepatic vein, and the third day after that, leeches were applied to the haemorrhoidal veins. The 10oz of blood is an estimate of the quantity I could extract. But I give thanks first to God, then to the hartshorn decoction, and finally to the venesection. I was quite restored to strength, for now I could take food. Previously nothing but fluid was welcome. I used steeled wine with scurvy-grass juice, and Foreest's scheletyrbic syrup. Once a week I was purged with holy powder, rhubarb infusion and diasereos. I was often wretchedly afflicted with toothache. I was completely cured with oil of hazel wood. Then I was wretchedly troubled by itching of the scrotum with excoriation. I was cured by our sarsaparilla decoction with antiscorbutic herbs. God did all this, to whom alone be all honour and glory for ever and ever. Amen.

[Case 156]

[p. 153] 8 [XXX] 16–.[1] Long-standing headache. Baronet Puckering,[2] aged about 44 years more or less: attacked by headache, worst in the morning and around the evening hours. He feels relief at night though, when he lies on his back with his head hanging down a little. *I undertake, with thanks to divine favour, to make a cure in this way:*[3]

℞: pills – of peony 1dr, amber, Ruffus's each 1sc, *Fernel's for headache* 2sc.[4] Make 15 pills with betony water. Take 2 at bedtime, 3 in the morning.

When these were finished I prescribed the application of leeches to the haemorrhoidal veins. This had the happy and desired result, for he was completely freed from the headache. Then he used the following opiate:

℞: sliced sassafras wood 6dr, powdered cinnamon, sweet flag each ½oz. Infuse in bugloss water 12oz for twenty-four hours, then boil, reduce to half. To the strained liquid add *conserves of chicory and bugloss flowers each ½oz, Venice treacle 1dr, alkermes, hyacinth confection each ½dr, prepared steel 1oz, diatrion santalon, diambra, sweet diamoschum each ½dr, bezoar stone ½sc, prepared hartshorn, prepared pearls each 2sc. Make an opiate with syrup of preserved citrons. Swallow the amount of a large hazelnut of the above opiate, morning and bedtime.*[5]

After catching cold he fell into a nightly quotidian fever; purged thus:

℞: diasereos syrup 2oz, expressed rhubarb 1dr, cream of tartar 1sc, betony water 2oz. Make a draught.

---

1 These crosses appear in Hall's manuscript.
2 Sir Thomas Puckering of Warwick Priory (cf. Case 135). Died in Sussex but buried in St Mary's, Warwick, where there is a monument by Nicholas Stone, master mason to Wren. Puckering left instructions and £200 for this monument. He also left money for the poor in six Warwickshire parishes.
3 Ruland the Elder, 'Centuria VI', *Curationum* […] *centuriae*, p. 437.
4 Fernel's for headache] See Case 23, n. 6.
5 Du Chesne, *De priscorum philosophorum* […] *materia*, p. 358.

He retained it for half an hour then vomited some, but still had four stools. The next day, for cough and phlegm:

℞: maidenhair syrup, **[p. 154]** hyssop each 1oz, magisterial scabious syrup ½oz. Make a linctus with a pleasing taste.

He regained his voice, and brought up large amounts of phlegm with a decoction of china with the capillary herbs, snails, yellow sandalwood, ivory shavings and hartshorn shavings, and a julep of the aperient decoction with syrup. For the fever:

℞: cordial water frigida Saxoniae 2 spoonfuls with 3 spoonfuls of this julep:

℞: magisterium of pearls 1dr, scabious water 1oz, syrup of cloves 1oz, alkermes confection 1sc.

He was freed from the fever. Afterwards he used Dr Lapworth's[1] preserve to maintain health:

℞: conserve of betony flowers, clove-gillyflowers each 1oz, conserve of citron peel 6dr, extract of sweet flag 1dr, powdered winter-cherry rind 2½sc, peony seeds 1dr, oil of cinnamon 4 drops. Make a preserve with sufficient betony syrup. Take the amount of a nutmeg.

He used this often with success and told me so, and on that account I wished him to take it. For the spleen:

℞: magisterial plaster for the spleen 1½oz, magisterial diachylon 6dr, caranna dissolved in vinegar of squills 4dr, white hellebore root 2sc, oil of rosewood 1sc. Mix. Make a plaster. Spread it on soft leather, cover with silk, sew together. Apply to the region of the spleen.

He was freed from all symptoms. As a precaution he had a fontanelle in the left brachial [vein]. *Praise God alone, he escaped entirely from the pain and associated circumstances.*[2]

---

1 Probably Dr Edward Lapworth MD, Oxford (Raach 1962: 62); there was also a William Lapworth MA (Cantab.) in Warwick (Raach 1962: 62).
2 Ruland the Elder, 'Centuria II', *Curationum* […] *centuriae*, p. 85.

[Case 157]

[p. 155] Heat and roughness of the tongue. Alderman Tyler:[1] complained of heat and roughness of the tongue. I helped him quickly with the following:

R: magisterial scabious syrup, brooklime, watercress, prepared scurvy-grass juice each ½oz, coltsfoot, liquorice, corn poppy each 1oz. Mix. Take often with a liquorice stick.

Cured.

[Case 158]

Suffocation of the womb. Alderman Smith's daughter,[2] a spinster aged about 22 years: fell into a fit of the mother with convulsions of the eyes and darkened vision because of diminished periods and grief. During the attack she was tortured by spasm and twisting of the neck, and palpitations of the heart with fever so that her whole bed shook hither and thither. By my advice, during an attack (because the attacks are lessening at intervals) I prescribe water for the womb, 3 spoonfuls dripped into her mouth. Afterwards fumigate the room with burning horse hooves. She recovered quickly from the attack. For prevention:

R: powdered castor ½dr, foetidae pills 1dr. Make 7 pills, gild them.

She was rightly purged, and freed from her symptoms. Finally:

R: castor powder ½dr, extract for the womb 1dr. Make 9 pills: 3 at bedtime, in the morning 2.

---

1 Richard Tyler, Alderman of Stratford-upon-Avon (1566–1636). Son of a butcher in Stratford. In 1588 he married an heiress, Susanna Woodward. Tyler was paid for providing arms in that Armada year. Elected a burgess in 1590. His death in the parish register was recorded as Mr Tyler, gent.

2 Margaret Smith of Stratford-upon-Avon (1599–?). Daughter of an alderman, probably Francis Smith, a mercer. In 1623 she married Paul Sylvester of Burford (cf. Case 125, her daughter Hester).

It was with these few that she regained complete health unexpectedly and very speedily, nor did this illness ever reappear.[1]

[Case 159]
Cure of smallpox. The only son of Reverend Holyoak[2] who compiled the most learned dictionary: seized by continual burning fever, lower backache, cough. I said they were the precursors **[p. 156]** of measles,[3] nor did my opinion fail me, for the next day they appeared on his face after he took the following potion:

> ℞: diascordium 1dr, coral tincture, bezoar stone each 3gr, in fennel water, with the desired result, for he was freed from pain in the back and stomach, and [the pocks] began to spring out.[4]

To preserve the eyes:

> ℞: *waters of plantain, eyebright, roses each 1dr, camphor 1sc, saffron 2gr. Mix. make eyedrops and anoint the eye often with a fine feather.*[5]

To preserve the throat and gullet, *I ordered him to gargle continuously with goat's or cow's milk, mixed at the same time with plantain water. This is a supreme remedy for the mouth and throat when the exanthematous signs show themselves.*[6] *In a case like this, pomegranate syrup is a secret, to protect the lungs, chest and throat from measles, despite the simultaneous presence of laboured breathing and cough. I therefore instructed him to lick this eclegma without a break:*

---

1 Ruland the Elder, 'Centuria I', *Curationum* [...] *centuriae*, p. 63.
2 Thomas Holyoak of Southam (1616–75). Son of Francis, rector of Southam. Attended Queen's College, Oxford, and became chaplain there, then rector of Birdingbury. Served in the royal army at the siege of Oxford. In 1647, forced out of his living, he practised medicine in Warwick. From 1660 he was rector of Whitnash. Buried in St Mary's, Warwick.
3 The MS has measles changed to smallpox in the heading, but not in the text.
4 the pocks] A good sign, as the body was expelling the dangerous humours.
5 Amatus Lusitanus, *Curationum medicinalium centuriae quatuor*, p. 232.
6 Foreest, *De febribus ephemeris et continuis*, p. 98.

℞: *sweet syrup of pomegranates 2oz, barley sugar 3dr, syrups of rose infusion, mulberries each ½oz, cold diatragacanth in tablets 3dr. refined flour 2sc. Make an eclegma.*[1]

But this was not to hand, so he used magisterial scabious syrup, maidenhair fern, liquorice each 1oz, with happy effect. *For the sense of smell*:

℞: *a little best rose vinegar with wheat bread, applied to the nostrils.*[2]

His food before night was barley made in this fashion:

℞: *wheat barley 1 handful,*[3] **[p. 157]** *sweet almonds 2oz. Make barley water to 1 pint. Sweeten with violet sugar and use in place of food.*

To make more spots appear through the skin, he used a decoction of liquorice, figs and common barley for greater expulsion. He stayed warm in bed and I ordered that he have a sufficiently bright fire in his bedroom.[4] To drink: a ptisane. These, praise God, rightly cured him.

[Case 160]
Wandering gout. 10 April. A gentleman of the Count of Northampton:[5] had severe pain now in one and then the other knee, so that he scarcely walked for pain. He has at some times been attacked by retention of urine. His name if I am not mistaken was Peter Hugges, a Welshman, aged 34. He was quickly freed, by these few ministrations:

---

1 Foreest, *De febribus ephemeris et continuis*, p. 98.
2 Amatus Lusitanus, *Curationum medicinalium centuriae quatuor*, p. 232.
3 Mostly I have translated *p.* as pinch (*pugillum*), but handful is also possible and seems more likely here.
4 Foreest, *De febribus ephemeris et continuis*, p. 99.
5 Cooke did not give this patient's name, describing him only as 'the Lord of Northampton's gentleman'. On this basis Lane identified him as William Beale. Five lines into the Latin text, Hall named the patient 'Peterus Hugges Wallicus' – Peter Hugges the Welshman. He was perhaps seen on one of Hall's visits to Ludlow. There are no more details for Hugges, and the consultation cannot be dated.

℞: pills – sine quibus, foetidae each 1dr, opoponax 2sc, powder of alhandal trochees 1sc, saltpetre 15gr. Make pills, gild them. Take pill about ten o'clock in the evening, 4 in the morning about seven o'clock, for three days.

He was truly purged.

℞: oxycroceum plaster, diachylon with gum each 1oz, oil of bricks 1dr. Make a plaster. Apply to the painful area.

He was freed. 27 December: for prevention:

℞: caryocostinum electuary ½oz, cream of tartar 1sc, diasereos syrup 1oz, betony water 4oz. Mix.

℞: pills, sine quibus 1dr, foetidae 1½dr, alhandal trochees 1sc. Make 10 pills. Give 5 per dose.

He was completely freed, praise God.

[Case 161]
Roundworms. 28 December. Mrs Bovey,[1] a gentlewoman of Kings Coughton aged 46: attacked by anal itching and roundworms. She was quickly cured in this way:

℞: pills – hiera with agaric 2dr, Ruffus's 1dr, foetidae 1sc. Make 15 pills. **[p. 158]** Take 2 at bedtime, 3 in the morning.

When these were finished, *give one roll, either 1dr or weighing more*:

℞: *Macedonian parsley seeds, wormseed each 4sc, pomegranate rind, burnt hartshorn each ½dr, white dittany, choice rhubarb, cloves each 1sc, cinnamon 2dr, saffron 1sc. Mix. Make a powder and make rolls 1dr in amount, with sufficient sugar.*[2] She is to use a lard suppository, followed by an enema of milk and unrefined sugar. Take the above rolls for fifteen days.

She was completely freed from the itching and worms.

---

1 Margaret Bovey of Kings Coughton (*c.* 1570–?). Daughter and heiress of William Harrison of Worcestershire. Married John Bovey of Kings Coughton, an eldest son. His will in 1637 mentions no children. His widow Margaret inherited Kings Coughton House, land and money.

2 Amatus Lusitanus, *Curationum medicinalium centuriae quatuor*, p. 313, *ponderans*.

[Case 162]

1633. Scorbutic fever. Lady Browne of Radford,[1] aged 49, 1 January: suffered for a long time from long-established scurvy, now tortured by a continual burning scorbutic fever. These symptoms trouble her: palpitation of the heart, wind in the stomach and bowels. Even when she passes wind or belches, she feels only a little relief. Her mouth is perpetually dry although she is satisfied with a small amount to drink. *She has a changing pulse, weak, unequal and often wormlike, so that I judge it more to crawl than to beat.*[2] *She has less heat in a scorbutic than an intense acute fever, and it is less associated with thirst and restlessness. Or, if the heat is worse, anxiety still recurs at intervals and troubles her over her heart, and the pulse is slow and unequal. One distinguishes these fevers carefully from other continual fevers by this: if thick* **[p. 159]** *reddish urine with thick, reddish, heavy and uneven sediment are added, and thirst is less than matches the degree of putrefaction* (as in her case) *this sign is much more convincing.*[3] When she rises from bed she feels faint, *so that it seems she is going to die on the instant. At that time the pulse feels rather stronger and larger than before, without doubt because there is the greatest need, and because the heart is attempting to expel the corrupt vapours which trouble it.*[4] *The smallness of the pulse warned me and I advised the lady not to fear that she would fall out of bed, because the descent is easy and with support. This is a common consequence of this mischief, because it arises from an exhalation of vapours released by internal putrefaction, and breathes out as high as the heart and its container, with wind.*[5] *The wind could be felt in either side of the belly*[6] (she complained of pain in the sides). *The source of scurvy in the spleen produces a flatulent melancholy, since the regions of the hypochondria encircle the spleen. The melancholy bubbles up in the meseraic*

---

1 Elizabeth, Lady Browne of Radford Semele (cf. Case 106). Still grieving for her daughter, who died in childbirth.
2 She ... beat] Sennert, *De scorbuto tractatus*, p. 88.
3 She ... convincing] Sennert, *De scorbuto tractatus*, pp. 129–130.
4 Sennert, *De scorbuto tractatus*, p. 88.
5 The ... wind] Eugalenus *De scorbuto morbo*, p. 297.
6 The wind ... belly] Martini, 'De scorbuto', in Sennert, *De scorbuto tractatus*, p. 603.

veins around the pancreas and putrefies as if it were fermenting.[1] *The winds spread out neither in the front nor back part of the body, indicating that they are affecting the stomach, constricting the precordium, obstructing freedom of respiration. She is attacked by most severe winds from the stomach, limbs and muscles, either continuously or breaking out at intervals.*[2]

[The patient], *pleading and demanding help from me, was freed through God's grace and mercy*[3] **[p. 160]** *by the following few devices in a few days,*[4] and from torments of the belly and fainting and constipation within twenty-four hours. NOTE: *She was very thirsty and drank often, but not large draughts. Her tongue was covered in cracks due the acrid nature of the vapours rising from putrefaction.*[5]

An enema:

> ℞: the common decoction for an enema 12oz, unrefined sugar 4oz, fresh butter 2oz. Mix.

She had two stools. But before I prescribed the administration of the enema, she swallowed the following electuary:

> ℞: liberans powder 1dr in barberry conserve an hour before the enema, and at bedtime bezoar stone 5gr. Repeat the above electuary in the morning.

The enema was repeated, which resulted in three stools with great relief. NOTE: All the heat ought to be removed with enemas, because they force the wind to rise. [Take] hartshorn jelly in broth containing antiscorbutic herbs. At bedtime:

> ℞: cordial water frigida Saxoniae 1oz, Foreest's scheletyrbic syrup.

---

1 The … fermenting] Alberti, 'De Schorbuti historia', in Sennert, *De scorbuto tractatus*, p. 403.

2 The winds … intervals] Martini, 'De scorbuto', in Sennert, *De scorbuto tractatus*, p. 603, continuing directly from the previous Martini borrowing.

3 The patient … mercy] Ruland the Elder, 'Centuria III', *Curationum* […] *centuriae*, p. 219.

4 by … days] Ruland the Elder, 'Centuria III', *Curationum* […] *centuriae*, p. 218.

5 Eugalenus, *De scorbuto morbo*, p. 312.

She was purged thus on the third day:

℞: manna 1oz, expressed rhubarb 1dr, tartar 1sc, Foreest's scheletyrbic syrup 1oz, chicory water 3oz. Four stools.

She used the hartshorn decoction when thirsty, and with these she
becomes heartily healthy. The cause was from grief at the death of
her only daughter, who died after giving birth. This daughter was
a phoenix of her sex, devoutly pious, as well structured as anyone
(I name her always to honour her). So I leave her with God.

[Case 163]

[p. 161] Stone, lower backache, fever. Lady Rainsford:[1] tortured
by the stone, fever and thirst, about 62 years old. She was cured
with the following, so that now she is healthy. She is modest, pious,
kindly and well-deserving of everyone. She was most devoted to
reading the Holy Scriptures, and was experienced in the French
and Italian languages.

℞: hellebore powder 1dr, Cyprus turpentine 2dr. Mix. Give 5 pills
from 1dr.

℞: oils – of scorpions 1oz, of sweet almonds 2dr. Mix. Rub on the
back.

℞: emollient decoction 12oz, lenitive electuary, diaphoenicon each
1oz, loosening rose syrup 3oz. Mix. Make an enema: two stools.

After six hours had passed, I administered another [enema]
from the prepared decoction: sugar 4oz, butter 4oz. Make it. But
NOTE: I prescribed the following to be taken every third hour:

℞: liberans powder 1dr, syrup of corn poppies ½oz, sufficient posset
ale.

The night was restful.

---

1 Anne, Lady Rainsford of Clifford Chambers (1571–?). Daughter of Sir Henry
Goodere, an anti-recusant and patron of Michael Drayton. Ben Jonson and John
Donne were among his guests. Married Henry Rainsford *c.* 1595 (cf. Case 80). He
was knighted in 1603; three sons. No record of her death.

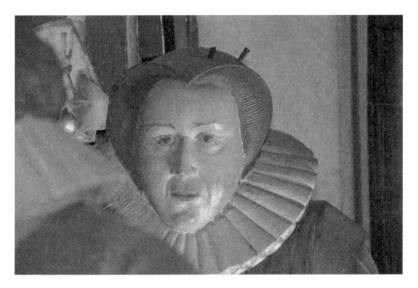

38 Effigy of Anne, Lady Rainsford (1571–?), St Helen's Church, Clifford Chambers. She was the dedicatee for Michael Drayton's 64-sonnet series *Idea*, published in 1594. Drayton had been a page in the household of her father, Sir Henry Goodere of Polesworth. Two years later she married Sir Henry Rainsford. Hall clearly admired her for her piety, intellect and kindness. He treated her for a stone (Case 163)

℞: powdered rhubarb 2dr, fumitory water 8oz. Boil, reduce to 4. To the strained liquid add cream of tartar 1sc, diasereos syrup 2oz. Make a draught: five stools.

An enema of linseed oil the next day, at bedtime:

℞: liberans powder 2sc, prepared hartshorn 1sc, coral tincture ½sc.

And so in the morning she was cured, praise God the three and one.

[Case 164]

Scorbutic arthritis. 1 February 1633. The Bishop of Worcester, Dr Thornborough,[1] about 86 years old: tortured for a long time

---

1 John Thornborough, Bishop of Worcester (1551–1641). At Oxford he was noted for fencing, dancing and womanising. Friend of Simon Forman, the famous

by scorbutic arthritis. *The deceptive appearance of the arthritis misled and toyed with his physicians,*[1] who were experienced and learned in traditional medicine. I enquired more thoroughly concerning the arthritis, whether it was fixed or wandering, then about his urine and finally the blotches. *The Reverend Father revealed that blackish blotches had appeared on his legs a few days earlier, which* **[p. 162]** *changed to a yellow colour, which confirmed scurvy.*[2] I found his urine now red, now turbid, frequent change being a sign of scurvy. *As far as I can recall from memory, it* changed daily: *either thick, bluish, red or white, appearing to be clearing or turbid, with or without sediment.*[3]

Blotches: *What is thick and heavier sinks to the legs, where it causes various blotches which are at first ruddy, not dissimilar to those left by flea bites. They break out bluish and purple, then turn black. Both the larger ones, and the smaller ones similar to flea bites,*[4] *occur more frequently on the legs, since nature is accustomed to banish vicious humours to the less noble and more distant parts.*[5] Wakefulness; a restless night: *They are harassed by wakefulness because of salty and bitter windy humours rising to the head, and if they sleep, they are terrified.*[6]

What affected the bishop was this. His son, a knight, had stabbed with his sword one of the bishop's servants the previous summer, for borrowing money and then asking for the debt to be cancelled. His son's rage was inflamed when his head was wounded with a sword, his clothes stained with blood. Then, anger turning to fury, his son drew his sword and stabbed [the servant] through the chest, so that he never said another word. The bishop fainted

---

astrologer. Anti-recusant. Became Bishop of Worcester in 1617. Married three times. Several scandals in his family: he divorced his first wife; one son killed himself. The bishop granted Hall a pew in Holy Trinity Church. Buried in Worcester Cathedral.

1 Eugalenus, *De scorbuto morbo*, p. 97.
2 Eugalenus, *De scorbuto morbo*, p. 167.
3 Eugalenus, *De scorbuto morbo*, p. 100.
4 Sennert, *De scorbuto tractatus*, p. 82.
5 Sennert, *De scorbuto tractatus*, p. 83.
6 Sennert, *De scorbuto tractatus*, p. 111.

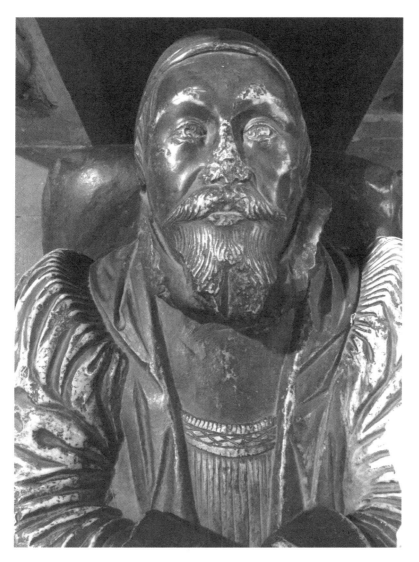

39 Tomb of John Thornborough, Bishop of Worcester (1551–1641), in Worcester Cathedral. Thornborough was 86 when Hall treated him for scurvy and arthritis (Case 164). He was troubled by terrible nightmares in which he imagined his son (who had murdered one of the bishop's servants) being hanged.

on hearing this, and seeing the servant (whom he especially loved) rolling in blood. When he recovered, he was seized in his imagination with severe melancholy **[p. 163]** and fear of the execution of his son (as he thought in his delirium) for murder. Because of grief and fear of the punishment (he dreamed at night that his son had been hanged) he was woken in terror by the sight of his execution. Following this he was troubled by severe melancholy so that he could neither eat nor sleep. This was the cause of these tears and the illness.

He now complained of pains in his knees and elsewhere. I told him he did not suffer from a simple gout but a wandering scorbutic arthritis, *for it often accompanies the arthritis of scurvy* which is called wandering scurvy, *because it does not stay in one place until the weakening of the illness but, wandering it seizes* now the knee, then the foot with *or without swelling.* There was a lot of such swelling in the knee and around the ankle, in the foot similar swelling to dropsy, though it did not yield to the fingers as in a true dropsy, nor *was it a true arthritis as described by early authorities,* for that does not change its place, now in the knees and then in the feet, hither and thither. *It takes possession of the limb which was first seized in order to weaken it. It has its roots in thin, watery, bitter humours ready for movement and apt for changing place.*[1]

I warned that I could alleviate but never cure it, because he was weakened by age. He replied, 'the old should be visited, the young cured'. But because his nights were sleepless and his days troubled, he instructed me to try to give some alleviation, for 'to live so is to die'. I prescribed the following in the name of God, omitting purgation because of his weak strength and since he had been purged before: **[p. 164]** A jelly of hartshorn shavings, antiscorbutic herbs, veal bones and partridge, made with raisins and dates. To the strained liquid I added a little tincture of saffron and alkermes with

---

1 Sennert, *De scorbuto tractatus*, p. 102.

sugar candy for sweetening, acceptable to the palate, fragrant to the nose, and suitable for the stomach. I wished him to take prepared scurvy-grass juice three times a day. *I prescribed live worms to be placed on the painful swellings*, seeing that I have applied them successfully in other cases, *for they leap up, curl around, bend down, dwindle away, and die.*[1] I have observed this as in Eugalenus's experience: *it is most appropriate for livid swellings because it dissipates and removes all swelling and hardness in three or four days.*[2] Wormwood powder and egg as before.

A bath for the feet before he used the poultice:

℞: brooklime 10 handfuls, sufficient beer. Boil and make a bath, bathe the feet in it morning and evening.

After the bath the night was more restful than for a long time. *He was gripped by sleep more closely than before.*[3] Then I reduced our antiscorbutic water, seeing he took [another] antiscorbutic water. He used scurvy-grass juice as before, and jelly. He also took antiscorbutic beer. These, praise God, freed him completely from the pain and swelling of his feet. The next month I contrived to visit him. He was walking vigorously and thanked me greatly. Praise to almighty God most high.

[Case 165]

[p. 165] Very severe vomiting, wind in the stomach, difficulty of breathing, constipation of the belly, scurvy. 1633. Mr Simon Underhill,[4] a gentleman about 40 years old: complained of the

---

1 Horst, *Observationum* […] *libri quatuor*, p. 350.
2 Eugalenus, *De scorbuto morbo*, p. 136.
3 Echoing Cicero, 'Somnium Scipionis, Book VI', *De re publica*.
4 Simon Underhill of Idlicote (1589–1664). Youngest son of Sir Hercules Underhill, lived all his life at Idlicote. Hercules's father had sold New Place to William Shakespeare. Married Elizabeth, a widow and heiress. No record of any children. Lane dated the consultation to 1629 based on Hall's estimate of age ('about 40 years') and the patient's baptism in 1589. Hall also gave a consultation date of 1633, which Cooke omitted. I prefer Hall's date for the consultation.

above symptoms, which are true signs of scurvy. For the causes, see Eugalenus, pages 238–240, 242,[1] and Daniel Sennert, *Tractatus de scorbuto*, pages 115, 612, 721.[2] This causes very loose bowel movements:

℞: jalap 1sc, cream of tartar ½sc, sufficient Cyprus turpentine. Make 3 pills.

He was wholly purged. For the difficulty in breathing, take:

℞: pleres archonticon powder 2dr, scurvy-grass conserve 2oz, alkermes confection 1sc. Mix. Dose: the amount of a nutmeg, an hour before meals. Repeat often.

He also used diacrocuma, up to 2dr before dinner. He improved a great deal, so it was unexpected when he turned up at my home, brought to me in a carriage. He said he would rather die here or be cured, for he much preferred that to living like this. 'For', he said, 'to continue to live like this is to die.' During the night of 7 March, wind from the stomach reached his head, like a pain. He asked for something to control it:

℞: red Pannonian powder 2sc with syrup of violets, from a spoon.

The rest of the night was restful. In the morning: an enema of a decoction of brooklime, watercress, scurvy-grass and nettle. I took 12oz of the decoction, Holland powder 1dr, diaphoenicon 1oz, diaturbith powder with rhubarb 1½dr. Mix. Make an enema. He discharged many cannon blasts and farts. Before the enema I wished him to swallow scurvy-grass conserve 3dr, red Pannonian powder 1sc.

On the 9th day:

℞: prepared scurvy-grass juice 8oz, syrups of brooklime and watercress each 2oz.

---

1 Eugalenus, *De scorbuto morbo*, pp. 238–240, 242–243.
2 Sennert, *De scorbuto tractatus*, pp. 115–116; Martini, 'De scorbuto', in Sennert, *De scorbuto tractatus*, pp. 612–613, 721–722.

He used steeled wine, pleres archonticon electuary after meals, and antiscorbutic beer all the time. Within fourteen days he was healthy again. Praise God.

[Case 166]

[p. 166] Fit of the womb, convulsion of the arms and left cheek, with fainting. 22 February. Mrs Swift,[1] a gentlewoman, spinster, modest, well-conducted, of excellent structure, a relative of Baron Brooke of Warwick Castle: wretchedly attacked by suffocation of the womb, spasm of the mouth, convulsions in the hands and arms. She was properly purged by an experienced physician and consulted many in vain. Then I hastened to the aid of this desperately ill gentlewoman in the name of God, thus:

> ℞: bryony decoction with feverfew ½lb, hiera picra powder 2dr, Holland powder 1dr. Make an enema: two stools with relief.

I gave water for the womb 1oz but she vomited, then at once the following pills:

> ℞: extract for the womb 1sc, bryony dregs ½sc. Make 3 pills, gild them.

After half an hour she vomited phlegm and black acid bile again, and complained of heat in the stomach, as if it were being scalded. I directed her to drink clear cold water, up to ½ pint. She vomited again at once. Again I repeated the draught of water, so that as it reached the heat of her stomach, she vomited. Then I directed it repeated once more. She retained it, and was much better. For the convulsion:

> ℞: Martiatum ointment ½oz, oils of sassafras and amber each 5 drops. Mix. Rub on to the neck.

---

1 Fulca Swift of Warwick Castle (1613–54). Daughter of Sir Francis Swift and related to the Greville family. Lived in the Warwick Castle household. Married James Horsey *c.* 1629; one daughter, Dorothy, an infant when James died in 1630. Fulca, according to her epitaph, 'lived many years a widow'.

To the umbilicus: a plaster of caranna with five grains of civet and musk in the middle on cotton-wool, and hartshorn shavings with a little bryony dregs and arum. Continue for several days. She used *Ruland's sneezing powder.*[1] **[p. 167]** She had slight fainting attacks, up to twice an hour, previously four to six. At bedtime:

> ℞: best musk 5gr, cinnamon, cloves, nutmeg each 1sc. Make gilded pills with alkermes confection.

These completely cured her, praise God.

[Case 167]

Burning fever, scorbutic dropsy. Mrs Fiennes,[2] a gentlewoman (whom I name always with respect), born of noble stock: seized by a burning fever with thirst and loss of strength three days after giving birth. The midwife in attendance wished to give her posset ale with lemon juice and wood-sorrel, and a morsel of chicken with wood-sorrel juice, so she ate it. They cooled her stomach too much. She fell into a dropsical swelling with swelling of the right leg and thigh, so that she was unable to move for pain. The midwife applied a plaster of red lead and instructed it to be tightly fastened round. The pain and swelling increased and finally she asked me to attend. When I saw the hard swelling, I diagnosed scorbutic dropsy. For the differences between a dropsical and a scorbutic swelling, see Daniel Sennert, *Tractatus de scorbuto*, page 623.[3] She was weakened by a slight hemiplegia and almost choked with phlegm. *I help the desperately ill gentlewoman in great measure with the skill of my hands and by calling on divine aid, in this way:*[4] First, so that she was not choked by abundance of phlegm, I prescribed a linctus of this sort:

---

1 Ruland the Elder, 'Centuria II', *Curationum [...] centuriae*, p. 125.
2 Frances Fiennes of Broughton Castle (1586–1632). Hall had attended her first confinement, and on this occasion saw her soon after the birth of her third child. A midwife had also treated her.
3 Martini, 'De scorbuto', in Sennert, *De scorbuto tractatus*, p. 623.
4 Ruland the Elder, 'Centuria VII', *Curationum [...] centuriae*, p. 505.

℞: syrups of hyssop, brooklime, watercress, magisterial scabious each 1oz.

She licked it often with a liquorice stick, with the desired result.

An enema:

℞: mallow, brooklime, watercress, scurvy-grass each 1 handful, **[p. 168]** fennel, parsley roots each 2oz, tops of elder ½ handful. Boil in sufficient water to 12oz. To the strained liquid add unrefined sugar 4oz.

She was very well purged of wind and phlegm, and thus the next day was rightly purged with the desired result. At bedtime:

℞: red Pannonian powder ½dr, prepared hartshorn ½sc, alkermes confection 1sc. Take it with lemon juice.

That night she was soaked in sweat. The powder was repeated in the morning during a faint for, when she wished to move from a bed or chair, she fell from diminished strength into a faint. This too is sign of scurvy that should not be disregarded. To restore strength I gave this electuary:

℞: scurvy-grass conserve 2oz, pleres archonticon powder ½oz. Mix. Give the amount of a nutmeg three hours before she rises.

Because I was hindered by much business, I could not stay with her longer. I asked her to send a servant to me the next day. He reported that she had almost been choked by phlegm during the night. I sent back the prepared syrup for phlegm again, and our antiscorbutic water as for the bishop. Take 6 spoonfuls in the morning and at bedtime. These restored her very well, praise God, beyond the expectation of her friends who thought death was at the doors.

An enema every other day:

℞: elder buds 1 handful, scurvy-grass, watercress, brooklime each ½ handful, entire fresh nettles 1 handful, parsley, fennel roots each 1oz. Boil in sufficient water. **[p. 169]**

259

℞: of the strained liquid 12oz, diacatholicon 1oz, diaturbith powder with rhubarb 2dr. Make an enema: three stools.

She also had a restorative of snails and earthworms, hartshorn shavings and saffron with antiscorbutic herbs as for the Bishop of Worcester, and chicken and partridge with cinnamon. She had an antiscorbutic beer of this sort:

℞: elder buds, leaves of betony, agrimony, scabious, wormwood each 1 handful, watercress, brooklime each 2 handfuls, blessed thistle, fumitory, wall germander each ½ handful, watercress, brooklime each 2 handfuls, scurvy-grass 4 handfuls, juniper berries ½lb. Infuse sliced and bruised in uncooked beer mash, 5 gallons. Boil, reduce to four gallons. *Combine these powders in a little knot*[1] and boil with the above. Afterwards boil again, and hang on a string in the barrel, coriander, anise seeds each ½oz, liquorice 1oz, sarsaparilla 2oz, sassafras 1oz, skin of winter cherries ½oz. Stand for fourteen days, then take a draught on an empty stomach, and before lunch and dinner and when retiring to bed.

The following ointment from the beginning, for contraction of the leg:

℞: oil of worms, chamomile, of castor each 1oz, goose, chicken fat each ½oz, marsh-mallow ointment 2oz, juice and leaves of scurvy-grass, brooklime, watercress each 1oz, sufficient wax. Make an ointment.

She used this ointment with the desired result, for within the space of three days she could walk without a stick. **[p. 170]** Take 4oz of this, every day:

℞: *scurvy-grass, watercress equal parts, brooklime half a part. Pound in a stone mortar and boil in milk, not pouring in a large amount of liquid.*[2]

The drink as before. Take an enema twice weekly:

---

1 Horst, *Observationum* […] *libri quatuor*, p. 141.
2 Sennert, *De scorbuto tractatus*, p. 168.

℞: *urine of a prepubescent boy 12oz. In this boil leavening 1 ½oz, fennel, anise, dill seeds each 1 ½oz, purified honey 1oz. Make an enema.*[1]

Then she was revived, restored to her previous health by the will of God alone, beyond the hope of friends.[2]

[Case 168]

Scorbutic dropsy, difficulty of breathing, swelling of the feet, yellow jaundice, swelling of the belly and sides. 12 March 1633. Mr Fortescue,[3] a gentleman, Catholic, of Cookhill aged 38: given to *frequent heavy drinking*,[4] *of very good build, sanguine by nature, fairly fat though compact.*[5] He fell into scorbutic dropsy from drunkenness, with difficulty in breathing, hard swelling of the belly, scrotum, feet, wind in the hypochondrium. yellow jaundice had spread over his whole body. He complained of these, and when I came I prescribed the following defence:

℞: laxative senna powder, diaturbith powder with rhubarb each 2sc, chicory syrup with rhubarb 1oz, sufficient posset ale. Make a draught: eight stools.

13th:

℞: pills – stomach, Ruffus's, sine quibus each 1sc. **[p. 171]** Make 5 pills: six stools.

14th: Venesection to 7oz. 15th:

℞: polypody of the oak, liquorice each 1oz, chicory root ½oz, shoots of brooklime, scurvy-grass, watercress, fumitory, lesser centaury each ½ handful, senna leaves 3oz, sliced agaric 6dr, rhubarb 2dr,

---

1 Willich, *Urinarum probationes*, p. 321.
2 Ruland the Elder, 'Centuria VII' *Curationum* [...] *centuriae*, p. 530.
3 Sir Nicholas Fortescue of Cookhill Priory, Worcestershire (*c.* 1595–1633). Came of a recusant family. Nicholas inherited the estate in 1605 and was knighted in 1618. Married Prudence Wheatley of Norfolk; seven children (Hall records two occasions when he treated his daughter, Martha; cf. Cases 41 and 153). His grandson John was an active Royalist.
4 frequent ... drinking] Foreest, *De febribus ephemeris et continuis*, p. 94.
5 of ... compact] Foreest, *De febribus ephemeris et continuis*, p. 113.

cream of tartar 1dr, chamomile flowers, elderflower buds each 2 pinches, fennel, carrot seeds each 1½dr, cinnamon, cloves, peel of winter cherries each 1dr, zedoary ½dr, saffron ½sc, stoned raisins 3oz. Make an infusion in 8 pints spring water overnight. In the morning boil, reduce by a third. Take 8 spoonfuls daily, resulting in five stools each day.

18th:

℞: pills – aggregative, for the stomach, Ruffus's each ½dr, prepared gamboge 14gr. Make 10 pills for 2 doses. Five stools from 1 dose.

After meals:

℞: diambra 2dr, rose sugar 2oz. Dose: ½ spoonful. The restorative as for Mrs Fiennes, page 169 and page 164.

He was purged every third day. *To assuage thirst, instead of beer he frequently used a decoction of sassafras infusion, made in this way*:

℞: *shavings of sassafras wood 1oz, of liquorice root 2oz, fennel seeds 2dr, small raisins 1½oz. Place in a pewter flask and pour on boiling water 6 pints. Close very well and allow to cool in a cold place.*[1]

He used diacrocuma up to 2dr. Every morning on five mornings, and after meals:

℞: pleres archonticon powder 2dr, sugar 1oz. Dose: ½ spoonful.

24th: He was purged with the above pills as on the 18th: eight stools. *A decoction of guaiacum, prepared in this way*:

℞: *guaiacum wood broken into chips 1lb, water 9 pints. Boil, reduce to a half. Near the end of cooking, I added dried bindweed 1 handful, inner cinnamon 2oz, raisins with seeds 2oz. Make a decoction.* **[p. 172]**

I ordered this to be poured, hot, into another glass jar, into which I poured 3 pints of good wine. I advised drinking this syrup hot, 9oz in the morning, in the evening 6oz, and to cover himself properly with the bedcovers, to elicit sweat.[2] His diet was drying. Every third day, an enema of urine and

---

1 Horst, *Observationum* […] *libri quatuor*, pp. 141–142.
2 Valleriola, *Observationum* […] *libri sex*, p. 89.

leavening as for Mrs Fiennes, page 170. He was purged weekly with the following bolus:

℞: jalap 1sc, cream of tartar 1dr, tamarind electuary ½oz. Make a bolus. Seven stools.

These removed the swelling completely.

I do not know by what fate, but on 3 April he fell into a fever. He had two attacks of rigors and shivering for six hours, then was hot for three. He was purged again with the above bolus: five stools, large and watery. This freed him from the fever. Next he used the above antiscorbutic beer with meals, and this powder after meals:

℞: red Pannonian powder, powders, diambra, sweet diamoschum each dr, distilled anise oil 3 drops, white sugar 4oz. Mix. Make a powder. Dose: the amount that can be held on six pennies.[1]

In this way he was completely restored in six weeks.[2] *Praise, honour and glory be to God, for ever.*[3]

[Case 169]
Long-standing scurvy with sweating. Mr Kimberley,[4] a gentleman about 26 years old: suffered from tiredness of the whole body for a long time. He has better appetite than digestion and is disfigured by jaundice. He is seized by lower back pain, weakness of the legs,

---

1 the amount ... pennies] Approximately 7 grams, or 11 grains.
2 In ... weeks] Ruland the Elder, 'Centuria VII', *Curationum* [...] *centuriae*, p. 523.
3 Praise ... ever] Ruland the Elder, 'Centuria VII', *Curationum* [...] *centuriae*, p. 524.
4 Apart from the name, we know only that Hall saw this patient at the age of 26. Lane identified him as either Gilbert (born 1590) or William (born 1592), giving dates of consultation in 1616 or 1618. However, Hall treated his Mr Kimberley with two remedies reproduced almost word for word from Horst's *Observationum* published in 1625. The consultation must have been after that date, making both Gilbert and William unlikely candidates. Lane's notes also mention William, Robert and Justinian Kimberley, sons of Robert, a shoemaker in Bromsgrove. Justinian was born in 1601, so would have been 26 in 1627, a feasible date. There is no positive evidence and the patient is left unidentified and the consultation undated.

stabbing pain in the head especially near the ear. Urine: frequent small changes, **[p. 173]** sometimes thick, more recently clear like spring water. He was weighed down by slight shaking in the limbs, attacked by pains in the legs, headache and swelling of the gums, afflicted by pain and swelling of the fingers, attacked by wandering hypochondriac pain and wind, disfigured by morphew,[1] with many other signs of scurvy. He took much from physicians, to no avail, and used natural baths without profit. He was purged often and used a sweating decoction, but to no purpose.

I returned him to health with these few following. 1 May:

R: diatartar 2oz. He received a small spoonful every day, resulting in four stools.

He was pleasantly purged in the body on each day. He definitely took 4oz of the expressed juice of the following plants at three or four o'clock in the morning when sweating was expected, and at four o'clock in the afternoon. Mix with sufficient sugar and cinnamon 1dr.[2]

R: *scurvy-grass, watercress each ½lb, brooklime 4oz. Bruise and express, add cinnamon 1dr, sufficient sugar.*

He also used this kind of antiscorbutic beer:

R: bark of ash, tamarisk, capers each 2oz, horseradish 6oz, wormwood, fumitory, germander, blessed thistle, celandine plants each ½ handful, betony, scabious, spleenwort, valerian, nettles each 1 handful, watercress, brooklime each 2 handfuls, scurvy-grass 4 handfuls.

Put the following in a bag and boil with the beer:

[p. 174] R: bruised juniper berries 6oz, winter-cherry skins ½oz, sarsaparilla, 2oz, sassafras ½oz, liquorice 1oz, anise, caraway, cloves, coriander seeds each ½oz, nutmegs 2. Afterwards hang the bag by a string in a barrel for 4 gallons of beer. Before you add the brewers' yeast pour in juice of short-stemmed apples 1 pint,

---

1 A non-specific illness of the skin, associated with freckles or scaliness, but nowhere well defined.

2 Wier, 'De scorbuto', in Sennert, *De scorbuto tractatus*, pp. 324–325.

prepared scurvy-grass juice 2 pints, white wine 1 pint. Add the yeast by the rule of practice and close at the right time in a suitable vessel. Keep for use as the ordinary drink.

For swelling of the fingers, place a living worm on the swollen finger as for the bishop, page 164. He was purged with these pills:

℞: pills – hiera with agaric, mastic, stomachic, imperial, Ruffus's each ½dr. Make lot, 5 [pills] from 1dr. Five stools from 1dr.

13 May:

℞: *9 worms bruised in a mortar with 2 spoonfuls of white wine, pressed through a cloth. Add the rest of the wine to these, so that you have 1 pint of wine in all. Drink 3 spoonfuls morning, mid-day and afternoon.*[1]

He was purged every third day.

℞: pills – aggregative 1dr, stomachic ½dr, prepared gamboge gum 14gr. Make 10 pills: from 5, five stools.

Day by day he was restored to health. He drank the prepared beer, and every day before the drink:

℞: steeled electuary 4oz, scurvy-grass conserve 2oz. Mix. Dose: the amount of a nutmeg, and he is to take exercise for an hour. Then take **[p. 175/** a draught of the beer.

The beer was repeated twice, and the steeled electuary used for fifteen days. After meals: scurvy-grass conserve 1oz, bugloss ½oz, pleres archonticon powder 2dr. Mix: the amount of a nutmeg after meals. Every fourth to sixth day he was purged with the following morsels, called *purgative morsels of mechoachan*:

℞: *conserve of violets 1oz, powder for cold diatragacanth 1½dr, turbith gum, best white mechoachan each ½dr, diagrydium with prepared fennel oil 2dr* (I use diagrydium prepared with sulphur fumes, or Horst's with oil of fennel) *sugar dissolved in fennel water 14oz, cinnamon oil 6 drops, anise oil 4 drops. Make sweetmeats in morsels.*[2] From 7dr, eight stools.

---

1 Horst, *Observationum* [...] *libri quatuor*, p. 350.
2 Horst, *Observationum* [...] *libri quatuor*, p. 293.

He took the beer for three months. *By these, through divine power and the medicines, he has been freed from the most ill-omened and intense pain in his parts so that one year later, he has never again relapsed into this sad and bitter mischief of the joints.*[1] He gave great thanks to God and to me, and he calls me father because I saved him from the jaws of death. He recovered completely.

[Case 170]
Roundworms. Mrs Edith Stoughton,[2] a gentlewoman: wretchedly attacked by melancholy and worms day and night. I cured her as for Mrs Bovey above. She was quickly freed and perfectly cured.

[Case 171]
[p. 176/ Scurvy, paralysis, fit of the mother, fainting. Mrs Wilson,[3] a gentlewoman aged 34, respected, as devoutly pious as anyone: went to Bristol for the restoration of her health, because she felt tortured by the stone. She drank the water of St Vincent's Spring with excessive greed, up to thirteen pints in one day, in order to expel the stone. As a result her body became excessively cooled and she fell into a paralysis. She took herself at once to Bath, was purged by Dr Lapworth,[4] and used the baths. She recovered. She returned home in wet and stormy weather, and was distressed by a fit of the mother at night, with fainting and a slight paralysis on the left side. She asks my advice. *Being summoned, I invoked the holy will and employed aids of these kinds.*[5]

---

1 Ruland the Elder, 'Centuria III', *Curationum* [...] *centuriae*, pp. 179–180.
2 Edith Stoughton of St John's, Warwick (1616–44). Daughter of Anthony Stoughton, who owned various lands in Warwickshire and had built a 'noble mansion' just outside Warwick. Married 1635 to Thomas Young of Worcestershire; three children. Thomas died 1657. Edith died at Warwick aged 27.
3 Mrs Wilson (?–1642). No definite identification. Possibly the wife of Thomas Wilson, the vicar of Stratford. Seven children. She had travelled to Bristol and Bath for treatment.
4 Dr Edward Lapworth MD of Oxford (Raach 1962: 62).
5 Ruland the Elder, 'Centuria VII', *Curationum* [...] *centuriae*, p. 523.

℞: clear aloes 2dr, trochiscated agaric, choice powdered rhubarb each 1dr, bark of caper root, winter cherry, tamarisk each 1sc, arum, bryony dregs each ½sc, castor 1½sc, cream of tartar ½dr, amber spirit 4gr. Make 6 pills with sufficient fumitory syrup for as many drachms. Take 3 pills at bedtime: four stools the next day.

[p. 177] For wind in the stomach:

℞: diambra powder 1dr, chymical oils of sage, nutmeg, cloves each 4 drops, sugar dissolved in rose water 2oz. Make rolls. Take after meals.

For the paralysis:

℞: rosemary powder, oil of amber each, with which anoint the neck, rubbing on lightly at the back and front.

For fainting:

℞: pleres archonticon powder ½dr, best sugar 2oz. The dose should be ½ spoonful.

Using these freed her at once from the fainting and palpitations of the heart. It is a powder worth gold and she always carries it with her. She used guaiacum decoction:

℞: *guaiacum 8oz, its bark, rosemary,* sassafras and sarsaparilla wood each 1oz, leaves of betony, sage, lavender, germander each 1 pinch, *roots of elecampane, peony, iris, dried citron rind each 1oz, spring water 6 pints. Infuse for twenty four hours in a hot place. Then boil in a closed vessel and sweeten with sugar, and flavour with diambra powder ½dr. Take 6oz in the morning and sweat, and again in the afternoon about four o'clock without sweating.*[1]

An enema of the common decoction, carminative seeds and Holland powder, and she used Cyprus turpentine often, in the form of pills. She was freed by these, praise God, from the paralysis, fainting and the fit of the mother, praise God alone, from deadly illnesses.

---

1 Sennert, *Medicina practica*, pp. 654–655.

[Case 172]

[p. 178/ Continuous vomiting, stomach ache, lower backache, numbness of the feet. Mrs Wagstaffe,[1] a gentlewoman of Warwick, widow, about 48 years old: weighed down by continuous vomiting, stomach ache and headache as if stabbed and transfixed by daggers, lower backache and numbness of the feet.

℞: the chymical cup 6dr: three vomits, two stools.

For the heartburn:

℞: fresh conserve of roses 1oz, Gabrieli's aromatic rose powder 1sc, *London treacle* 1dr.[2] Mix for 2 doses.

For the back:

℞: oil of scorpions 2dr, sweet almond oil 2oz. Mix.

The night was restful, and she was well relieved of the torments. The next morning, inject an enema:

℞: marsh-mallow root 1oz, pellitory of the wall 2 handfuls, melilot, mallow, chamomile flowers each 1 handful, linseed, fenugreek seeds each ½oz, fennel 2dr. Boil in sufficient water.

℞: of the strained liquid 10oz, cassia extract for enemas 1oz, fresh sweet almond oil 2oz, chicken or goose fat 1oz.

Make an ointment for the side:

℞: *marsh-mallow ointment 2oz, sweet almond oil ½oz. Dissolve and mix at the fire for an ointment, with which anoint the side. Cover it with a cloth smeared with warm butter,*[3] twice a day.

For wind she used:

℞: rosemary, bugloss conserves each 1½oz, clove-gillyflower 1oz, preserved elecampane root, preserved ginger each ½oz, aromatic rose powder 1½dr, alkermes confection ½oz. **[p. 179]** Make an

---

1 Cf. Case 47. Hall had treated her previously. She was the widow of Thomas Wagstaffe, and continued to manage the family estates.

2 *Pharmacopoeia Londinensis*, p. 90.

3 Ruland the Elder, 'Centuria III', *Curationum* [...] *centuriae*, p. 181.

electuary with syrup – regis, or of apples. Dose: the amount of a nutmeg after meals.

After meals take this roll:

R: diambra powder ½dr, sweet diamoschum 1sc, chymical oil of anise 3 drops, sufficient sugar dissolved in borage water. Make rolls.

She was purged with diatartar twice a week. I removed the wakefulness in this way:

R: alabaster or populeon ointment ½oz, Paracelsus's laudanum dissolved in rose water 10gr. Rub on the temples.

With these very few aids and with the help of God, I his unworthy servant soon restored her to health.[1] Praise God, three and one. 1634.

[Case 173]
Cure of stomach ache, dimness of vision, deafness, palpitations of the heart. Mrs Cookes,[2] a gentlewoman, 48 years more or less, of a slender build: complains of stomach ache, dimness of vision, tinnitus, deafness, cold in the head, palpitations of the heart. All of these symptoms seem to be due chiefly to hypochondriac winds springing from obstruction and a diseased state of the spleen so that the general function is affected directly and the nobler subsequently, the pure head and heart suffering by consent. To bring on a weak crisis so that [her body] performs its functions, **[p. 180]** the [winds] should first be purged again, starting in an easy way with the following decoction:

R: sarsaparilla 2oz, colchicum 1½oz, guaiacum, liquorice each 1oz, senna 2oz, polypody of the oak 2oz, dodder ½oz, elecampane 6dr, agaric, rhubarb each 2dr, seeds of anise, caraway, coriander each ½oz. Soak in 4 pints spring water in a closed vessel for twenty-four hours, then boil. Cover the vessel so that no steam escapes.

---

1 Ruland the Elder, 'Centuria VIII', *Curationum* [...] *centuriae*, p. 566.
2 No definite identification. Possibly the wife of William Cookes of Snitterfield. They had four children. Alice Cookes died in 1624.

℞: ½ pint of this decoction, magisterial syrup for melancholy 4oz. The dose may be from 2 to 4oz.

She was properly purged. Next:

℞: steeled electuary 1½oz, of tamarinds 1oz. Mix. Dose: ½oz, and she is to take exercise, and twice a week she was purged with the following pills:

℞: pills – stomachic, sine quibus each ½dr, of peonies, ground-pine each 1sc. Make 12 pills, 3 at bedtime.

Then take the electuary as for Mrs Fiennes, page 168. For the deafness, blessed thistle water, properly double distilled, was dripped into her ears. These freed her within a few days, praise God.

[Case 174]

Spitting up blood. Nurse Deacle of Bengeworth,[1] aged 29: discoloured by spitting blood from an eroded vein in the lungs, weakened and disfigured by yellow jaundice. The erosion is due to bile, for *from the lungs* **[p. 181]** *blood can be produced in many ways, either from an opening in a pulmonary vessel, or excessive thinning or even erosion. It is agreed that a vessel opened because of blood, and much hot corrosive blood broke out in this woman.*[2] *Moreover, the expulsion of much thin, highly coloured blood mixed with froth indicates with full confidence the production of blood being driven out when a vessel has been opened, and more so if any pain appears in or near the chest with a troublesome cough (Hippocrates: 'anyone who spits out frothy blood is bringing it up from the lungs'). What comes from the chest is discharged with pain because this part is full of organs and nerves. The flesh of the lungs is loose, soft and spongy; the lungs are fed with entirely clean, finely golden and vaporous blood.*[3] *I freed her quickly with the aid of divine mercy, and with the following:*[4]

---

1 No reliable identification. Possibly a midwife, but there is no record of her licence from the bishop.

2 from ... woman] Valleriola, *Observationum* [...] *libri sex*, p. 218.

3 Moreover ... blood] Valleriola, *Observationum* [...] *libri sex*, pp. 217–218.

4 Ruland the Elder, 'Centuria III', *Curationum* [...] *centuriae*, p. 203.

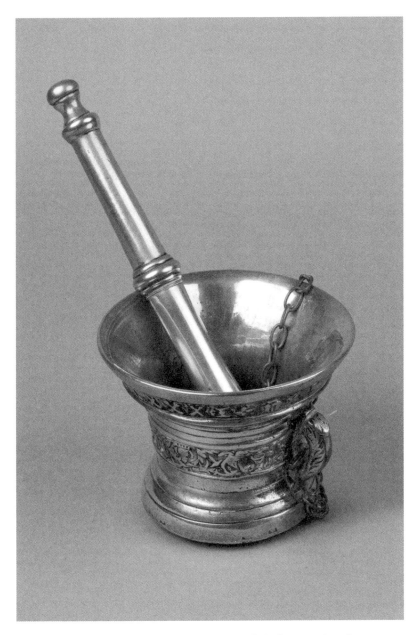

40 A seventeenth-century pestle and mortar. Grinding powders for
medicinal components was a job for an apothecary rather than a physician.
It is likely that Susanna Hall helped to grind some of the ingredients needed
for her husband's medicines.

℞: simple oxymel 4oz, maidenhair syrup 2oz. Mix: for two mornings.

She was purged with the following prepared medicine:

℞: powdered rhubarb 1½dr, loosening rose syrup 1oz, plantain water 4oz, maidenhair syrup 1oz. Mix.

She was properly purged, then bled, **[p. 182]** then [treated with] astringents:

℞: *haematite stone finely ground and washed with plantain water 1dr (it has wonderful power in stopping bleeding)*[1] *red coral, prepared bole Armeniac each 3dr,* sealed earth 1½dr, simple diaireos powder 1dr *(which ought to be mixed with astringents for administration to the chest). Make a fine powder. Dose: 1½dr per dose in barley water, decoctions of plantain and knotgrass.*[2] Take on an empty stomach, and *Croll's frog spawn water*[3] at bedtime. Continue the course for several days.

An emollient enema every third or second day:

℞: *mallows, marsh mallows, violets, beets, mercury each 1 handful,* plums 5, fat Carian figs 12, melon seeds with the husks bruised 1oz, anise and fennel seeds each 1dr, barley with the husk, *rye bran each 1 pinch. Make a decoction of everything in sufficient milk whey for 12oz. In the strained liquid dissolve catholicon 1oz, cassia extract for enemas 5dr, brown sugar 2oz. Make an enema.*[4]

These cured her, with the aid of almighty God most high.

[Case 175]
Fit of the mother, melancholy. Mrs Edith Stoughton,[5] a gentlewoman: wretchedly afflicted with melancholy. **[p. 183]** Her periods had not yet started at 17 years of age. She was tortured by a fit of the mother so that *she did not wish to live, does not know how to die.*[6]

---

1 haematite ... bleeding] Valleriola, *Observationum* [...] *libri sex*, p. 190.
2 red ... knotgrass] Valleriola, *Observationum* [...] *libri sex*, pp. 149–150.
3 Croll, *Basilica chymica*, p. 276.
4 Valleriola, *Observationum* [...] *libri sex*, p. 144.
5 Cf. Case 170. Hall saw her when she was aged 17, and noted her mental instability.
6 Burton 2001: 346 [quoting Seneca].

She is easily angered by her closest friends. She thinks that they say all kinds of things about her, and constantly shouts that her father is coming to kill her. At night she mutters and often declares that her father is coming with many others to murder her. She has been purged by an experienced physician, nonetheless her father entreats my advice. *He asked firmly that I should not fatigue her with many remedies, of which she was exceedingly weary. I replied that a cure would be difficult, for her constitution and temperament had resulted in a melancholic state. Accordingly I did not wish to make many promises, but I judged that a cure could be started with a pleasant and supportive remedy.*[1]

First of all, her bowel movements should be freed with an emollient clyster, dispelling wind but not cooling the humours:[2]

> ℞: *chicken broth (in which cook sorrel, pimpernel, borage, hyssop) 1 pint, common oil 2 ½oz, salt of tartar 1dr. Make an enema, repeat for two days.*

Then she was purged in this way:

> ℞: *the above broth 5oz, cream of tartar 4sc, oil of vitriol 5 drops.*[3] Make a potion. *Thus the natural humours will be restored to obedience.*[4]

Next the left brachial vein should be opened. She was purged again **[p. 184]** the next day, then leeches were applied to the haemorrhoidal veins. *She should be purged again with softening purgative medications (so as not to dry out the body) and preferably use stronger potions than pills, because pills are more drying.*[5] I therefore wished her to use *Rodrigo de Fonseca's helleborated apple.*[6] She was rightly purged: Dose: hellebore 1dr cooked in an apple, afterwards remove and give the apple. *Humours should be diverted from the brain, the principal parts strengthened with bindings and stronger clysters:*[7]

---

1 Platter, *Observationum* […] *libri sex*, p. 67.
2 Bruele, *Praxis medicinae*, p. 30.
3 Fonseca, *Consultationes*, pp. 83–84.
4 Bruele, *Praxis medicinae*, p. 30.
5 Bruele, *Praxis medicinae*, p. 30.
6 Fonseca, *Consultationes*, p. 68.
7 Bruele, *Praxis medicinae*, p. 30.

℞: vitriolated conserves of roses, borage, bugloss each 1oz, preserved citron peel, red speedwell conserve each ½oz, electuary powders – of gems, laetificans each 2sc, prepared emeralds 1sc, alkermes confection 1dr, powder for cold diamargiton, cold diatragacanth each 1½dr. Make an electuary with apple syrup. Dose 1dr before meals. Dispel the winds with the powder on page 33.

She used the following wine:

℞: *the opening roots each 1oz, bark of caper root 1oz, sassafras wood 1½oz, wormwood and ground-pine leaves each 1½ handfuls, shoots of spleenwort, balm, germander each 1 handful, borage, bugloss, scabious flowers* **[p. 185]** *each 2 pinches, broom leaves 1 pinch, fennel seeds 1oz, caraway seeds 2dr, silphium seeds 1dr. Crush, put in a barrel in which juniper wood chips have been placed. Pour on 30 pints white wine. Close well and store in a cellar until used. Eight days after soaking, I wished her to drink 9 pints of it in which was infused rhubarb 6dr, senna leaves 2oz, mechoacan ½oz, dodder, cinnamon each ½oz, cloves 1dr. Store the wine like this because it is another purgative. Drink the purgative wine in the morning two hours before eating, taking it with a few spoonfuls of chicken broth at the same time, for three days. Afterwards, on the fourth day, take a draught of the purgative wine.*[1]

'After purging, strengthen the heart and brain', as the saying is. NOTE: *We add moistening matter to all medications since melancholy comes mostly from excessive dryness.*[2] When I was strongly pressed about sleeplessness I gave simple diacodium 1 spoonful as she went to bed. I repeated it the next night because it promotes sweating and brings on sleep. She is to use tartar often, *for crystal tartar has great power to subdue* **[p. 186]** *melancholy and dark humours, as it draws to itself certain vinegary properties. An experiment can be made with sharp vinegar, for if one places four pints of very sharp vinegar and 1oz wine tartar in a container, water or phlegm are distilled at the fire without any dryness, because the tartar draws the acid spirits of the vinegar to itself by sympathy.*[3]

---

1 Platter, *Observationum* […] *libri tres*, p. 67.
2 Bruele, *Praxis medicinae*, p. 30.
3 Fonseca, *Consultationes*, p. 53.

Thus she was freed from a most severe and long-standing illness, through the unique grace of almighty God most high.[1]

[Case 176]

Cure of scurvy. 1 January 1634. Master Thomas Underhill,[2] first-born son, of Loxley, aged about 12 more or less: suffered the previous year from malignant fever with visible scabs. Then he fell into the measles and was incompletely cured, the cause of the scurvy. When he asked my advice he was weighed down by swelling of the right side around the false and floating ribs without pain or discoloration, so that I diagnosed swelling of the liver. He was so thin you would have thought him a skeleton, melancholic, with black crusted ulcers appearing on his legs. From these symptoms and unproductive vomiting, erratic fever and aversion to food I judged that he suffered from long-established scurvy. Nor did my opinion fail me, for his urine was red as **[p. 187]** in burning fever, though without much thirst or desire to drink. *His pulse was small, weak and unequal, hard to feel with the fingers,*[3] which is a clear sign of established scurvy, and he said *he was more tired than ill.*[4] *The parents asked me earnestly to disregard nothing which I thought relevant to the good health of their son. I made clear to the parents as I was duty-bound,*[5] that the cure would be long and difficult. I start the cure in this way:

> ℞: crystal tartar 2dr, diatrion santalon powder 1dr, Holland powder 2dr. Mix. Make a powder for four days: three or four stools each day without discomfort. Anoint the affected area with *Valleriola's Fidum ointment*[6] and diacalchitys for the ulcers, then cream of tartar

---

1 Ruland the Elder, 'Centuria III', *Curationum* [...] *centuriae*, p. 160.
2 Master Thomas Underhill of Loxley (1622–after 1679). Aged about 12 when his anxious parents brought him to Hall in 1634. Eldest child of Thomas and Elizabeth (cf. Case 132). Thomas later served in the King's Life Guards. Lived in London with his uncle, Sir John Underhill. Unmarried. William Dugdale in *The Antiquities of Warwickshire* states that he was a Royalist.
3 Eugalenus, *De scorbuto*, p. 125.
4 he ... ill] Eugalenus, *De scorbuto*, p. 148.
5 The ... duty-bound] Eugalenus, *De scorbuto*, p. 288.
6 Valleriola, *Observationum* [...] *libri sex*, p. 234.

for three days: 1dr in the morning and an hour later our steeled wine 4oz, with essence of fumitory and germander ½oz, (following Baudouin Ronsse, page 259, in Sennert's book *De scorbuto*, in octavo)[1] brooklime syrup 2oz, watercress 1oz, prepared scurvy-grass juice 6oz. Mix. Dose: 4 spoonfuls and he is to take exercise, resulting in two stools and one vomit.

The first day he vomited phlegm. On the third day: diacrocuma ½oz in the morning, and afterwards steeled wine. Every third day he was purged with *Du Chesne's diatartar* ½ spoonful,[2] cooked in an apple under ashes. He used our antiscorbutic beer. I ordered Foreest's ammoniac plaster applied to the spleen. To drink, always, at any time:

℞: scurvy-grass juice ½lb, brooklime, watercress syrups each 1½oz, for three mornings.

He did not omit the steeled wine with scurvy-grass juice and brooklime and watercress syrup for the whole month. **[p. 187b]** He was purged with Rivière's ammoniac pills.[3] Make 3 pills from ½dr. Take 1 pill every third day, resulting in two or three stools. He was purged at bedtime and in the morning. For the painful swollen side: an ointment of magisterial splenic ointment 1oz, marsh-mallow ointment ½oz, morning and evening. He used our antiscorbutic beer, all others being prohibited. After using the above pills for two days he fell into a painful swelling of the feet, so that he could not sleep at night nor move his feet any more, and he almost fainted from every slight movement of the legs. When I came, I gave red Pannonian powder ½sc, magisterium of corals ½sc, bezoar stone 3gr to strengthen the stomach. I prescribed the following decoction for his legs:

---

1 Ronsse, 'Scorbuto commentarius', in Sennert, *De scorbuto tractatus*, p. 259.

2 Du Chesne, *De priscorum philosophorum* [...] *materia*, p. 330; the recipe is also to be found in the *Pharmacopoea dogmaticorum*, possibly *pulvis melangogus Quercetani*, p. 126, to which it is similar.

3 Rivière's ammoniac pills] Du Chesne, *Pharmacopoea dogmaticorum*, pp. 120–121.

℞: brooklime 4 handfuls, wormwood, melilot, chamomile, sage each 1 handful. Make a bath in sufficient beer, use twice daily without a break.

He was completely freed from the swelling and pain within three days. He was purged with pills – Ruffus's, stomachic and hiera with agaric each [XXX].[1] Make 6 pills, give one at bedtime. Finally when his legs were well cured, he was tortured by wretched pain in the right upper arm. He was freed within twenty-four hours by Fidum ointment, besides never missing the steeled wine except on days of purgation.

He swallowed the following powder, the amount that can be held on twelve [pennies],[2] after food:

℞: pleres archonticon powder ½oz, sugar 2oz. Mix.

He was very powerfully purged twice weekly with Rivière's pills as above: 2 pills some time in the morning, resulting in three or four stools.

℞: ammoniac pills 1dr, prepared gamboge gum 9gr, sine quibus ½oz.

By this method, praise God, he was cured.

[Case 177]

[p. 188] Mr John Trapp,[3] minister, second to none for manifest piety and learning, having just passed the thirty-third year of his age, melancholic by nature and devoted to books. Last year he fell into a hypochondriac melancholy and splenic pain with related scorbutic symptoms, evident from difficulty in breathing after

---

1 These crosses appear in Hall's manuscript.
2 twelve pennies] Approximately 14 grams, or 1 drachm and 2 grains.
3 John Trapp, schoolmaster of Stratford-upon-Avon (1601–60). Came of a yeoman family. Went to Oxford, MA in 1624. Master at the grammar school from 1622. Married Mary Gibbard; four children. Vicar of Weston from 1636. Chaplain to the Parliamentary forces, captured by Royalists in 1643. Returned to Stratford in 1660.

slight movement of the body, palpitations of the heart rushing headlong like the motion of wind to the heart so that it instilled a fear, by no means trifling, of weakness. When the wind dispersed, he felt better after a short time. *Finally he was constantly consumed by a slow erratic fever, loss of appetite and feebleness of spirit and unaccustomed faintness, from which everyone concluded that he was wasting away.*[1] After he finished his sermon on Sunday his strength was exhausted. He could hardly speak. I, however, having observed the sudden change of the urine and uneven pulse and from being aware of his customary way of life, declared that he suffered from atrophic scurvy, *the more so because with these he had worrying troubles in his precordium at intervals.*[2] *In agreement with the sufferings from this atrophy, his body was often more tired than ill, so that he complained of nothing more than weariness of the body.*[3] When first assaulted by this illness he used common medicines to no purpose, and at last asked my help and advice. *With these few remedies, without any annoyance, nausea or unpleasant taste of medicines, we rescued this learned young man from the jaws of death entirely, quickly and pleasantly, and restored him to health. He lives very well, enjoying good health.*[4] To God thrice greatest be praise and glory for ever. Amen. 11 March 1635:

℞: vitriolated tartar 4sc cooked in an apple under the ashes.

This produced a greater quantity of urine, coloured indeed like spring water. He had two stools. 12th:

℞: mercurius dulcis 20gr, vitriolated tartar 1sc, prepared gamboge gum 3gr. Give as before: four stools.

[p. 199] 14th: crystal tartar 1dr: one stool. He held our pectoral rolls in his mouth at night, for cough and catarrh. 15th:

---

1 Potier, *Insignium curationum*, p. 33.
2 Eugalenus, *De scorbuto morbo*, p. 311.
3 Eugalenus, *De scorbuto morbo*, p. 117.
4 Potier, *Insignium curationum*, p. 4.

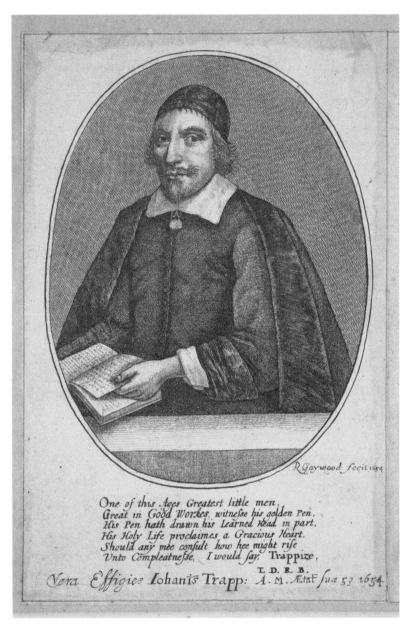

One of this Ages Greatest little men,
Great in Good Workes, witnesse his golden Pen.
His Pen hath drawn his Learned Head, in part.
His Holy Life proclaimes a Gracious Heart,
Should any mee consult how hee might rise
Vnto Compleatnesse, I would say, Trappize,

I. D. R. B.
Vera Effigies Iohanis Trapp: A. M. Ætat sua 53 1654

R Gaywood fecit 1654

41 John Trapp, a schoolmaster at the King's New School, Stratford-upon-Avon from 1624. He was 53 when this portrait was made in 1654. Hall treated him on 11 March 1635 for melancholy and pain in the spleen (Case 177). Hall also treated his third child of ten, Lydia (Case 114).

℞: our steeled wine 4oz, with Foreest's scheletyrbic syrup 3oz: on the first day 2 spoonfuls, on the second 4 spoonfuls.

He exercised for two hours. To strengthen the spleen:

℞: *large raisins ½lb. Boil in good wine to the consistency of a poultice, sift through a sieve and mix with rosemary*, bugloss conserves each ½oz, powders of laetificans, *aromatic roses, cold diamargiton, diacinamomu each 2sc, sweet-smelling aloe wood ½dr*, preserved citron peel, cinnamon powder each *1dr*, finely powdered prepared steel filings ½oz (prepared with sulphur following Du Chesne)[1] *oriental saffron 1sc. Mix. Take the amount of a chestnut in the morning.*[2]

19th:

℞: magisterial syrup for melancholy 2oz, bugloss water 2oz, finely powdered tartar 1dr. Mix.

He evacuated four times. The next day he used steeled wine as before. 2 April: Purged as before, *by which he evacuated four times.*[3] In three days he finished the steeled wine.

7th: Purged, cream of tartar 1dr. He now had our antiscorbutic beer. When the electuary was finished, he took 6 spoonfuls of the following water:

℞: our snail water, simple frog water each 4oz, alkermes confection 2sc, pearled manus Christi ½oz, Foreest's scheletyrbic syrup 2oz, our *antiscorbutic water* 6oz, *splenitic* 2oz.[4] Mix.

This water was consumed and drunk. He asked for the electuary again, in which he said there was the greatest hope of a cure. He said it was worth gold. He used the electuary again for eight days. Every fourth day he was purged, but complained of bitterness

---

1 large ... Chesne] Du Chesne, *Pharmacopoea dogmaticorum*, pp. 243–244.
2 oriental ... morning] Hartmann, *Praxis chymiatrica*, p. 133. As Hartmann says, this is based on a recipe in Solenander, *Consiliorum medicinalium*, p. 221, but Hall's wording matches Hartmann more closely. There are slightly different versions in Holler, *De morbis internis*, p. 371, and Horst, *Observationum [...] libri quatuor*, p. 259.
3 Torrella, 'De dolore in pudendagra', in Luisini, *De morbo Gallico omnia*, p. 472.
4 Dornkrell, *Dispensatorium novum*, pp. 33–36.

in the mouth. Our chymical cup: 5dr. He was freed and again returned to the use of the electuary. These by God's will freed him from all pain, and cured him rightly and properly and he thanked me greatly. Praise God.

[Case 178]

[p. 200] The [2nd] Earl of Northampton,[1] about 32 years old, following his hunting dogs on a swift steed in cold and rainy weather: caught a cold and was wretchedly attacked by a sudden windy pleurisy and abdominal colic, *very like a true pleurisy. It caused a small degree of coughing, restlessness, fever, thirst and painful distension.*[2] Being at hand when he returned home, I prescribed this enema:

> ℞: common decoction for an enema ½ pint, diaphoenicon, diacatholicon each 1oz, Holland powder 2dr. Make an enema: three stools with a large amount of wind, with the desired result for the pain eased.

At this point he felt a pricking pain in his chest, to banish which:

> ℞: *marsh-mallow ointment 2oz, sweet almond oil ½oz. Dissolve and mix at the fire for an ointment, with which I anointed the chest and sides. I placed over it a folded cloth smeared with warm butter.*

The pain diminished,[3] the night was restful, *and he was seized by heavier sleep than was his custom.*[4] During the day he used these proven syrups frequently:

> ℞: magisterial scabious, maidenhair, liquorice, hyssop syrups each 1oz. Take often with a liquorice stick.

---

1 Cf. Case 137. Hall knew the family and had treated him before. A keen hunter, he became Master of the Leash to Charles I.

2 Feyens, *De flatibus*, p. 121.

3 marsh mallow … diminished] Ruland the Elder, 'Centuria III', *Curationum […] centuriae*, p. 181.

4 and … custom] Cicero, 'Somnium Scipionis, Book VI', *De re publica*.

At night he held one of our pectoral rolls in his mouth. In the morning I wished him to be anointed again. He was completely freed from the pain and sat down to eat in his dining room.[1]

---

1 Hall's Latin manuscript includes an abbreviation *tr̃s c* at the very end. This might mean *terminus curae* referring only to this one report, or *terminus curarum* referring to the whole manuscript. If Hall deliberately chose to end his *Little Book of Cures* at this point, then it was in a surprisingly low-key and abrupt fashion.

Appendix I
John Hall's working library

These books have been used as references for this edition. They are not necessarily the editions owned by John Hall. The dates following the publication details give the range for the editions to which Hall might have had access. If no date range is given, there is evidence that Hall used the specific edition listed.

Adams, Thomas, *Mystical Bedlam: or, the World of Mad-Men* (London: Clement Knight, 1615).

Amatus Lusitanus, *Curationum medicinalium centuriae quatuor, quarum duae priores ab auctore sunt recognite, duae posteriores nunc primum edite* (Basel: Froben, 1556). 1556–57.

Amatus Lusitanus, *Curationum medicinalium centuriae duae, quinta videlicet ac sexta* (Venice: Valgrisius, 1560). 1557–80.

Béguin, Jean, *Tyrocinium chymicum e natura fonte et manuali experimentia depromptum* (Königsberg: Iohannes Fabricius, 1618). 1608–34.

Bernard de Gordon, *Lilium medicinae inscriptum: de morborum prope omnium curatione* (Lyons: Rovillius, 1574). 1557–80.

Bruele, Walter, *Praxis medicinae theorica et empirica familiarissima* (Leiden: Plantin, Raphelangius, 1599). 1621–32.

Burton, Robert, *The Anatomy of Melancholy*, ed. Holbrook Jackson (New York: New York Review of Books, 2001). Numerous editions of this work were available in Hall's lifetime.

Cardano, Girolamo, *Ars curandi parva, tomus I* (Basel: Officina Henricpetriana, 1564). 1524–1621.

Castro, Rodrigo de, *De universa mulierum medicina, pars secunda, sive praxis* (Hamburg: Froben, 1604). 1603–28.

College of Physicians of London, *Pharmacopoeia Londinensis*, 2nd edn (London: John Marriot, 1618).

Collegium Medicum (Augustana), *Pharmacopoeia Augustana* (Augsburg: Kruger, 1613).

Crato, Johannes, *Consiliorum et epistolarum medicinalium … liber: … nunc primum a Laurentio Scholzio … in lucem editus* (Frankfurt: Wechel, Marnius et Aubrius, 1591). 1591–1611.

Crato, Johannes, *Consiliorum et epistolarum medicinalium … liber quintus: nunc primum labore et studio Laurentii Scholzii … in lucem editus* (Frankfurt: Wechel heredes, Marnius et Aubrius, 1594). 1591–1619.

Crato, Johannes, *Consiliorum et epistolarum medicinalium, liber secundus: nunc primum studio et opera Laurentii Scholzii … in lucem editus* (Hanover: Wechel, Marnius et haeredes Aubrii, 1609). 1592–1609.

Crato, Johannes, *Consiliorum et epistolarum medicinalium … liber tertius: nunc primum labore et industria Laurentii Scholzii … in primum editus* (Hanover: Wechel, Marnius et heredes Aubrii, 1609). 1592–1609.

Crato, Johannes, *Consiliorum et epistolarum medicinalium … liber sextus: nunc primum studio et opera Laurentii Scholzii … in lucem editus* (Hanover: Wechel, haeredes Marnii, 1611).

Crato, Johannes, *Consiliorum et epistolarum medicinalium … liber quartus: nunc primum studio et labore Laurentii Scholzii … in lucem editus* (Hanover: Wechel, haeredes Aubrii, 1614). 1593–1619.

Croll, Oswald, *Basilica chymica* (Frankfurt: Marnius et heredes Aubrii, 1609). 1600–34.

da Monte, Giovanni Battista, *Consultationum medicinalium centuria prima* (Venice: Valgrisius, 1556). 1554–69.

da Monte, Giovanni Battista, *Consultationes medicae* (Basel?: n.p., 1583).

Donne, John, *Devotions upon Emergent Occasions: and Severall Steps in my Sicknes* (London: Thomas Jones, 1624).

Dornkrell, Tobias, *Dispensatorium novum continens descriptiones et usum praecipuorum medicamentum* (Ultzen: Cröner, 1600). 1600–23.

Du Chesne, Joseph, *De priscorum philosophorum verae medicinae materia, praeparationis modo, atque in curandis morbis, praestantia* (Geneva: Vignon, 1603). 1593–1630.

Du Chesne, Joseph, *Diaeteticon polyhistoricon* (Frankfurt: Schönwetter, 1607).

Du Chesne, Joseph, *Pharmacopoea dogmaticorum restituta* (Frankfurt: Schönwetter, 1607).

Dunus, Thaddaeus, *De curandi ratione per venae sectionem liber quartus* (Zurich: Frosch, 1579).

Eugalenus, Severinus, *De scorbuto morbo liber* (Leipzig: Michael Rantzenberger, 1604). 1588–1624.

Fernel, Jean, *Therapeutices universalis seu medendi rationis libri septem* (Lyons: Sebastianus Honoratus, 1571).

Fernel, Jean, *Consiliorum liber* (Lyons: Soubron et Du Prez, 1597). 1579–1627.

Feyens, Jean, *De flatibus humanum corpus molestantibus* (Geneva?: in Officina Sanctandreana, 1592). 1582–92.

Fonseca, Rodrigo de, *Consultationes medicae singularibus remediis refertae* (Venice: Ioannis Guerilius, 1620). 1611–25.

Foreest, Pieter van, *Observationum et curationum medicinalium de febribus ephemeris et continuis libri duo* (Antwerp: Plantin, 1584). 1584–1614.

Hartmann, Johann, *Praxis chymiatrica* (Leipzig: Grossius, 1633).

Horst, Gregor, *Observationum medicinalium singularium libri quatuor* (Ulm: Saurius, 1625).

Houllier, Jacques, *De morbis internis libri II* (Frankfurt: Wechel, 1589). 1570–1623.

John of Gaddesden, *Praxis medica, rosa anglica dicta* (Augsburg: Michael Manger, 1595).

Liébault, Jean, *Thresor des remedes secrets pour les maladies des femmes* (Paris: Jacques du Puys, 1585).

Luisini, Luigi, *De morbo Gallico omnia quae extant apud omnes medicos* (Venice: Zilettus, 1566). 1566–67.

Penot, Bernard, *De denario medico, quo decem medicaminibus, omnibus morbis internis medendi via docetur* (Berne: Ioannis le Preux, 1608). 1608–18.

Platter, Felix, *Praxeos: tractatus de functionem laesionibus* (Basel: Conrad Waldkirch, 1602). 1602–25.

Platter, Felix, *Praxeos: tractatus secundus de doloribus* (Basel: Conrad Waldkirch, 1603). 1603–25.

Platter, Felix, *Praxeos: tractatus tertius et ultimus de vitiis* (Basel: Conrad Waldkirch, 1608). 1608–25.

Platter, Felix, *Observationum in hominis affectibus plerisque, corpori et animo, functionem laesione, dolore, aliave molestia et vitio incommodantibus: libri tres* (Basel: Conrad Waldkirch, 1614). 1586–1614.

Potier, Pierre, *Insignium curationum, et singularium observationum centuria prima* (Bologna: Nicolai Tebaldini, 1622). 1622–32.

Potier, Pierre, *Pharmacopoea spagirica* (Bologna: n.p., 1622). 1622–25.

Ranzau, Henrik, *De conservanda valetudine liber in privatum librorum suorum usum* (Antwerp: Plantin, 1584). 1553–84.

Rondelet, Guillaume, *Methodus curandorum omnium morborum corporis humani in tres libros distincta* (Paris: Carolus Macaeus, 1574). 1553–67.

Rueff, Jacob, *De conceptu et generatione hominis, et iis quae circa hec potissimum consyderantur, libri sex* (Zurich: Frosch, 1554). 1554–87.

Ruland the Elder, Martin, *Balnearium restauratum, in quo curantur morbi tam externi quam interni* (Basel: n.p., 1579). 1556–1613.

Ruland the Elder, Martin, *Curationum empyricarum et historicarum, in certis locis et notis personis optime expertarum, et rite probatarum, centuriae decem* (Lyons: Pierre Ravaud, 1628). 1577-1628.

Ruland the Younger, Martin, *De morbo Ungarico recte cognoscendo et foeliciter curando* (Leipzig: Jacobus Apellius, 1610). 1600–10.

Sennert, Daniel, *De scorbuto tractatus* (Wittenberg: Zacharia Shürer, 1624).

Sennert, Daniel, *De febribus libri IV* (Wittenberg: Vidue et haeredes Zachariae Shüreri, 1628). 1605–33.

Sennert, Daniel, *Medicina practica* (Lyons: Pierre Ravaud, 1629). 1620–34.

Solenander, Reiner, *Consiliorum medicinalium* (Hanover: Wechel, Marnius, heredes Aubrii, 1609). 1558–1609.

Taranta, Valesco de, *Epitome operis perquam utilis morbis curandi* (Lyons: Ioan. Tornaesius: Gulielmus Gazeius, 1560).

Valleriola, François, *Observationum medicinalium libri sex* (Lyons: Gryphius, 1573).

Vettori, Benedetto, *Exhortatio ad medicum recte, sancteque medicari cupientem: medicatio empirica singulorum morborum* (Venice: Erasmus, Valgrisius, 1550). 1550–51.

Vittori, Leonello, *De aegritudinibus infantium tractatus* (Venice: Erasmus, Valgrisius, 1557). 1550–62.

Willich, Jodocus, *Urinarum probationes* (Basel: Henricpetri, 1582).

Appendix 2

Early modern glossary of medical and pharmaceutical terms

This glossary includes many of the medical and pharmaceutical words and phrases (other than remedies) used in the *Little Book of Cures*. Rather than attempt to explain them myself, or to use present-day definitions, I have relied on English medical texts of Hall's period, mostly using ones that give information on the causes as well as the appearance of illnesses. The intention is to give the reader some further insight into the early modern understanding of these terms. I have resorted to Latin texts (with my own translations when necessary) only when I could find nothing more appropriate in English.

Abdominal swelling: 'Ascites is that, when great store of winds, but greater of water, is gathered together in that place, which doth lie between the guts and the syphach [peritoneum]' (Bruele 1599: 319).

Bastard tertian fever: 'is caused, when choler is mixed for the most part with fleame [phlegm] [...] in this feaver also the time of the fits doth exceed twelve hours [...] the signes of concoction do appear more slowly, neither is there such great heate [...] as in the exquisite tertian' (Barrough 1624: 234).

Bleeding from the mouth: 'Blood is oft voyded from the gummes, and mouth itselfe, and then the spittle is of a bloody colour and very little voyded out and that without a cough; if it doe come from the throat [...] it is voyded by hemming, not by cough [...] but if the blood doth come from the lungs, then is the blood foamy [...] as oft as blood is voyded because some great veine is burst, then plenty of blood is cast up' (Bruele 1599: 198).

Catarrh: 'is a distillation commonly taken, and is a deflux of humours and excrements from the head or braine into the other parts of the body' (Bruele 1599: 151).

Cold: 'a cold distemper simply, without the fluxe of any cold humour. This paine in the head is caused of outward cold, as when the aire is very cold, especially when one tarrieth in it long time bareheaded' (Barrough 1624: 5).

Colic: 'a continuall passione of the bowel which is called colon, and there follows it a difficulty of voiding excrements, and wind at the lower parts' (Bruele 1599: 309).

Consent: 'a pain by propriety is when the cause [...] is in the part pained, as when the head-ach comes from humors in the head [...] when it proceeds of vapors sent up from the stomach or any other part it's called head-ach by consent or sympathy' (Anon. 1657: sig. L3).

Continual burning fever: 'if choler do putrifie and rot within the vessels, it causeth a continuall tertian, or burning fever' (Barrough 1624: 214).

Diarrhoea: 'a copious and great fluxe of the wombe [*sic*] without exulceration and inflammation. It is caused through weakness of the instruments that belong to digestion, also through abundance of nourishment and meat that is moist and vicious, and through corruption of the same meate. Moreover, gnawing and biting of those things that are contained in the belly' (Barrough 1624: 119).

Difficulty of breathing: asthma: 'caused when as grosse and clammy humors begotten in abundantly into the gristles or lappets of the lungs, or that there be some other swelling in it, like a botch' (Barrough 1624: 81).

Dropsy of the chamber pots: diabetes: 'Latini urinae

incontinentiam, urinae fluorem, urinam involuntariuam, hydropem matellae, vel aquam intercutem ad matulam vocant' [in Latin they call it incontinence of urine, flowing of urine; involuntary urination, dropsy of the pot; or dropsical water in the chamber pot] (Ruland the Elder 1628: 152).

Dysentery: 'an exulceration and inflammation of the bowels [...] caused through exulceration of the bowels which sometims chanceth through outward causes, as of cold, heate, and moistnesse [...] drinking of pernicious and naughtie medicines [...] eating of fruit' (Barrough 1624: 123).

Epilepsy: 'a convulsion, drawing and stretching of all the parts of the whole body, but not continually [...] there be three differences in this sicknesse or disease. The first is caused when this sicknesse cometh only of disease in the braine, as it chanceth when grosse or clammy fleame or sharpe choler doth stop the passage of the spirit in the ventricles [...] secondly it is caused through an evill affect in the mouthe and stomacke, that is, when the braine laboureth to drive away the vapours and humours that ascend up to it from the stomacke. Thirdly [...] when the patient feeleth a thing like unto a cold aire, coming from some member and creeping up to the braine' (Barrough 1624: 40).

Erratic fever: 'are such feavers as be contrary to [those which come justly at their appointed time] because they keep no certaine and juste time nor any order of fits, nor the intermission between them, as be those feavers which ingender of melancholy' (Barrough 1624: 216).

Excessive quantity of urine: diabetes is 'a continuall disease about the reines, causing much thirst; and also whatsoever is drunk, even as it is taken it is pissed out againe. The disease is ingendred of weaknesse of the retentive vertue of the reines' (Barrough 1624: 165).

Exercise: 'Qui hoc electuarium assumit exercitio utatur' [Whoever takes this electuary – medicine mixed with honey – should take exercise] (Crato 1609: 379).

Flux of the reds: 'Uteri fluor in Latin, fluxe of the matrice in English, is a continuall distillation, and flowing out for a long time, of the whole body purging itselfe [...] for some is red as bloud purified [...] if pure blood come forth, as in the cutting of a veine, you must take good heede that some erosion and gnawing be not ingendred in the wombe' (Barrough 1624: 188).

Flux of the whites: 'fluxe of the matrice [...] is a continuall distillation and flowing out for a long time of the whole body purging itself. That which is voided out doth represent such forme and colour as the humour that doth abound in the bodie [...] some white, which cometh of fleame' (Barrough 1624: 188).

Frenzy: 'a disease where the mind is hurt, and doth onely differ from madnesse [...] for that a feaver is joyned with the frenzie, and therefore the frenzie may be called a continuall madnesse and fury joyned with a sharpe feaver' (Barrough 1624: 21).

Generalised dropsy: anasarca: 'a passion, that it is not without plenty of watery humours, because the blood-breeding faculty is vitiated [...] anasarca is a scattering of phlegmy humours over the whole body [...] the whole body increaseth most unnaturally, for it is all over swelled' (Bruele 1599: 319).

Giddiness: 'a disease wherein the patient doth imagine that his head is turned round about [...] through the inordinate moving of windy vapours and spirits contained in certaine parts of the braine [...] caused either of the braine itselfe being distempered and evill affected, or of the mouth of the stomacke offending the braine' (Barrough 1624: 18–19).

Gonorrhoea: 'excretion and shedding of seede or sperme against the patients will, and without sicknesse of the yard. It is caused through imbecilitie and weaknesse of the retentive virtue in the vessels containing the sperm [...] this disease chanceth not only to men, but also to women, and in women it is hard to cure' (Barrough 1624: 178–179).

Gout: 'the joynt-gout is a feeblenesse of the joynts, and pain coming upon them at certain distances of time; for the most part it is caused by a flux, which winds itselfe betweene the ligaments, filmes, and tendones of the joynts' (Bruele 1599: 380).

Haemorrhoids: 'an unfolding and spreading abroad of the veines of the well. Of these some be blind, which do swell, and do send out none, or very little blood; some be open, which be set wide open abroad certaine times, and do send forth blood. The haemorrhoids are caused through dreggie and melancholy blood, when there is abundance thereof, which the liver sendeth to those veins' (Barrough 1624: 135).

Heartburn: 'caused by sharpe and biting humours, which doe sticke about the mouth of the stomacke, whereby the appetite is abated, and they are in more paine before meate than after' (Bruele 1599: 239).

Heart palpitations: 'panting and trembling of the heart [...] caused of all such things as do trouble and affect the heart above nature' (Barrough 1624: 92).

Hectic fever: 'when heate is kindled in the sound, hard and fleshie parts of mans bodie [...] like to a hote vessel; for as the vessell doth heate the water that is poured into it: so also the feaver hectic' (Barrough 1624: 215).

Hemiplegia: 'the palsy possessing one side' (Anon. 1657: sig. G3).

Hypochondriac melancholy: 'The hypochondriacal or windy Melancholy is often caused by the overboyling of dreggish blood, which was settled neere unto the stomack, or gristles of the short ribs, by a distemper of the liver, stomacke, or miseraical veins; hence it is that grosse and burnt humours are carryed up to the principall seate of the braine, and so doe disquiet it and stirre up melancholy' (Bruele 1599: 34).

Jaundice: 'a shedding either of yellow choler or of melancholy all over the body [...] many times the jaundice is caused and doth chance when the blood is corrupted without fever, of some outward occasion, and is made cholericke' (Barrough 1624: 81).

Liver obstruction: 'caused of vapours and grosse windinesse, hard to digest. But sometime it is caused of grosse and vicious humours in the ends of the veines, springing from the flat part of the liver, by which veines nourishment is sent to the liver from the stomach and bowels' (Barrough 1624: 141).

Lyentery: 'in this disease the bowels do not hold the meate, but they let it slide away before it be changed and perfectly digested, even in the same forme and likenes that it was eaten [...] it is caused oftentimes through a grievous fluxe disenteria by name going before, which causeth deepe exulceration of the bowels' (Barrough 1624: 121).

Magisterium: 'magistral syrup is a particular syrup prescribed by a skilful physitian to his patient for a particular disease' (Anon. 1657, sig. I1).

Malignant fever: 'Cum vero ab aliis causis ortum habet, morbus malignus vel febris maligna vocatur' [When it is caused by outward causes, it is called a pestilent fever, or plague] (Bruele 1599: 412).

Mass: 'by mass, alwaies understand the composition brought into such a thickness, that you may easily with your fingers make it into pills' (Culpeper 1649: 198).

Melancholy: 'an alienation of the mind, troubling reason [...] without a feaver, and is chiefly engendred of melancholy occupying the mind [...] sometime it is caused of the common vice of melancholy bloud being in all the veines of the whole body [...] oftentimes onely the bloud which is in the brain is altered [...] sometime is engendred through inflammation, and evill affect about the stomacke and sides' (Barrough 1624: 45).

Mother: 'is a running back of the wombe, or of maligne vapors bredded in the wombe, unto the higher parts, whereby the bowels, midriffe, and stomacke, are sometimes so crushed, that they cannot be widened by breathing' (Bruele 1599: 372). See also 'Suffocation of the womb'.

Nosebleed: 'oftentimes bleeding at the nose is caused by nature, which doth by this means expell the excrements, and that which is troublesome to the body [...] sometime it is caused by the evil affection of the veins [or] the veines bleed because some gnawing humour hath got thereinto; also: haemorrhagia [...] doth signify bleeding at the nose [...] through which for the most part nature doth expel the superfluous blood in many' (Bruele 1599: 142–143).

Obstructed menstruation: 'The menstruis are wont to be suppressed and stopped against nature, either through overmuch grossenesse, or slendernesse. For fat folk are more without bloud than other folke, and they have lesse and streighter [narrower] veines [...] but those that are leane and slender [...] have no superfluous blood in them' (Barrough 1624: 188).

Omphacine: 'Omphacy, unripe, it signifies properly the juyce of unripe grapes' (Anon. 1657: K1).

Pain in the side of the head: 'Hemicrania is a painfull evil remaining in one halfe of the head, either on the right halfe or on the left [...] in English is called the migrime. This paine cometh be fits, and some the griefe is felt within the skull, in some within deepe in the braine, and in some other night to the temples [...] this paine is caused by ascending and flowing of many vapours or humours either hote or colde, either by the veines or arteries, or both' (Barrough 1624: 17).

Passing blood: 'a disease of the reines, through the which thin wheyish blood is pissed. It is caused through weeknesse of the reines [...] or [...] through amplitude of the reines [or] through breaking of a vein in the reines [or] through gnawing of the veines by sharpe humours flowing from above' (Barrough 1624: 158).

Phthisis: 'a kind of consumption' (Anon. 1657: L1).

Pleurisy: 'an inflamation of the thinne and small skinne which clotheth the ribs on the inner side [...] whereby it appeares that every paine of the side is not a pleurisy [...] if the pain be great because of windines, this is a bastard pleurisy, then are they without a fever' (Bruele 1599: 186).

Quartan fever: 'An intermitting quartane is ingendred of melancholy petrified and rotted without the vessels. It is so named because it ceasseth two days, and returneth againe the fourth day' (Barrough 1624: 215).

Quiet day(s): 'the day that the sicke hath not his fever' (Barrough 1624: 233). Other examples showing that it refers to treatments on the middle day between attacks of a tertian fever are found in Platter and Ruland (Platter 1614: 268; Ruland the Elder 1628: 683).

Quotidian fever: 'caused of sweete fleam [phlegm] being putrified and rotten without the vessels: and is so called, because it returneth every day' (Barrough 1624: 215).

Rheum from the eyes: 'an inflamation of the tunicle or membrane growing close unto the eye [...] there cometh withall a tumor of the eye, redness and a loading paine [...] sometimes the eye is swollen to the cheeks, and store of tears fall from them caused by vehement paine, and pricking of the eye' (Bruele 1599: 126–127).

Saltpetre: 'said to be beneficial in Ungaric fever' (Du Chesne 1607: 244).

Scurvy: 'a stopping of the spleen hindering thereby the course of melancholy, whiche mingling with the rest of the bloud infecteth all the body with vile wasting corruption, the grosse part whereof falling downe, staineth the legs with spots like unto pomgranats, and the thinner part being carried up defileth the tender gums with sharpe fretting and loathsome growing out of the flesh' (Banister 1587?: 1).

Sore throat: 'The squinancy is an inflamation of the throate, or the highest parts of the gullet, hindering breathing and swallowing, when as the fault is neyther in the brest nor lungs. This disease doth threaten present danger by strangling because [...] a man is deprived both of breath and sustenance' (Bruele 1599: 160).

Spasm of the mouth (*tortura oris*): 'if it be from moisture, it is a kind of palsie; if through dryness, then a kind of cramp; and is commonly a sign of death' (Anon. 1657: sig. N4).

Stone: 'the stone of the reines happeneth oftener to men of perfect age than to children. The cause [...] is continuall crudity and rawnesse of the stomach, whereby abundance of grosse and earthy humours is heaped up together, and burning or fierie heate about the reines parcheth the humours, and knits them together, and hardeneth them into a stone' (Barrough 1624: 161).

Suffocation of the womb: 'is nothing else but a drawing back of it up to the upper parts. It is caused through the stretching out of it, which is ingendred of fulnesse that followeth after the retention and stopping of the menstruis. For in a woman, the wombe when it is reached and stretched out, it runneth not to another place like a wandring beast, but is drawne backe through the extension' (Barrough 1624: 189). See also 'Mother'.

Tenesmus: 'a continuall desire to go to the stool or siege, which the patient cannot deferre nor eschue [*sic*], and yet he avoydeth nothing, except it be a little blood' (Barrough 1624: 126).

Tertian fever: 'a pure and exquisite tertian is caused when choler doth putrifie and rot within the vessels. It is so called, because it ceaseth one day, and cometh again the third day' (Barrough 1624: 215).

Tympany: 'a kind of dropsy [...] when there is greater store of wind than water, whereby the abdomen is stretched beyond meas-ure, then it is called *tympanites*, and than rather a noyse of wind then water, is perceived if the belly be strooke' (Bruele 1599: 319).

Ulcer at the mouth of the bladder: 'The bladder is exulcerate either through some bile, or botch, or swelling [...] or by eating and gnawing of a fluxe [...] there followeth this sharpe pain of the bladder [...] when the ulcers be foule and filthie, there commeth forth dreggie and slimie matter' (Barrough 1624: 171).

Ungaric fever: 'Inter febres malignas, et quidem non raro pete-chiales, est febris illa, quae vulgo morbus Ungaricus [...] dicitur' [Among the malignant fevers, and indeed not rarely those with rashes, is the fever commonly called the Ungaric disease] (Sennert 1628: 543).

Uterine wind: 'The wombe is puffed up through cold, or humors corrupt in it, or through abortion or sore travell in childbirth the dore of it being shut, or a clod of bloud being in it, and stopping it' (Barrough 1624: 196).

Wheat barley: 'called […] in Latin Hordeum nudum of other some Hordeum mundum. It maye be called in Englishe wheate barley because it hath no mo huskes on it then wheat hath' (Turner 1548: second part, sig. 16v).

Wind and phlegm in the stomach: 'windinesse is engendred through flegmaticke humours in the stomack, or else through meates dissolved into vapors through want and debilitie of heate' (Barrough 1624: 114).

Worms: 'There be three kinds of worms. The first be round and long, named Teretes. The second be broad, called therefore Lati. The third are called Ascarides. The first kind […] be round and hand breadth in length […] often in the slender and small guts, and they go into the stomach, and therefore are voided often by the mouth […] peculiar to infants and children. The second kind […] be broad and long like a gard or band […] Ascarides be thin and short like small worms. They be found most commonly in the right gut, and in the end of the fundament. All […] are engendred and caused of crude, raw, grosse and flegmaticke matter and through inconvenient rottennesse' (Barrough 1624: 132).

Bibliography

Adams, T. (1615). *Mystical Bedlam: or, the World of Mad-Men* (London: Clement Knight).

Amatus Lusitanus (1556). *Curationum medicinalium centuriae quatuor* (Basel: Froben).

Anon. (1657). *A Physical Dictionary or: an Interpretation of such Crabbed Words and Terms of Art as are derived from the Greek or Latin* (London: John Garfield).

Anon. (1990), 'Dendrochronological results for Hall's Croft', Shakespeare Birthplace Trust.

Banister, R. (1587?). 'A Discourse of the Scorby, translated out of Wyers observations', in Richard Banister, *A Treatise of One Hundred and Thirteene Diseases of the Eyes with some Profitable Additions* (London: Thomas Man and William Brome).

Barrough, P. (1624). *The Method of Physick, containing the Causes, Signes and Cures of Inward Diseases in Mans Body*, 6th edn (London: Richard Field).

Bearman, R. (1994). *Shakespeare in the Stratford Records* (Stroud: Sutton).

Beier, L.M. (1987). *Sufferers and Healers: The Experience of Illness in Seventeenth-century England* (London: Routledge and Kegan Paul).

Betts, T., and Betts, H. (1998). 'John Hall and his epileptic patients – epilepsy management in early 17th-century England', *Seizure*, 7, 411–414.

Brinkworth, E.R.C. (1972). *Shakespeare and the Bawdy Court of Stratford* (London: Phillimore).

Bruele, W. (1599). *Praxis medicinae theorica et empirica familiarissima* (Leiden: Plantin, Raphelangius).

Bucknill, J.C. (1860). *The Medical Knowledge of Shakespeare* (London: Longman).

Burton, R. (2001). *The Anatomy of Melancholy*, ed. Holbrook Jackson (New York: New York Review of Books).

Churchill, W. (2012). *Female Patients in Early Modern Britain* (Farnham: Ashgate).

Cooke, J. (1648). *Mellificium Chirurgiae, or the Marrow of Many Good Authors, wherein is briefly and faithfully handled the Art of Chirurgery* (London: Samuel Cartwright).

Cotta, J. (1619). *A Short Discoverie of Severall Sorts of Ignorant and Unconsiderate Practisers of Physicke in England* (London: John Barnes).

Crato, J. (1609). *Consiliorum et epistolarum medicinalium, liber secundus: num primum studio et opera Laurentii Scholzii … in lucem editus* (Hanover: Wechel, Marnius et haeredes Aubrii).

Croll, O. (1609). *Basilica chymica* (Frankfurt: Claudius Marnius).

Culpeper, N. (1649). *A Physical Directory: or, a Translation of the London Dispensatory made by the Colledge of Physicians of London* (London: Peter Cole).

Donne, J. (1624). *Devotions upon Emergent Occasions: and Severall Steps in my Sicknes* (London: Thomas Jones).

Du Chesne, J. (1607). *Pharmacopoea dogmaticorum restituta* (Frankfurt: Schönwetter).

Du Chesne, J. (1607). *Tractatus duo quorum prior inscribitur diaeteticon polyhistoricum, alter vero pharmacopoea dogmaticorum restituta* (Frankfurt: Schönwetter).

Eccles, M. (1963). *Shakespeare in Warwickshire* (Madison, WI: University of Wisconsin Press).

Eugalenus, S. (1604). *De Scorbuto morbo liber* (Leipzig: Lantzenberger).

Fernandez-Florez, A. (2010). 'On the Practice of John Hall in the Field of Dermatology in the 17th Century', *Clinics in Dermatology*, 28, 356–363.

Greer, G. (2007). *Shakespeare's Wife* (London: Bloomsbury).

Hall J. (1635). 'Curationum Historicarum et Empiricarum, in certis locis et notis personis expertarum et robatarum, libellus', Egerton MS 2065, British Library.

Hall, J. (1657). *Select Observations on English Bodies: or, Cures both Empiricall and Historicall performed upon very eminent Persons on desperate Diseases*, trans. and ed. James Cooke (London: John Sherley).

Hall, J. (1679). *Select Observations on English Bodies of Eminent Persons in Desperate Diseases: First Written in Latin by Mr John Hall, Physician*, ed. J. Cooke (London: Benjamin Shirley).

Halliwell-Phillipps, J.O. (1886). *Outlines of the Life of Shakespeare*, 6th edn, 2 vols (London: Longmans Green).

Houllier, J. (1611). *De morbis internis libe* (Paris: Perier).

Hughes, A. (1994). 'Religion and Society in Stratford upon Avon, 1619–1638', *Midlands History*, 19, 58–84.

Ingleby, C.M. (1885). *Shakespeare and the Enclosure of Common Fields at Welcombe, being a fragment of the private diary of Thomas Greene, town clerk of Stratford upon Avon, 1614–1617* (Birmingham: Robert Birbeck).

Jones, P.M. (2000). 'Medical Libraries and Medical Latin 1400-1700', in Wouter Bracke and Herwig Deumens (eds), *Medical Latin from the Late Middle Ages to the Eighteenth Century* (Brussels: Koninklijke Academie voor Geneeskunde van België), 49–68.

Joseph, H. (1964). *Shakespeare's Son-in-law John Hall: Man and Physician* (Hamden, CT: Archon).

Lane, J. (1996). *John Hall and His Patients: The Medical Practice of Shakespeare's Son-in-law* (Stratford-upon-Avon: Sutton).

Leong, E., and Pennell, S. (2007). 'Recipe Collections and the Currency of Medical Knowledge in the Early Modern Medical Marketplace', in Mark Jenner and Patrick Wallis (eds), *Medicine and the Market in England and its Colonies, c.1450–c.1850* (Basingstoke: Palgrave Macmillan), 137–140.

Leong, E., and Rankin, A. (eds) (2011). *Secrets and Knowledge in Medicine and Science, 1500–1800* (Abingdon: Routledge).

Liébault, J. (1585). *Thresor des remedes secrets pour les maladies des femmes* (Paris: du Puy).

Mackinnon, L. (2015). 'His Daughter Susanna Hall', in Paul Edmondson and Stanley Wells (eds), *The Shakespeare Circle: An Alternative Biography* (Cambridge: Cambridge University Press), 71–85.

Malone, E. (1821). *The Plays and Poems of William Shakespeare … Comprehending a Life of the Poet*, 21 vols (London: n.p.).

Marcham, F. (1931). *William Shakespeare and his Daughter Susannah* (London: Grafton).

Marshall, P. (2012). *Reformation England 1480–1642*, 2nd edn (London: Bloomsbury).

Mitchell, C.M. (1947). *The Shakespeare Circle: A Life of Dr John Hall* (Birmingham: Cornish).

Moran, B.T. (2005). *Distilling Knowledge: Alchemy, Chemistry and the Scientific Revolution* (Cambridge, MA: Harvard University Press).

Moschowitz, E. (1918). 'Dr John Hall: Shakespeare's Son-in-law', *Bulletin of the Johns Hopkins Hospital*, 19, 148–152.

Nagy, D.E. (1988). *Popular Medicine in Seventeenth Century England* (Bowling Green, OH: Bowling Green State Popular Press).

Newton, H. (2014). *The Sick Child in Early Modern England, 1580–1720* (Oxford: Oxford University Press).

Pearce, J.M.S. (2006). 'Dr John Hall (1575–1635) and Shakespeare's Medicine', *Journal of Medical Biography*, 14, 187–191.

Pelling, M., and Webster, C. (1979). 'Medical Practitioners', in C. Webster (ed.), *Health, Medicine and Mortality in the Sixteenth Century* (Cambridge: Cambridge University Press), 165–236.

Penot, B. (1608). *De denario medico, quo decem medicaminibus, omnibus morbis internis medendi via docetur* (Berne: Ioannis le Preux).

Platter, F. (1602). *Praxeos seu de cognoscendis, praedicendis, praecavendis, curandisque affectibus homini incommodantibus tractatus: de functionum laesionibus* (Basel: Waldkirch).

Poynter, F.N.L., and Bishop, W.J. (1951). *A Seventeenth-century Doctor and his Patients: John Symcotts, 1592?–1662*, Publications of the Bedfordshire

Bibliography

Historical Record Society Vol. XXXI (Streatley: Bedfordshire Historical Record Society).

Raach, J.H. (1962). *A Directory of English Country Physicians 1603–1643* (London: Dawson).

Rondelet, G. (1574). *Methodus curandorum omnium morborum corporis humanis in tres libros distincta* (Paris: Macé).

Ruland the Elder, M. (1628). *Curationum empyricarum et historicarum, in certis locis et notis personis optime expertarum et rite probatarum, centuriae decem* (Lyons: Pierre Ravaud).

Schoenbaum, S. (1987). *William Shakespeare: A Compact Life*, rev. edn (Oxford: Oxford University Press).

Sennert, D. (1624). *De Scorbuto tractatus* (Wittenberg: Schürer).

Sennert, D. (1628). *De Febribus Libri IV* (Wittenberg: Vidue et Haeredes Zacharia Schürer).

Sennert, D. (1631). *Opera omnia ... tomus I* (Paris: Apud Societatem).

Shakespeare, W. (2005). *The Complete Works*, ed. Stanley Wells, Gary Taylor, John Jowett and William Montgomery (Oxford: Clarendon Press).

Siraisi, N. (1990). *Medieval and Early Renaissance Medicine: An Introduction to Knowledge and Practice* (Chicago: University of Chicago Press, 1990).

Slack, P. (1979). 'Mirrors of Health and Treasures of Poor Men: The Uses of the Vernacular Medical Literature of Tudor England', in C. Webster (ed.), *Health, Medicine and Mortality in the Sixteenth Century* (Cambridge: Cambridge University Press), 237–273.

Stratford-upon-Avon Corporation Chamberlain's Accounts 1585–1619, BRU4/1, Shakespeare Birthplace Trust.

Taplin, J. (2018). *Shakespeare's Country Families: A Documentary Guide to Shakespeare's Country Society* (Warwick: Claridges).

Thornborough, J. (1635). 'Grant by John Thornborough, Bishop of Worcester, April 1635', ER78/7, Shakespeare Birthplace Trust.

Turner, W. (1548). *The First and Second Partes of the Herball ... set out with the Names of the Herbes* (Birchmann: Cologne).

Valesco de Taranta (1560). *Epitome operis perquam utilis morbis curandis Valesci de Taranta in septem congesta libros* (Lyons: Tornæsius and Gazeius).

Valleriola, F. (1573). *Observationum medicinalium libri sex* (Lyons: Gryphius).

Wear, A. (2000). *Knowledge and Practice in English Medicine 1550–1695* (Cambridge: Cambridge University Press).

Index of names and works

Index of names and works

Luisini, Luigi
 De morbo Gallico omnia 37, 97, 280,
 285
Lynes, Humphrey, the elder 196n.
Lynes, Humphrey, the younger
 196n.
Lynes, Joan, née Richardson (Case
 126) 196–7

Malone, Edmond 58
Manning, Elizabeth 91n.
Mansfeldt, Ernst von 99n.
Marcus Aurelius 51
 De vita sua 77
Markham, Mary 126n.
Markham, Thomas 126n.
Martini, Matthaeus
 'De scorbuto' 38–9, *39*, 79, 149,
 170–3, 181–5, 199, 248–9, 256,
 258
Montagnana, Pietro da 61, 141, 154
Morley, Sir John 171n.
Morrys, John 3
Morrys, Matthew 3
Morrys, Susanna 3
Murden, Mary (later Lady Harvey),
 see Harvey, Lady Mary, née
 Murden
Murden, Mary, of Moreton Murrell
 (Case 107) 174, *175*
Murden, Richard 133n., 174n., *175*

'Mr Nash's serving maid' 20, (Case
 6) 85–6
 see also Nash, Anthony
Nash, Anthony 85n., 103–4n.
Nash, Elizabeth, née Hall (later
 Elizabeth, Lady Barnard) 6,
 19–21, 25, 93n., 103–4n., (Case
 36) 111–14, *112*, 190n.
Nash, Mary, née Bough 19, (Case
 30) 103–4
Nash, Thomas 25, 57, 103–4n., 111n.
Nason, Elizabeth, née Rogers 138n.
Nason, John 4, *4*, (Case 67) 138

Nidd, John 29
Norbury, John 148n.
Northampton, Elizabeth Compton,
 née Spencer, 1st Countess 19,
 (Case 1) 77–80, 82, 86, 88n.,
 (Case 95) 159–61, 167, pl. 2
Northampton, Mary, née
 Beaumont, 2nd Countess 19,
 60, 62–3, 208n., 210, (Case 144)
 222–5
Northampton, William Compton,
 1st Earl 19, 77n., (Case 2) 80–2,
 82, 83n., 86n. 93n., 95n., (Case
 64) 135–6, (Case 68) 138–9,
 (Case 79) 149, (Case 83) 152–3,
 208, 210, 246n., pl. 2
Northampton, Spencer Compton,
 2nd Earl 66, (Case 137) 208–12,
 210, 222n., 246n., (Case 178)
 281–2

Occo, Albert
 Pharmacopoeia Augustana 37, 45,
 141

Pakington, Dorothy, née Smith
 141n., 142
Pakington, Sir John 61, (Case 71)
 141–2, (Case 85) 154, pl. 2
Palmer, Jane, née West (Case 54)
 130
Palmer, John 130n.
Paracelsus 11, 15, 144, 194, 202, 269
Pargetter, Christopher 220n.
Parker (Mr) (Case 52) 128–9
 see also Parker, Henry
Parker, Henry 128n.
Peers, Clare, née Benlow 70, (Case
 123) 193–4
Peers, Philip 193n.
Peers, Thomas 193n.
Penell (Mr), *see* Pennell, Edward
Pennell, Edward (Case 97) 161–2
Pennell, Margaret, née Greville
 161n.

Index of names and works

Index of names and works

Index of places

page numbers in italics refer to illustrations

313

Index of places

Leicester 6, 145
Leicestershire 118n., pl. 2
  Elmesthorpe 218n.
London 1–3, 7–10, 16–18, 46–7, 58,
    80n., 93n., 112, 128n., 154,
    216, 222n., 275n., pl. 3
  Blackfriars 3
  British Library and Museum 18,
    50, 54
  College of Physicians 1–3, 18, 32,
    284
  Little Britain 54
  Middle Temple 122n., 149n.
  St Gregory by St Paul's 38
  St Paul's Cathedral 38
  Southwark, *see* Surrey
  Westminster Abbey 95n.
Low Countries 62, 167, pl. 3
  Delft pl. 22
Ludlow (and Ludlow Castle) 78,
    80–3, 86, 95n., 246n.,
    pl. 2

Middlesex
  Acton 7

Norfolk 26n.
Northamptonshire 111n.
  Abington 111n.
  Castle Ashby 80n.
  Hardingstone 214n., 215
  Northampton 59, 214
Norwich 9–10
Nottinghamshire 126n.

Oxford 47, 66, 211, 222n., 245n.,
    266n.
  University 83n., 162n., 174n.,
    211n., 236n., 243n., 251n.,
    277n.
  Balliol College 115n., 133n.,
    236n.
  Bodleian Library 47
  Magdalen College 185n.
  Queen's College 245n.

Oxfordshire 187n., pl. 2
  Banbury 19
  Broughton Castle 258n.
  Burford 195, 244n.
  Charlbury 190n.
  Walcot 190n.

Shrewsbury 167
Stratford-upon-Avon 1–27, 30, 44–7,
    57, 81, 83, 85, 87, 92n., 93n.,
    96, 101, 103–4n., 115n., 130n.,
    135, 138, 141, 148n., 150,
    152n., 154, 162, 165n., 181n.,
    183n., 191, 195n., 196–8, 203,
    215, 216, 220n., 226, 230,
    234–5, 240n., 244n., 266n.,
    277n., pl. 2
  Bear Inn 85, 103–4n., 165n.
  Bridge Street 85n., 103–4n., 165n.
  Clopton House 181n.
  Ecclesiastical Court *4*
  Gospel Bush 8–9
  Hall's Croft 6–7, *7*
  Holy Trinity Church *2*, 6, 12–14,
    14, 25–6, *26*, 115n., 136n.,
    152n., 252n.
  King's New School 277n., 279
  New Place 2, 6, *8*, 93n., 136n.,
    255n.
  St Mary's 136n.
  Stratford Old Town 6, 7, 152,
    200n.
  Welcombe 8, 197n.
Surrey
  Mitcham 92n.
  Southwark 78
Sussex 171n., 187n., 242n.
  Ladyholt 171n.

Wales 80, 82, 149, 152, 246
  Glamorgan 236n.
Warwick 18–19, 54, 122, 141n., 147n.,
    195n., 206n., 242n., 243n.,
    245n., 266n., 268
  Warwick Castle 257

314

Index of places

Index of ailments and treatments

page numbers in italics refer to illustrations

Index of ailments and treatments

Index of ailments and treatments

Index of ailments and treatments

phthisis 103–4, 294

pigeon, *see* animal products

pike's jaw, *see* animal products

pimples, *see* skin disorders

pine leaves 114

   see also ground-pine; nuts

pistachio, *see* nuts

placenta ('retained and corrupted products of conception') 234

plantain 107, 120, 121, 125, 146, 164, 180, 191, 203, 209, 212, 214, 216, 221, 231, 245, 272

pleres archonticon, *see* archonticon

pleurisy 210, 281–2, 294

plume alum, *see* alum

plums 272

polypydy of the oak (fern) 104, 109, 136, 153, 158, 162, 173, 185, 199, 218, 261, 269, pl. 21

pomegranate 61, 83, 108, 125, 128, 212, 214, 220–1, 245, 246–7, pl. 14

poppy 94, 97, 117, 121, 149, 176, 194, 211–12

   corn 152, 231, 244

   field 99, 148, 189, 224

   white 211

   wild 120

populeon (ointment) 114, 131, 221, 224–5, 269

pork fat, *see* animal products

posset ale 87, 106, 117, 131, 137, 149, 151, 223–4, 233, 250, 258, 261

powder of worms, *see* worms

pregnancy 15, 62, 97, 134, 134n., 156, 156n., 157, 157n., 200–1, 220, 222

prepared steel, *see* steel and steeled preparations

puerperal fever, *see* fever

purslane 94, 148, 180, 195, 203, 211

pustules, *see* skin disorders

pyrethrum 103, 113, 115, 183, 196

quartan fever, *see* fever

quince 180

   see also oils

quinsy 208–12

quotidian fever, *see* fever

radish 105, 171, 220, 231

raisins 84, 93, 115, 126, 134, 142, 158–9, 165, 173, 185, 205, 207, 212, 254, 262, 280

realgar (arsenic) 129

red lead (oxide), *see* lead

respiratory complaints 21–2, 83–5, 92–5, 115–16, 118, 126–9, 132–3, 139–40, 165–6, 168–71, 198–201, 226–7, 255–7, 261–3, 277–82, 289

'retained products of conception', *see* placenta

rheum 77–81, 86, 98, 124, 152, 295

rhodium wood 190

rhubarb 16, 79, 81, 85, 89, 92, 99–100, 109, 111, 114–15, 118, 120–21, 123, 130, 138–9, 148–9, 152–4, 158–9, 162–6, 173–4, 176, 182, 185–6, 190, 202, 207, 209, 213, 218–19, 231, 233, 240–2, 247, 250–1, 256, 260–1, 267, 269, 272, 274, pl. 12

rock alum, *see* alum

rocket seed 98

rooster, *see* animal products

rose 89, 99, 109–10, 120, 128, 176, 178, 191, 197, 199, 203, 205, 212, 214, 280

   conserve 84, 91, 108, 121, 148, 152, 161, 222, 268, 274

   damask 170, 179, 190, 199

   honey 136, 140, 144, 164, 180, 191, 201, 209, 212, 220

   juice 85, 163, 203, 213, 227, 240, 241

   julep 105, 108, 220

   ointment 221

330

Index of ailments and treatments

stomach conditions 91 101, 106, 133,
143, 147, 163–4, 172–4, 181,
220, 234, 289, 292–3 295
abscess 89
ache 87, 153–4, 161, 204–5, 208,
218, 268–70
pain 83–4, 138, 198, 200–1, 245
wind 21, 87–8, 103–4, 121–2,
132–3, 149–51, 153–4, 174–6,
187, 198–201, 236–9, 248–50,
255–7, 261–7, 288, 297
see also abdominal pain; pain in
the side; inflammation and
swelling
stone 188–9, 237–8, 250–1, 295–6
see also kidneys
strawberry 99, 109
styrax 84, 114, 115, 129, 166, 167, 181,
201, 241
'suffocation of the mother', *see*
uterine conditions
'suffocation of the womb', *see* uterine
conditions
sugar 62, 79, 81, 85, 90, 92, 94, 98,
101, 104, 107, 109–10, 114,
119, 121, 126, 131–2, 141, 163,
169, 176, 179, 184–7, 195–7,
202, 215, 218–19, 221, 223,
227, 230, 233, 235, 237, 247,
250, 262, 264–5, 267, 269,
277
'best' 153, 199, 267
brown 92, 180, 272
'candy' 81, 84, 88, 115–16, 134,
154, 203, 205, 254–5
lavender 207
red 140, 151
rose 92, 94, 110, 116, 121, 123–4,
176–7, 181, 186, 203, 211, 229,
262, 267
unrefined 108, 236, 247, 249, 259
violet 98, 139, 246
white 94, 104, 138, 197, 211, 216,
263
see also barley sugar

sulphur 84, 137, 177, 265, 280
balsam 226
flowers of 85, 108, 118, 129, 198,
217, 226
'live' 124, 185
rock 90
see also oils
sulphuric acid 199
sweet flag 80, 93, 104, 114–15, 119,
132, 158, 170, 190, 196, 199,
207, 209, 242–3
swallows' nest, *see* animal products
swelling, *see* inflammation
'syrup of the five roots' 130

tacamahacca powder 170
tamarind 176, 185, 193–4, 198, 213,
227, 263, 270
tamarisk 109, 119, 122–3, 190, 199,
264, 267
tapsi valentia 225
tarragon 145
tartar 201, 250, 274, 275, 280
crystal 90, 173, 191, 238, 274, 278
vitriolated 168, 278
see also cream of tartar; salt of
tartar; oils
tenesmus 88, 180–1, 296
see also bowel disorders
tertian fever, *see* fever
testicles 130, 149–51
thirst 98–9, 108, 134, 143, 145,
149–52, 168–71, 184, 205,
248–51, 258, 262, 275, 281,
290
throat conditions, *see* inflammation
and swelling; sore throat
tinnitus 269–70
see also auditory ailments
tiredness 21, 198–200, 263–6, 275,
277–8
tobacco 106, 198
tongue 144, 164–5, 167–8, 220–2,
244, 249
see also inflammation and swelling